Advances in Psychiatry

Advances in Psychiatry

Edited by

CHITTARANJAN ANDRADE

OXFORD
UNIVERSITY PRESS

OXFORD
UNIVERSITY PRESS

YMCA Library Building, Jai Singh Road, New Delhi 110001

Oxford University Press is a department of the University of Oxford. It furthers the University's objective of excellence in research, scholarship, and education by publishing worldwide in

Oxford New York
Athens Auckland Bangkok Bogota Buenos Aires Calcutta
Cape Town Chennai Dar es Salaam Delhi Florence Hong Kong Istanbul
Karachi Kuala Lumpur Madrid Melbourne Mexico City Mumbai
Nairobi Paris Sao Paolo Singapore Taipei Tokyo Toronto Warsaw

with associated companies in

Berlin Ibadan

Published in India
By Oxford University Press, New Delhi

ISBN 0 19 564985 0

Typeset by Excellent Laser Typesetters
Printed in India at Rashtriya Printers, Delhi 110032
and published by Manzar Khan, Oxford University Press
YMCA Library Building, Jai Singh Road, New Delhi 110 001

Preface

Research in psychiatry is progressing at an explosive pace and, the availability of textbooks and journals notwithstanding, practising clinicians and academicians alike experience difficulties in keeping abreast of the developments in the field. This is because standard textbooks require to be comprehensive in scope, and therefore do not have the space to provide an in-depth coverage of specialized topics; in contrast, while journal articles indeed do address specialized topics in moderate detail, they are similarly limited by space constraints. This is where a book on advances in psychiatry enters the picture; it provides a detailed and relatively comprehensive discussion on specially selected subjects. As a result, clinicians and academicians obtain the opportunity to update their knowledge in emerging disciplines, and in areas of super-specialization other than their own.

In this volume, eight chapters address focussed topics that range from schizophrenia to eating disorders, and from neuropsychology to psychopharmacology. The ninth chapter presents a pot pourri of themes on various subjects that are likely to be of interest to psychiatrists. The topics covered in these chapters are theoretical, practical or both. All authors are internationally renowned experts in their respective disciplines.

I take this opportunity to thank my panel of authors, all of whom submitted manuscripts of such excellence that my job as an editor was a pleasant one.

CHITTARANJAN ANDRADE

Bangalore
July, 1999

Contents

Contributors

Alan J. Gelenberg, MD
Department of Psychiatry
University of Arizona
Health Sciences Center
Tucson
Arizona, USA

Brett Mensh, MD, PhD
Department of Biological Psychiatry
New York State Psychiatric Institute
Department of Psychiatry
College of Physicians and Surgeons
Columbia University
New York, USA

Cameron S. Carter, MD
Departments of Psychiatry and Psychology
University of Pittsburgh
Pittsburgh
Pennsylvania, USA

Chittaranjan Andrade, MD
Department of Psychopharmacology
National Institute of Mental Health and Neurosciences
Bangalore, India

Chris P. L. Freeman, MBChB, FRC Psych, MPhil
Department of Psychiatry
Royal Edinburgh Hospital
Edinburgh
Scotland, UK

Deanna M. Barch, PhD
Departments of Psychology and Psychiatry
Washington University, St Louis
Missouri, USA

Georgios Petrides, MD
Research Department
Long Island Jewish Hillside Hospital Medical Center
Albert Einstein College of Medicine
Department of Psychiatry
State University of New York at Stony Brook
New York, USA

Harold A. Sackeim, PhD
Department of Biological Psychiatry
New York State Psychiatric Institute
Department of Psychiatry
College of Physicians and Surgeons
Columbia University, Department of Radiology
College of Physicians and Surgeons
Columbia University
New York, USA

Joseph Levine, MD, MSc
Western Psychiatric Institute and Clinic
Stanley Center for the Innovative Treatment of Bipolar Disorder
Special Studies Center at Mayview State Hospital
University of Pittsburgh Medical Center
Pittsburgh
Pennsylvania, USA

K. N. Roy Chengappa, MD, FRCPC
Western Psychiatric Institute and Clinic
Stanley Center for the Innovative Treatment of Bipolar Disorder
Special Studies Center at Mayview State Hospital
University of Pittsburgh Medical Center
Pittsburgh
Pennsylvania, USA

Kavitha Vijayalakshmi, MD
Department of Psychiatry
National Institute of Mental Health and Neurosciences
Bangalore, India

Kirstine Postma, MSc
Department of Psychiatry
Royal Edinburgh Hospital
Edinburgh
Scotland, UK

Max Fink, MD
Research Department
Long Island Jewish Hillside Hospital Medical Center
Albert Einstein College of Medicine
Department of Psychiatry
State University of New York at Stony Brook
New York, USA

Mitchell S. Nobler, MD
Department of Biological Psychiatry
New York State Psychiatric Institute
Department of Psychiatry
College of Physicians and Surgeons
Columbia University
New York, USA

Prabha S. Chandra, MD
Department of Psychiatry
National Institute of Mental Health and Neurosciences
Bangalore, India

R. Raguram, MD
Department of Psychiatry
National Institute of Mental Health and Neurosciences
Bangalore, India

Robert L. DeLaPaz, MD
Department of Radiology
College of Physicians and Surgeons

Columbia University
New York, USA

Ronald L. Van Heertum, MD
Department of Radiology
College of Physicians and Surgeons
Columbia University
New York, USA

Sarah H. Lisanby, MD
Department of Biological Psychiatry
New York State Psychiatric Institute
Department of Psychiatry
College of Physicians and Surgeons
Columbia University
New York, USA

Vishwajit L. Nimgaonkar, D Phil, MRC Psych
Departments of Psychiatry and Human Genetics
University of Pittsburgh
School of Medicine and Graduate School of Public Health
Pittsburgh, USA

Chapter 1

Progress in Psychiatric Genetics: Focus on Schizophrenia and Bipolar Disorder

VISHWAJIT L. NIMGAONKAR

OVERVIEW

Several interrelated developments over the past three decades have resulted in major advances in the field of human genetics; these advances have already begun to impact upon research into the genetics of psychiatric disorders. This chapter initially presents general strategies for identifying genes that are responsible for human diseases. The ethical implications of genetic studies are discussed next. Finally, the relevance of psychiatric genetic research is examined, using schizophrenia and bipolar disorder as examples. Recent developments in these fields are reviewed and their clinical ramifications explained. It is concluded that psychiatric disorders place unusual demands on the geneticist, but may ultimately reward sustained efforts.

THE IDENTIFICATION OF GENETIC ABNORMALITIES THAT CAUSE HUMAN DISEASES

The aim of human genetic studies is deceptively simple: to identify the mutations in a gene which cause the disease of interest. The

Acknowledgements: This work was funded in part by grants to Dr Nimgaonkar from the Fogarty International Center (#R03 TW00730), the National Institute of Health (#MH 01489, MH 56242 and MH 53459) and the Stanley Foundation.

effort is hampered by the fact that the majority of the estimated 100,000 genes in the human genome have not yet been identified or localized. Therefore, an indirect approach is necessary: investigators attempt to identify the chromosomal location rather than the identity of the gene or the nature of the mutations. This is effected through the identification of 'anonymous' genetic polymorphisms (*genetic markers)* which segregate along with the disease in question. The function of such genetic markers need not be known; it is only necessary that their chromosomal location be available. The identification of a marker which segregates with the disease in the family or in the population can thus provide key information about the likely location of the disease gene.

The next step, known as *positional cloning*, involves the identification of other markers in the region. By screening such markers, investigators progressively narrow down the region of interest. The final step is the identification of mutations in a gene in this region, which completely discriminate persons with the illness from unaffected individuals. Accidents of nature, such as cytogenetic abnormalities, may assist and speed up the process of disease gene identification. In most cases, however, the quest is arduous and requires a search throughout the genome. The search is thus dependent on the availability of both informative clinical samples and relevant markers.

The positional cloning effort is heavily dependent upon sophistication and ingenuity in the laboratory. The entire investigation additionally depends upon competent statistical support. Since this method of investigation does not require a knowledge of the pathogenesis of the disease, the strategy is also known as *reverse genetics.*

Recent advances in the genetics of human disease have been much assisted by the availability of detailed genetic maps as well as thousands of genetic markers identified as part of a systematic world-wide effort. The known genetic markers are variations in the coding sequence of deoxyribonucleic acid (DNA) and can be assayed directly; indirect methods for identifying genetic markers, such as serological assays for blood group types or human leucocyte antigen (HLA) variants, are therefore unnecessary. The chromosomal location and methods for assaying the markers are available on computerized public databases, ensuring ease of access and replicability (Dib *et al.*, 1995; Collins *et al.*, 1997).

Another key development is the *polymerase chain reaction*. This allows rapid and economical amplification of relatively small regions of the gene (Saiki *et al*., 1988). Amplified fragments can then be manipulated, separated electrophoretically, and visualized.

The automation of genetic screening strategies has shortened the screening process considerably. Ingenious methods for detecting and screening mutations have often simplified the last stage in the hunt for disease genes (Gejman and Gelerenter, 1993; Inazuka *et al*., 1997). Working in tandem with such laboratory developments are sophisticated and ongoing refinements of computing techniques. Thanks to these advances, it is feasible to conduct large scale genetic studies rapidly and economically.

Linkage and Association

These terms describe complementary approaches to gene mapping. Consider the situation in which the researcher seeks to identify the gene responsible for a particular trait. When a variant (allele) of a genetic marker segregates with that trait in a family, it is said to be *linked* to the trait. Linkage implies that the marker gene and the gene underlying the trait are physically or geographically close. The concept of linkage is used in the initial efforts to localize or *map* a disease gene. The process involves the examination of diverse genetic markers among members of a family tree (pedigree) chosen on the basis of an affected member or proband. The aim is to identify a variant of the marker which is inherited along with the trait in the pedigree. The inheritance pattern of the marker is compared with the inheritance pattern of the trait in the pedigree, and the chance of a random association between the two is expressed as a *lod score*. To insure against spurious results, correct specification of the mode of inheritance of the trait as well as of the marker is necessary. Linkage studies are necessarily conducted in families.

In contrast, *association* usually describes a phenomenon at the population level. It assumes that a disease mutation arose in a founding member of the population currently under investigation. The mutation may have been passed down to the progeny along with an allele at a neighbouring gene located on the ancestral chromosome. A non-random association between the mutation and the marker allele may thus be expected at the population level among the cases who are descendants of the affected founder. This phenomenon is known as *linkage disequilibrium* (Nimgaonkar, 1997).

The strength of the association between the disease mutation gene and the marker allele gene (situated on the same chromosome, at a neighbouring locus) decays in succeeding generations. This is a result of meiotic crossovers between the two loci, consistent with Mendel's laws. The rate of decay increases with greater physical distance between the marker and the disease gene, and with increased number of generations since the introduction of the mutation into the population (Jorde, 1995). Nevertheless, the linkage disequilibrium may be exploited to localize disease genes if suitable genetic markers are available (Mourant *et al.*, 1978). It is only necessary to compare a representative sample of cases with ethnically matched, unaffected and unrelated controls (Cooper and Clayton, 1988). Detection of an association implies that the marker gene itself is the disease gene or that an allele of the marker gene is in linkage disequilibrium with the disease gene mutation (Suarez and Hampe, 1994).

Because of the effects of decay with time, the requirements for physical proximity between the marker and disease genes are more stringent for association studies than for linkage analysis. Since markers with the required density are not currently available, two options are available. In the first option, linkage analyses are initially used to localize the region of the genome harbouring the disease gene. Association studies are then used for fine mapping (Gershon *et al.*, 1998). This two-stage approach proved highly successful for Huntington's disease (Kieburtz *et al.*, 1994). In the second option, the association approach is used primarily by selecting *candidate genes* as markers (Gurling, 1985). Candidate genes are those which encode proteins that have been implicated in the pathogenesis of the disease; such proteins might have previously been identified in non-genetic investigations. The success of this method is crucially dependent on the choice of candidate genes.

The different techniques that are described here have been exploited in several hundred genetic studies. The most dramatic results have been obtained with the so-called monogenic diseases such as cystic fibrosis (Kerem *et al.*, 1989). Progress has been slower with more common disorders such as diabetes mellitus, probably because these disorders do not follow the simple Mendelian patterns of inheritance. The polygenic model best explains complex patterns of inheritance. The model proposes the presence of several disease genes, the interaction between which results in the liability to the disease (Falconer, 1965). This model also proposes a threshold of liability, beyond which the illness occurs (Gottesman and Shields, 1967). The threshold can be attained in an individual by combinations of alleles at various disease-predisposing loci, with or without the presence of environmental factors, even though each allele individually may not be necessary or sufficient to produce the disease.

There are other, practical, difficulties in linkage and association studies of genetically complex disorders. Most disorders have a variable age of onset, making it difficult to assess the likelihood of illness in an as yet unaffected member of a pedigree. This uncertainty hampers traditional linkage analysis and necessitates the use of a *penetrance* estimate to assess the chances of illness in an unaffected member who carries an allele of a putatively linked gene. Many disorders such as Alzheimer's disease are associated with late onset; many disorders such as schizophrenia are also associated with reduced fertility. In both situations, it becomes difficult to obtain sufficiently large pedigrees for research.

Investigations into polygenic disorders have therefore required revisions of the traditional linkage analysis which presumes knowledge of the mode of inheritance. Most of such *model-free* analyses require investigation of only the affected members of pedigrees. The most popular strategy involves the study of nuclear families with two or more affected siblings. For markers that are not linked to the disease gene, pairs of affected siblings share two, one, or no parental alleles by descent in the proportion of 1:2:1. A significant alteration in this proportion is suggestive of linkage between the putative marker and the disease gene (Penrose, 1935). This 'identical by descent' analysis requires knowledge about the parental alleles (Green and Woodrow, 1977). If knowledge about the parental alleles cannot be obtained, examination of alleles 'identical by state' can be used among the affected siblings (Weeks and Lange, 1988). In this analysis, no assumptions are made about whether an allele shared between two siblings originated in the same parent. This method is less powerful than the 'identical by descent' analysis. Multipoint analysis, that is, simultaneous analysis of several neighbouring markers, can have a very high power (Kruglyak and Lander, 1995).

This *affected sib pair* strategy has several advantages over the conventional linkage analysis. It makes no assumptions about the mode of inheritance. Since only the affected members are included in the analysis, problems related to variable penetrance do not arise. Unlike conventional analysis, the affected sib pair strategy can also be used to identify individual gene loci in disorders with a presumed polygenic form of inheritance, provided the contribution from a given locus is relatively large (Suarez *et al.*, 1991).

The affected sib pair method has already yielded results in the genetic dissection of insulin-dependent diabetes mellitus (Davies *et al.*, 1994) and celiac disease (Zhong *et al.*, 1996). Though the regions of susceptibility have been identified, using this approach, it has not been possible to precisely localize any disease gene for complex genetic disorders. The limiting factor is the prohibitively large number of sib pairs that are required for a fine mapping effort (Risch and Merikangas, 1996). Therefore, investigators have resorted to association studies. For example, case-control association studies have been valuable for the identification of the HLA region as the prime disease susceptibility zone for insulin-dependent diabetes mellitus (Trucco, 1992; Trucco and Dorman, 1989).

Association studies using unrelated controls are accepted to have shortcomings. The studies can be hampered by biases in the selection of unaffected controls (Cooper and Clayton, 1988). With genetic case-control studies, a major difficulty is related to differing rates of ethnic admixture among cases and controls (Cox and Bell, 1989). If admixture between two or more populations with differing gene frequencies occurs at different rates among the cases and controls, spurious associations can occur (Suarez and Hampe, 1994).

To overcome such difficulties, Rubinstein and his colleagues proposed a hypothetical control group, comprising alleles which are *not* inherited by the proband from his/her parents (Rubinstein *et al.*, 1981; Falk and Rubinstein, 1987). Studies utilizing this strategy investigate a population-based, unselected sample of cases and their parents. This simple *haplotype relative risk* strategy ensures that both cases and controls come from the same genetic group. The ancestral chromosomal segment with the disease may be identified with an increased confidence by examining multiple markers at the region of interest (Jazwinska *et al.*, 1995). Under random mating conditions and single ascertainment, associations will only be detected if the marker and disease genes are *also* linked (Knapp *et al.*, 1993; Ott, 1989).

Other variations of the family-based association studies are under investigation. The most popular method is the Transmission Disequilibrium Test (Spielman *et al.*, 1994) which investigates preferential transmission of alleles from heterozygous parents to affected persons. Though family-based association studies which utilize strategies such as the Transmission Disequilibrium Test are appealing, their use may be restricted in conditions (such as Alzheimer's disease) which are associated with a late age of onset. Since these studies involve the investigation of two individuals (the parents) for every case, family-based associations studies are also more laborious than association studies using unrelated controls. Therefore, their utility for genetically complex disorders awaits further investigation.

Studies on Genetically Isolated Populations

A difficulty associated with the genetic research of polygenic or multifactorial diseases arises from the likelihood that several disease genes of small effect substantially alter disease susceptibility in large populations that are composed of many admixed ethnic groups. This difficulty has also been encountered in the genetic dissection of insulin-dependent diabetes mellitus and multiple sclerosis (Davies *et al.*, 1994; Bell and Lathrop, 1996).

A smaller number of genes may be involved in populations which are genetically isolated; that is, populations which are characterized by significant inbreeding. In such populations, disease genes may be passed to descendants through several lines of inheritance from an affected ancestor (Emery, 1986). Therefore, such genes may be present with greater frequency among affected individuals, and it may be possible to trace them back to a common, affected ancestor if genealogies are available. Linkage may be demonstrated by searching for excess sharing of alleles among affected, related individuals. This technique, known as *identity by descent analysis*, is powerful, and requires a relatively small sample. It is easy to scan the entire genome in such pedigrees using highly polymorphic genetic markers.

Studies among genetic isolates are ideal for recessive conditions in which the disease is manifested only when two copies of the abnormal gene are present in the individual. Examples of conditions studied in this manner include diastrophic dysplasia and cartilage-hair hypoplasia (Hastbacka *et al.*, 1992; Sulisalo *et al.*, 1993). This strategy has also been useful in Hirschsprung's disease, which has a complex pattern of inheritance (Puffenberger *et al.*, 1994). Recent success in the genetic dissection of asthma among the Hutterites, a genetically isolated North American community, also supports the use of the strategy (Ober *et al.*, 1997).

It is thus evident that a variety of strategies are available for the genetic dissection of complex diseases. The choice of technique will necessarily be dictated by the circumstances, but a combined approach is likely to be the most successful (Ghosh, 1995). Recent computational advances will be of immense benefit. Such advances include the multipoint mapping of multigenic traits in affected sib pairs (Kruglyak and Lander, 1995), incorporation of a variety of familial groups in association studies (Thomson, 1995), and modeling of risk when more than one genomic region involved in susceptibility has been discovered.

Ethical Issues

Research into the genetics of human diseases has profound ethical implications stemming from the potential availability of predictive genetic tests and the recent advances in cloning technology. The ethical issues concerning genetic testing acquire added gravity in psychiatric contexts due to concerns about competence to consent, stigma associated with psychiatric illnesses, and limitations of the available treatments (Shore *et al.*, 1993).

While the rationale for genetic investigations is evident, individuals at high risk for illness may face adverse repercussions. For example, their marital choice may be narrowed; they may suffer a refusal of health insurance and worse, this refusal of insurance may extend to their relatives. Thus, an individual may unwittingly suffer from a predictive genetic test performed by a relative; and, a relative may suffer from such a test conducted on the patient. For their part, insurance companies claim that predictive information obtained through genetic testing is required for actuarial purposes. While the relative merits of arguments on the subject are debatable, the need for an informed public discussion cannot be denied. It goes without saying that the ethical and legislative decisions on the matter will be influenced by local religious and cultural forces. Therefore, ethical 'recipes' will need to be contextually evolved, and cannot be transplanted from one country to another.

Regrettably, the rate of scientific advance in genetics has far outpaced deliberations about ethical issues. Guidelines for genetic studies are under regular review (American Society of Human Genetics, 1996). Currently, the prime ethical requirement for genetic studies is a written informed consent (Parker, 1995). It has been suggested that individual consent should be supplemented by 'communal consent' to increase awareness of relevant issues (Foster *et al.*, 1997).

Status of Psychiatric Genetic Studies

Is it feasible to identify the gene(s) predisposing to psychiatric disorders? In view of past controversies about the very existence of psychiatric disorders, it is not surprising that grave doubts have been expressed (Horgan, 1993). These doubts have been fueled by inconsistent results, some of which are described in the sections that follow.

In defence of psychiatric genetic studies, there is little doubt that inherited factors play a significant role in the aetiology of conditions such as schizophrenia and bipolar disorder. Supportive evidence for a genetic basis of schizophrenia has come from family and adoption studies (Heston, 1966; Kety and Ingraham, 1992). Concordance, which is the risk for illness in a twin if the other twin is already ill, is significantly higher for schizophrenia among monozygotic twins (39 per cent) than among dizygotic twins (10 per cent) (Gottesman, 1991). Heritability, which is a measure of the proportion of the aetiology (at the population level) that is attributable to genetic factors, is estimated at 60–70 per cent for schizophrenia after the influences of a common environment are taken into account (Rao *et al.*, 1981; McGue *et al.*, 1983).

The genetic basis of bipolar disorder has similarly been supported by twin studies. For example, the concordance for bipolar disorder I was found to be 69 per cent among monozygotic as compared with 19 per cent among dizygotic twins (Bertelsen *et al.*, 1977). Similar monozygotic concordance figures were obtained from studies of monozygotic twins reared apart (Bertelsen, 1985). A review of family studies suggests that the morbid risk for bipolar disorder is elevated from about 1 per cent in the general population to 5.7–7.8 in first degree relatives of patients with bipolar I illness (Rice *et al.*, 1987; McGuffin and Katz, 1989).

It is likely that the infrequent replications of research findings, endemic to other fields of psychiatric research as well, are due to a failure to understand the complex mode of inheritance of most psychiatric disorders. These issues are discussed in the following sections.

Definition of Phenotype in Psychiatric Studies

A crucial but often overlooked aspect of psychiatric genetic research is the definition of the traits (phenotype) under consideration. A failure to use a valid definition of the trait is likely to result in unreliable findings. Many of the family studies of schizophrenia cited earlier did not use operationalized diagnostic criteria with demonstrated reliability and validity. While the more recent studies did use such criteria, the validity of these criteria for genetic studies cannot be presumed. Reassuringly, certain of the operationalized criteria have gained validity from reanalysis of previous as well as recent adoption studies (Kety and Ingraham, 1992).

In another novel strategy, the difference in concordance between monozygotic and dizygotic twins was investigated using different diagnostic criteria for schizophrenia (McGuffin *et al.*, 1984; Farmer *et al.*, 1987). From the genetic perspective, it was hypothesized that the most valid diagnostic scheme would yield the highest heritability values; for this purpose, greater heritability was defined as a greater monozygotic as compared with the dizygotic twin concordance rate. The Research Diagnostic Criteria (RDC; Spitzer *et al.*, 1977) yielded the highest heritability values, while Schneiderian First Rank Symptoms yielded much poorer results. DSM-III criteria yielded values comparable with RDC only when the following diagnoses were included along with schizophrenia: affective disorder with mood-incongruent delusions, atypical psychosis, and schizotypal personality disorder.

Such analyses have been extended to DSM-IIIR criteria, but not to DSM-IV criteria (Onstad *et al.*, 1991). Across diagnostic criteria, significant differences in monozygotic and dizygotic twin concordance rates have been observed for schizophrenia, but not for schizophreniform, schizoaffective or delusional disorders, or psychoses not otherwise specified (Franzek and Beckmann, 1998). Similar twin studies may thus be used to dictate the phenotype to be investigated in genetic studies of other psychiatric conditions.

Research Models for Schizophrenia and Bipolar Disorder

The modes of inheritance for both schizophrenia and bipolar disorder are controversial. Autosomal dominant and recessive modes of inheritance have both been suggested (Slater, 1958; Hurst, 1972; Bucher *et al.*, 1981; Goldin *et al.*, 1983; McGuffin *et al.*, 1994). More importantly, complex segregation analysis of published family and twin data has consistently rejected the monogenic models (Carter and Chung, 1980; Rao *et al.*, 1981; McGue *et al.*, 1983; Gershon *et al.*, 1998). Finally, the possibility of genetic heterogeneity cannot be excluded; that is, different genes may be involved in different populations (Baron, 1985).

Several features of schizophrenia support a polygenic or multifactorial model for the disorder. These features include absence of full concordance among monozygotic twins, gradation in severity of illness across affected individuals, sharp drop in the risk for illness from first to second to third degree relatives, increased risk for illness among relatives of more severely ill probands, and increased risk for illness among persons with a larger number of affected members in their pedigree (Emery, 1986). Recent analysis by Risch (1990) convincingly shows that the liability to schizophrenia is best explained by a few (three or four) loci, each of which increases the risk for schizophrenia (amongst siblings of an affected individual, as compared with unrelated individuals) by no more than 2–3 fold. This oligogenic model is consistent with the findings of illness frequency in first, second, and third degree relatives. A similar picture is emerging with respect to bipolar disorder.

It is important to note that none of the genetic factors necessarily has a large impact on risk. Thus, studies with small sample sizes may have insufficient statistical power to identify a significant result; this may be responsible for the failure of such studies to replicate a reported finding.

Given the uncertainties outlined above, it would be prudent to use a combination of approaches, with an emphasis on model-free analyses. As described subsequently, precisely these approaches are now yielding converging findings.

Review of Gene Mapping Studies of Schizophrenia and Bipolar Disorder

LINKAGE STUDIES

Some research teams have studied large, multi-generational families with several affected members, and have conducted linkage analysis using highly polymorphic DNA markers throughout the genome. Unfortunately, this strategy is hampered by several uncertainties; these include the variable age of onset of the illness, the possibility of genetic heterogeneity, the unknown mode of inheritance, and the unknown penetrance values (Baron *et al.*, 1990; Pauls, 1993). Not surprisingly, inconsistent results have emerged from the research that has been conducted. An initial report describing linkage to markers on chromosome 5q11–q13 among Icelandic and English pedigrees generated considerable excitement (Sherrington *et al.*, 1988). Unfortunately, linkage to these markers was rejected in studies of other Caucasian pedigrees (McGuffin *et al.*, 1990). In a similar vein, initial highly publicized studies of bipolar disorder suggested linkage to polymorphic DNA markers on chromosomes 11p15 and Xq28 (Egeland *et al.*, 1987; Baron *et al.*, 1987), but subsequent studies in the same populations failed to support the results (Kelsoe *et al.*, 1989; Baron *et al.*, 1993). The contradictory findings have fueled skepticism about the usefulness of psychiatric genetics.

More consistent results have begun to emerge from studies that have used the affected sib pair method. Recent reports have suggested linkage to markers on the short arm of chromosome 6 (6p21–pter) among nuclear families having probands with schizophrenia. This linkage was first detected in a large sample of Irish families (Wang *et al.*, 1995). Supportive evidence was subsequently obtained from an enlarged cohort of approximately 285 families (Straub *et al.*, 1995), and from studies conducted by other groups (Moises *et al.*, 1995; Schwab *et al.*, 1995; Lichter *et al.*, 1995). The failure of other studies to detect linkage on chromosome 6 may have been a result of the small samples studied (Kalsi *et al.*, 1995; Sasaki *et al.*, 1995). A recent consortium, which studied over 800 families, also provided some support for linkage in this region of chromosome 6, and indicated markers on chromosome 8 as well (Schizophrenia Linkage collaborative Group, 1996), Nevertheless, the linkage to the chromosome 6 markers accounts for only 20–30 per cent of the variance attributable to genetic factors (Maier *et al.*, 1996). Furthermore, the large region of susceptibility (20 cM) precludes the easy identification of the genes that predispose to schizophrenia. Clearly, even the study of large samples (as in the research discussed here) is inadequate for disease gene localization. Therefore, complementary methods are required.

A susceptibility locus for schizophrenia may also exist on chromosome 22q12–q13. An initial report using large US pedigrees (Pulver *et al.*, 1994) received support from a consortium which analyzed 574 families (Gill *et al.*, 1995). A pseudoautosomal telomeric locus for the schizophrenia susceptibility gene was also proposed (Collinge *et al.*, 1991), but the finding could not be replicated (d'Amato *et al.*, 1991).

The picture is more complex with bipolar disorder linkage studies, although consistencies are emerging. For example, linkage to markers on chromosome 21q22.3 (Straub *et al.*, 1994) has been supported by independent teams (Detera-Wadleigh *et al.*, 1996; Smyth *et al.*, 1997). Considerable interest has focused on chromosome 18 following reports of linkage in the pericentromeric region (Berrettini *et al.*, 1994). Another group has suggested linkage at Chromosome 18p11, which overlaps the pericentromeric region, and at another region 40 cM distally on chromosome 18q (Stine *et al.*, 1995). The latter finding has received support from independent studies (Coon *et al.*, 1996; Freimer *et al.*, 1996; McMahon *et al.*, 1997). The relative risk conferred by these loci is, however, likely to be small and may be obscured by a *parent of origin effect* (Stine *et al.*, 1995; Gershon *et al.*, 1996; Nothen *et al.*, 1996). This is a newly discovered phenomenon; for some diseases, it is not only the identity of the allele or the variant of a gene which is important, but also which parent passes it to the offspring. Such complexities may explain both the difficulty in localizing susceptibility genes and the absence of linkage in some studies (Kelsoe *et al.*, 1995; Pauls *et al.*, 1995; Detera-Wadleigh *et al.*, 1997a).

Other promising regions for bipolar disorder research include chromosome 4p16 (Blackwood *et al.*, 1996), chromosome 22q11 (Lachman *et al.*, 1997), chromosome 7p (Berrettini *et al.*, 1994), chromosome 12q23–q24 (Dawson *et al.*, 1995), chromosome 5q35 (Coon *et al.*, 1993), chromosome 11q22–q24 (Detera-Wadleigh *et al.*, 1997b) and chromosome 4q35 (Adams *et al.*, 1998). Reviewing these bewildering results, Risch and Botstein (1996) suggested that bipolar disorder is unlikely to be due to a single disease gene, and that its genetic aetiology may not be explainable merely by genetic heterogeneity. Besides suggesting stringent criteria for acceptance of linkage, they advocated analysis of pooled results using primary data from published studies. An earlier review, which reached similar conclusions, also underlined possible clinical heterogeneity (Merikangas *et al.*, 1989).

ASSOCIATION STUDIES

As discussed earlier, association studies make no assumptions about the mode of inheritance, and are also able to detect genes of small effect. For both these reasons, association studies could be considered to be useful in schizophrenia and bipolar disorder. Unfortunately, their promise has not yet been fulfilled. Several genetic markers had been used in early association studies (reviewed by McGuffin and Sturt, 1986). Numerous candidate gene polymorphisms were examined directly in recent studies (Detera-Wadleigh *et al.*, 1987; Nimgaonkar *et al.*, 1992; Nothen *et al.*, 1993; Sommer *et al.*, 1993). However, no robust associations with schizophrenia or its subtypes were demonstrated (McGuffin and Sturt, 1986; Owen, 1992). Even so, some studies suggested associations of small magnitude with the genes encoding the D3 dopamine and the 5-HT2A serotonin receptors, as well as the genes in the HLA region (Nimgaonkar *et al.*, 1992 and 1996b; Wright *et al.*, 1995; Williams *et al.*, 1996 and 1998). The associations in the HLA region involve the Class II region, which encodes HLA molecules involved in antigen presentation. The findings at the HLA DQB1 gene locus are particularly intriguing because they suggest a negative association; the prevalence of the allele HLA DQB1*0602 is reduced among cases, suggesting a protective effect of this marker (Nimgaonkar *et al.*, 1992, 1995 and 1996a). Another recent report describing an association at the hSKCa3 gene locus is also of interest because the polymorphism involves trinucleotide repeat expansions in the coding region of the gene (Chandy *et al.*, 1998). Such expansions have been implicated in the aetiology of Huntington's disease (Kieburtz *et al.*, 1994).

Replicated associations with bipolar disorder I at the tyrosine hydroxylase and serotonin transporter gene loci have been published (Leboyer *et al.*, 1990; Collier *et al.*, 1996b). Associations with trinucleotide repeat expansions are also under investigation (O'Donavan *et al.*, 1995). Like the linkage studies, these results have been replicated by some but not all groups (Meloni *et al.*, 1995; Collier *et al.*, 1996a; Bellivier *et al.*, 1997; Battersby *et al.*, 1997).

Genetically Isolated Populations and Psychiatric Disorders

Disequilibrium mapping studies among genetic isolates hold great promise as they may help identify regions of the genome that harbour disease susceptibility genes. A genome scan had been completed in a large Micronesian pedigree with many members diagnosed with schizophrenia, but convincing evidence of linkage did not emerge (Byerley *et al.*, 1997). In contrast, studies in a Costa Rican population with many members suffering from bipolar disorder suggested the presence of susceptibility genes on chromosome 18q (Freimer *et al.*, 1996).

Clinical Relevance

At present, the genetic studies reviewed here have limited clinical relevance. One clinical application relates to the operationalization of diagnostic criteria. As discussed earlier, twin studies have already suggested different levels of validity for diagnostic criteria for schizophrenia. Such genetically-determined characterization of validity could become more precise if specific genetic factors could be identified. Another application of the findings of genetic research is the identification of subgroups of diseases based on genetic aetiology. Such a classification has been applied to Alzheimer's disease, in which age at onset current provides a basis for subclassification.

If a consistently replicable finding emerges in psychiatric genetics, the rapid pace of scientific research is likely to ensure a rapid impact on therapeutics. Interventions at the levels of primary, secondary, and tertiary prevention are all conceivable.

Other Psychiatric Disorders

This review has focused on schizophrenia and bipolar disorder at the expense of other psychiatric disorders, such as major depression, alcohol and substance abuse, attention deficit disorder, dyslexia, and autism. These disorders are being intensively investigated at present. The investigations have evolved from initial simplistic assumptions of monogenic aetiology to a realization that more complex processes are involved. Therefore, model-free linkage analyses and family based association studies are increasingly being used. Sophisticated quantitative analyses are also being applied in the genetic investigation of normal traits such as intelligence and novelty-seeking (Fulker *et al.*, 1995; Fulker and Cherny, 1996).

IN CONCLUSION

The genetics revolution has entered a mature phase with the investigation of genetically complex disorders. Among these conditions, psychiatric disorders pose a unique challenge because of their complex inheritance patterns; results from this field of enquiry are likely to shed light on brain function. With growing awareness of the complexity of the task at hand, investigators are using more sophisticated techniques. These approaches have been rewarded with consistent evidence for schizophrenia susceptibility genes on chromosomes 6p21-pter and 21q12–q13. For bipolar disorder, there is support for susceptibility loci on chromosome 21q22. Though suggestive evidence for linkage on chromosome 18 has been obtained, unanimity has not been achieved. Plausible associations with tyrosine hydroxylase and serotonin transporter loci have not been replicated by all groups. These disparate findings illustrate the complex genetic aetiology of schizophrenia and bipolar disorder I, besides emphasizing the importance of recruiting additional samples.

It is very likely that during the next five years susceptibility genes for one or more psychiatric disorders will be identified.

The advances will lead to the following series of questions:

1. What is the role of the identified gene(s) in normal brain functioning?

2. How does the mutation lead to the abnormality under investigation?
3. How does the mutation interact with environmental factors in the pathogenesis?
4. Does the discovery help in the development of rational pharmacotherapy?
5. Can the disorder of interest be prevented through genetic counselling or by avoidance of the deleterious gene-environment interaction?

REFERENCES

Adams L. J., Mitchell P. B., Fielder S. L. *et al.* (1998). 'A susceptibility locus for bipolar affective disorder on chromosome 4q35', *Am. J. Hum. Genet.*, 62: 1084–91.

American Society of Human Genetics (1996). 'ASHG report: statement on informed consent for genetic research', *Am. J. Hum. Genet.*, 15: 471–4.

Baron M. (1985). 'The genetics of schizophrenia: new perspectives', *Acta. Psychiatr. Scand.*, 319: Suppl. 85–92.

Baron M., Risch N., Hamburger R. *et al.* (1987). 'Genetic linkage between X-chromosome markers and bipolar affective illness', *Nature*, 326: 289–92.

Baron M., Endicott J. and Ott J. (1990). 'Genetic linkage in mental illness: Limitations and prospects', *Br. J. Psychiatry*, 157: 645–55.

Baron M., Freimer N. F., Risch N. *et al.* (1993). 'Diminished support for linkage between manic depressive illness and X-chromosome markers in three Israeli pedigrees' (*see* commets), *Nature Genet.*, 3: 49–55.

Battersby S., Ogilvie A. D., Smith Cad *et al.* (1997). 'Haplotype Analysis of the Serotonin Transporter Gene in Mood Disorder', *Am. J. Hed. Genet.*, 74(6) 619.

Bell J. I. and Lathrop G. M. (1996). 'Multiple loci for multiple sclerosis', *Nature Genet.*, 13: 377–83.

Bellivier F., Laplanche J. L., Leboyer M. *et al.* (1997). 'Serotonin transporter gene and manic depressive illness: an association study', *Biol. Psychiatry*, 41: 750–2.

Berrettini W. H., Ferraro T. N., Goldin L. R. *et al.* (1994). 'Chromosome 18 DNA markers and manic-depressive illness: evidence for a susceptibility gene', *Proc. Natl. Acad. Sci. USA*, 91: 5918–21.

Bertelsen A. (1985). 'Controversies and consistencies in psychiatric genetics', *Acta. Psychiatr. Scand.*, 319: (Suppl.) 61–75.

Bertelsen A., Harvald B. and Hauge M. (1977). 'A Danish twin study of manic-depressive disorders', *Br. J. Psychiatry*, 130: 330–51.

Blackwood D. H., He L., Morris S. W. *et al.* (1996). 'A locus for bipolar affective disorder on chromosome 4p', *Nature Genet.*, 12: 427–30.

Bucher K. D., Elston R. C., Green R. *et al.* (1981). 'The transmission of manic depressive illness: II. Segregation analysis of three sets of family data', *J. Psychiatr. Res.*, 16: 65–78.

Byerley W., Polloi A., Dale P. *et al.* (1977). 'Genome-wide linkage analysis of a large schizophrenia pedigree ascertained from Palao, Micronesia', *Am. J. Med. Genet.*, 74: 559–60.

Carter C. L. and Chung C. S. (1980). 'Segregation analysis of schizophrenia under a mixed genetic model', *Hum. Hered.*, 30: 350–6.

Chandy K. G., Fantino E., Wittenkindt O. *et al.* (1998). 'Isolation of a novel potassium channel gene, hSKCa3 containing a polymorphic CAG repeat: a candidate for schizophrenia and bipolr disorder?', *Molecular Psychiatry* (in press).

Collier D. A., Arranz M. J., Sham P. *et al.* (1996a). 'The serotonin transporter is a potential susceptibility factor for bipolar affective disorder', *Neuroreport*, 7: 1675–9.

Collier D. A., Stober G., Li T. *et al.* (1996b). 'A novel functional polymorphism within the promoter of the serotonin transporter gene: possible role in susceptibility to affective disorders' (see comments), *Molecular Psychiatry*, 1: 453–60.

Collinge J., Delisi L. E., Boccio A. *et al.* (1991). 'Evidence for a pseudo-autosomal locus for schizophrenia using the method of affected sibling pairs', *Br. J. Psychiatry*, 158: 624–9.

Collins F. S., Guyer M. S. and Chakravarti A. (1997). 'Variations on a theme: Cataloging human DNA sequence variation', *Science*, 278: 1580–1.

Coon H., Jensen S., Hoff M. *et al.* (1993). 'A genome-wide search for genes predisposing to manic-depression, assuming autosomal dominant inheritance', *Am. J. Hum. Genet.*, 52: 1234–49.

Coon H., Hoff M., Holik J. *et al.* (1996). 'Analysis of chromosome 18 DNA markers in multiplex pedigrees with manic depression', *Biol. Psychiatry*, 39: 689–96.

Cooper D. N., and Clayton J. F. (1988). 'DNA Polymorphism and the study of disease associations', *Hum. Genet.*, 78: 299–312.

Cox N. J., and Bell G. I. (1989). 'Disease associations: Chance, artifact, or susceptibility genes?', *Diabetes*, 38: 947–50.

d'Amato T., Campion D., Gorwood P. *et al.* (1991). 'Linkage analysis using four RFLP markers of the pseudoautosomal region in schizophrenia', *Psychiat. Genet.*, 2: 30.

Davies J. L., Kawaguchi Y., Bennett S. T. *et al.* (1994). 'A genome-wide search for human type 1 diabetes susceptibility genes', *Nature*, 371: 130–6.

Dawson E., Parfitt E., Robert Q. *et al.* (1995). 'Linkage studies of bipolar disorder in the region of the Darier's disease gene on chromosome 12q23–24. 1', *Am. J. Med. Genet.*, 60: 94–102.

Detera-Wadleigh S. D., Berrettini W. H., Goldin L. R. *et al.* (1987). 'Close linkage of c-Harvey-ras-1 and the insulin gene to affective disorder is ruled out in three North Am. pedigrees', *Nature*, 325: 806–8.

Detera-Wadleigh S. D., Badner J. A., Goldin L. R. *et al.* (1996). 'Affected-sib pair analyses reveal support of prior evidence for a susceptibility locus for bipolar disorder on 21q', *Am. J. Hum. Genet.*, 58: 1279–85.

Detera-Wadleigh S. D., Badner J. A., Yoshikawa T. *et al.* (1997a). 'Initial genome scan of the NIMH genetics initiative bipolar pedigrees: chromosomes 4, 7, 9, 18, 19, 20, and 21q', *Am. J. Med. Genet.*, 74: 254–62.

Detera-Wadleigh S. D., Berrettini W. H., Yoshikawa T. *et al.* (1997b). 'Linkage disequilibrium detects a potential susceptibility locus for bipolar disorder at 11q2–24', *Am. J. Med. Genet.*, 74: 669.

Dib C., Faure S., Fizames C. *et al.* (1995). 'The final version of the Genethon Human Linkage Map', *Proceedings of the Cold Spring Harbor Mapping and Sequencing Symposium*, 298.

Egeland J. A., Gerhard D. S., Pauls D. L. *et al.* (1987). 'Bipolar affective disorders linked to DNA markers on chromosome 11', *Nature*, 325: 783–7.

Emery A. E. H. (1986). *Methodology in Medical Genetics: An Introduction to Statistical Methods*, 2nd ed., Edinburgh: Churchill Livingstone.

Falconer D. S. (1965). 'The inheritance of liability to certain diseases estimated from the incidence among relatives', *Ann. Hum. Genet.*, 29: 51–76.

Falk C. T. and Rubinstein P. (1987). 'Haplotype relative risks: an easy, reliable way to construct a proper control sample for risk calculations', *Ann. Hum. Genet.*, 51: 227–33.

Farmer A. E., McGuffin P. and Gottesman II (1987). 'Twin concordance for DSM-III schizophrenia: Scrutinizing the validity of the definition', *Arch. Gen. Psychiatry*, 44: 634–41.

Foster M., Eisenbraum A. and Carter T. (1997). 'Communal discourse as a supplement to informed consent for genetic research', *Nature Genet.*, 17: 277–9.

Franzek E. and Beckmann H. (1998). 'Different genetic background of schizophrenia spectrum psychoses: a twin study', *Am. J. Psychiatry*, 155: 76–83.

Freimer N. B., Reus VI, Escamilla M. A. *et al.* (1996). 'Genetic mapping using haplotype, association and linkage methods suggests a locus for severe bipolar disorder (BPI) at 18p22–q23', *Nature Genet.*, 12: 436–41.

Fulker D. W. and Cherny S. S. (1996). 'An improved multipoint (sib pair) analysis of quantitative traits', *Beh. Genet.*, 26: 527–32.

Fulker D. W., Cherny S. S. and Cardon Lr. (1995). 'Multipoint interval mapping of quantitative trait loci, using sib pairs', *Am. J. Hum. Genet.*, 56: 1224–33.

Gejman P. V. and Gelerenter J. (1993). 'Mutational analysis of candidate genes in psychiatric disorders', *Am. J. Med. Genet.*, 48: 184–91.

Gershon E. S., Goldin L. R., Badner J. A. *et al.* (1996). 'Detection of linkage to affective disorders in the catalogued Amish pedigrees: a reply to Pauls *et al.* (letter), *Am. J. Hum. Genet.*, 58: 1381–5

Gershon E. S., Badner J. A., Goldin L. R. *et al.* (1998). 'Closing in on genes for manic-depressive illness and schizophrenia', *Neuropsychopharmacol.*, 18: 233–42.

Ghosh S. (1995). 'Probability and complex disease genes', *Nature Genet.*, 9: 223–4.

Gill M., Vallada H. and Collier D. (1995). 'Sib pair analysis of D22S278 genotypes in 574 pedigrees', *Psychiat. Genet.*, 5: 13–14.

Goldin L. R., Gershon E. S., Targum S. D. *et al.* (1983). 'Segregation and linkage analyses in families of patients with bipolar, unipolar, and schizoaffective mood disorders', *Am. J. Hum. Genet.*, 35: 274–87.

Gottesman I. (1991). *Schizophrenia Genesis: The Origins of Madness*, New York: WH Freeman.

Gottesman II and Shields J. (1967). 'A polygenic theory of schizophrenia', *Proc. Natl. Acad. Sci. USA*, 58: 199–205.

Green J. R. and Woodrow J. C. (1977). 'Sibling method for detecting HLA-linked genes in disease', *Tissue Antigens*, 9: 31–5.

Gurling H. M. D. (1985). 'Candidate genes and favoured loci: strategies for molecular genetic research into schizophrenia, manic depression, autism, alcoholism and Alzheimer's disease', *Psychiat. Develop.*, 4: 289–309.

Hastbacka J., de la Chapelle A., Kaitila I. *et al.* (1992). 'Linkage disequilibrium mapping in isolated founder populations: diastrophic dysplasia in Finland', *Nature Genet.*, 2: 204–11, (published erratum appears in *Nature Genet.* (1992) 2: 343).

Heston L. L. (1966). 'Psychiatric disorders in foster home-reared children of schizophrenic mothers', *Br. J. Psychiatry*, 112: 819–25.

Horgan J. (1993). 'Eugenics revisited', *Scientific Am.*, 268: 122–32.

Hurst L. A. (1972). 'Hypothesis of a single-locus recessive genotype for schizophrenia', in Kaplan A. R. (ed.), *Genetic Factors in 'Schizophrenia'*, Springfield: Charles C. Thomas.

Inazuka M., Wenz H. M., Sakabe M. *et al.* (1997). ' A streamlined mutation detection system: multicolor post-PCR fluorescence labeling and single-strand conformational polymorphism analysis by capillary electrophoresis', *Genome. Res.*, 7: 1094–1103.

Jazwinska E. C., Pyper W. R., Burt M. J. *et al.* (1995). 'Haplotype analysis in Australian hemochromatosis patients: evidence for a predominant ancestral haplotype exclusively associated with hemochromatosis', *Am. J. Hum. Genet.*, 56: 428–33.

Jorde L. B. (1995). 'Linkage disequilibrium as a gene-mapping tool', *Am. J. Hum. Genet.*, 56: 11–14.

Kalsi G., Chen A., Brynjolfsson J. *et al.* (1995). 'Genetic linkage analysis of the putative chromosome 6p subtype of schizophrenia in 23 UK and Icelandic families', *Psychiat. Genet.*, 5 (suppl 1): S33.

Kelsoe J. R., Ginns E. I., Egeland J. A. *et al.* (1989). 'Re-evaluation of the linkage relationship between chromosome 11p loci and the gene for bipolar affective disorder in the Old Order Amish' (see comments), *Nature*, 342: 238–43.

Kelsoe J. R., Sadovnick A. D., Kristbjarnarson H. *et al.* (1995). 'Genetic linkage studies of bipolar disorder and chromosome 18 markers in North American, Icelandic and Amish pedigrees', *Psychiat. Genet.*, 5 (suppl. 1): S17–S18.

Kerem B., Rommens J. M., Buchanan J. A. *et al.* (1989). 'Identification of the cystic fibrosis gene: genetic analysis', *Science*, 245: 1073–80.

Kety S. S. and Ingraham L. J. (1992). 'Genetic transmission and improved diagnosis of schizophrenia from pedigrees of adoptees', *J. Psychiatric Res.*, 26: 247–55.

Kieburtz K., MacDonald M., Shih C. *et al.* (1994). 'Trinucleotide repeat length and progression of illness in Huntington's disease', *J. Med. Genet.*, 31: 872–4.

Knapp M., Seuchter S. A. and Baur M. P. (1993). 'The haplotype-relative-risk (HRR) method for analysis of association in nuclear families', *Am. J. Hum. Genet.*, 52: 1085–93.

Kruglyak L. and Lander E. S. (1995). 'Complete multipoint sib pair analysis of qualitative and quantitative traits', *Am. J. Hum. Genet.*, 57: 439–54.

Lachman H. M., Kelsoe J. R., Remick R. A. *et al.* (1997). 'Linkage studies suggest a possible locus for bipolar disorder near the velo-cardio-facial syndrome region on chromosome 22', *Am. J. Med. Genet.*, 74: 121–8.

Leboyer M., Malafosse A., Boularand S. *et al.* (1990). 'Tyrosine hydroxylase polymorphisms associated with manic-depressive illness', *Lancet*, 335: 1219.

Lichter J. B., Cardon L., Crow T. *et al.* (1995). 'Identification of susceptibility genes for schizophrenia', *Psychiat. Genet.*, 5 (suppl 1): S39.

Maier W., Albus M., Schwab S. *et al.* (1996). 'Evaluation of a susceptibility gene for schizophrenia on chromosome 6p', *Schizophr. Res.*, 18: 167.

McGue M., Gottesman II and Rao D. C. (1983). 'The transmission of schizophrenia under a multifactorial threshold model', *Am. J. Hum. Genet.*, 35: 1161–78.

McGuffin P., Farmer A. E., Gottesman II *et al.* (1984). 'Twin concordance for operationally defined schizophrenia: Confirmation of familiality and heritability', *Arch. Gen. Psychiatry*, 41: 541–5.

McGuffin P. and Sturt E. (1986). 'Genetic markers in schizophrenia', *Hum. Hered.*, 36: 65–88.

McGuffin P. and Katz R. (1989). 'The genetics of depression and manic-depressive disorder', *Br. J. Psychiatry*, 155: 294–304.

McGuffin P., Sargeant M., Hetti G. *et al.* (1990). 'Exclusion of a schizophrenia susceptibility gene from the chromosome 5q11–q13 region: new data and a reanalysis of previous reports' (see comments), *Am. J. Hum. Genet.*, 47: 524–35.

McGuffin P., Owen M. J., O'Donovan M. C. *et al.* (1994). *Seminars in Psychiatric Genetics*, London: Gaskell.

McMahon F. J., Hopkins P. J., Xu J. *et al.* (1997). 'Linkage of bipolar affective disorder to chromosome 18 markers in a new pedigree series', *Am. J. Hum. Genet.*, 61: 1397–1404.

Meloni R., Leboyer M., Bellivier F. *et al.* (1995). 'Association of manic-depressive illness with tyrosine hydroxylase microsatellite marker' (*see* comments), *Lancet*, 345: 932.

Merikangas K. R., Spence M. A. and Kupfer D. J. (1989). 'Linkage studies of bipolar disorder: methodologic and analytic issues. Report of MacArthur Foundation Workshop on Linkage and Clinical Features in Affective Disorders', *Arch. Gen. Psychiatry*, 46: 1137–41.

Moises H. W., Yang L., Kristbiarnarson H. *et al.* (1995). 'An international two-stage genome-wide search for schizophrenia susceptibility genes', *Nature Genet.*, 11: 321–4.

Mourant A. E., Kopec A. C. and Domaniewska-Sobczak K. (1978). *Blood groups and diseases*, Oxford: Oxford University Press.

Nimgaonkar V. (1997). 'In defense of genetic association studies', *Molecular Psychiatry*, 2: 275–7.

Nimgaonkar V. L., Ganguli R., Rudert W. A. *et al.* (1992). 'A negative association of schizophrenia with an allele of the HLA DQBI gene among African-Americans', *Schizophr. Res.*, 8: 199–209.

Nimgaonkar V. L., Rudert W. A., Zhang X. R. *et al.* (1995). 'Further evidence for an association between schizophrenia and the HLA DQBI gene locus', *Schizophr. Res.*, 18: 43–9.

——— (1996a). 'Negative association of schizophrenia with HLA DQBI*0602: evidence from a second African-American cohort', *Schizophr. Res.*, 23: 81–6.

Nimgaonkar V. L., Sanders A. R., Ganguli R. *et al.* (1996b). 'Association study of schizophrenia and the dopamine D3 receptor gene locus in two independent samples', *Am. J. Med. Genet.*, 67: 505–14.

Nothen M. M., Korner J., Lannfelt L. *et al.* (1993). 'Lack of association between schizophrenia and alleles of the dopamine D1, D2, D3 and D4 receptor loci', *Psychiatr. Genet.*, 3: 89–94.

Nothen M. M., Cichon S., Craddock N. *et al.* (1996). 'Linkage studies of bipolar disorder to chromosome 18 markers', *Biol. Psychiatry*, 39: 615

Ober C., Cox N. J., Parry R. R. *et al.* (1997). 'Genome-wide search for asthma susceptibility loci in the Hutterites', *Am. J. Hum. Genet.*, 61 (suppl.) : A213.

O'Donovan M. C., Guy C., Craddock N. *et al.* (1995). 'CAG repeats in schizophrenia and bipolar disorder', *Nature Genet.*, 10: 380–1.

Onstad S., Skre I., Torgersen S. *et al.* (1991). 'Subtypes of schizophrenia-evidence from a twin-family study', *Acta. Psychiatr. Scand.*, 84: 203–6.

Ott J. (1989). 'Statistical properties of the haplotype relative risk', *Genet. Epidemiol.*, 6: 127–30.

Owen M. J. (1992). 'Will schizophrenia become a graveyard for molecular geneticists?', *Psychol. Med.*, 22: 289–93.

Parker L. (1995). 'Ethical concerns in the research and treatment of complex disease', *Trends Genet.*, 11: 520–3.

Pauls D. L. (1993). 'Behavioural Disorders: Lessons in Linkage', *Nature Genet.*, 3: 4–5.

Pauls D. L., Ott J., Paul S. M. *et al.* (1995). 'Linkage analyses of chromosome 18 markers do not identify a major susceptibility locus for bipolar affective disorder in the Old Order Amish', *Am. J. Hum. Genet.*, 57: 636–43.

Penrose L. S. (1935). 'The detection of autosomal linkage in data which consists of pairs of brothers and sisters of unspecified parentage', *Ann. Eugenics*, 6: 133–8.

Puffenberger E. G., Hosoda K., Washington S. S. *et al.* (1994). 'A missense mutation of the Endothelin-B receptor gene in multigenic Hirschsprung's disease', *Cell*, 79: 1257–66.

Pulver A. E., Karayiorgou M., Wolyniec P. S. *et al.* (1994). 'Sequential strategy to identify a susceptibility gene for schizophrenia: report of potential linkage on chromosome 22q12–q13.1: Part 1', *Am. J. Med. Genet.*, 54: 36–43.

Rao D. C., Morton N. E., Gottesman II *et al.* (1981). 'Path analysis of qualitative data on pairs of relatives: application to schizophrenia', *Hum. Hered.*, 31: 325–33.

Rice J., Reich T., Andreasen N. C. *et al.* (1987). 'The familial transmission of bipolar illness', *Arch. Gen. Psychiatry*, 44: 441–7.

Risch N. (1990). 'Linkage strategies for genetically complex traits: II. The power of affected relative pairs', *Am. J. Hum. Genet.*, 46: 229–41.

Risch N. and Botstein D. (1996). 'A manic depressive history' (news), *Nature Genet.*, 12: 351–3.

Risch N. and Merikangas K. (1996). 'The future of genetic studies of complex human diseases', *Science*, 273: 1516–17.

Rubinstein P., Walker M., Carpenter M. *et al.* (1981). 'Genetics of HLA disease associations. The use of the haplotype relative risk (HRR) and the "Haplo-delta" (Dh) estimates in juvenile diabetes from three racial groups', *Hum. Immunol.*, 3: 384.

Saiki R. K., Gelfand D. H., Stoffel S. *et al.* (1988). 'Primer-directed enzymatic amplification of DNA with a thermostable DNA polymerase', *Science*, 239: 487–91.

Sasaki T., Bassett A. S., Honer W. G. *et al.* (1995). 'Evaluation of markers at 6p21–23 in Eastern Canadian schizophrenia families', *Psychiat Genet.*, 5 (suppl. 1): S34.

Schizophrenia Linkage Collaborative Group for Chromosomes 3, 6 and 8 (1996). 'Additional support for schizophrenia linkage on chromosomes 6 and 8: a multicenter study', *Am. J. Med. Genet.*, 67: 580–94.

Schwab S. G., Albus M., Hallmayer J. *et al.* (1995). 'Evaluation of a susceptibility gene for schizophrenia on chromosome 6p by multipoint affected sib pair linkage analysis', *Nature Genet.*, 11: 325–7.

Sherrington R., Brynjolfsson J., Petursson H. *et al.* (1988). 'Localization of a susceptibility locus for schizophrenia on chromosome 5', *Nature*, 336: 164–7.

Shore D., Berg K., Wynne D. *et al.* (1993). 'Legal and ethical issues in psychiatric genetic research', *Am. J. Med. Genet.*, 48: 17–21.

Slater E. (1958). 'The monogenic theory of schizophrenia', *Acta. Genetics and Statistics in Med.*, 8: 50–60.

Smyth C., Kalsi G., Curtis D. *et al.* (1997). 'Two-locus admixture linkage analysis of bipolar and unipolar affective disorder supports the presence of susceptibility loci on chromosomes 11p15 and 21q22', *Genomics*, 39: 271–8.

Sommer S. S., Lind T. J., Heston L. L. *et al.* (1993). 'Dopamine D4 receptor variants in unrelated schizophrenic cases and controls', *Am. J. Med. Genet.*, 48: 90–3.

Spielman R. S., McGinnis R. E. and Ewens W. J. (1994). 'The transmission/disequilibrium test detects cosegregation and linkage', *Am. J. Hum. Genet.*, 54: 559–60.

Spitzer R., Endicott J. and Robins E. (1977). *Research Diagnostic Criteria for a Selected Group of Functional Disorders*, 3rd ed., New York: New York State Psychiatric Institute.

Stine O. C., Xu J., Koskela R. *et al.* (1995). 'Evidence for linkage of bipolar disorder to chromosome 18 with a parent-of-origin effect', *Am. J. Hum. Genet.*, 57: 1384–94.

Straub R. E., Lehner T., Luo Y. *et al.* (1994). 'A possible vulnerability locus for bipolar affective disorder on chromosome 21q22.3' (*see* Comments), *Nature Genet.*, 8: 291–6.

Straub R. E., Maclean C. J., Walsh D. *et al.* (1995). 'A potential susceptibility locus for schizophrenia on chromosome 6p: evidence for genetic heterogeneity', *Psychiatric Genet.*, 5 (suppl. 1): S26–S27.

Suarez B. K. and Hampe C. L. (1994). 'Linkage and association', *Am. J. Hum. Genet.*, 54: 554–9.

Suarez B. K., Van Eerdewegh P. and Hampe C. L. (1991). 'Detecting loci for oligogenic traits by linkage analysis', *Am. J. Hum. Genet.*, 49: 14.

Sulisalo T., Sistonen P., Hastbacka J. *et al.* (1993) 'Cartilage-hair hypoplasia gene assigned to chromosome 9 by linkage analysis', *Nature Genet.*, 3: 338–41.

Thomson G. (1995). 'Mapping disease genes: Family-based association studies', *Am. J. Hum. Genet.*, 57: 487–98.

Trucco M (1992). 'To be or not to be ASP 57, that is the question', *Diabetes Care*, 15: 705–15.

Trucco M. and Dorman J. S. (1989). 'Immunogenetics of insulin-dependent diabetes mellitus in humans', *Crit. Rev. Immunol.*, 9: 201–45.

Wang S., Sun C., Walczak C. A. *et al.* (1995). 'Evidence for a susceptibility locus for schizophrenia on chromosome 6pter–p22', *Nature Genet.*, 10: 41–6.

Weeks D. E. and Lange K. (1988). 'The affected-pedigree-member method of linkage analysis', *Am. J. Hum. Genet.*, 42: 315–26.

Williams J., Spurlock G., McGuffin P. *et al.* (1996). 'Association between schizophrenia and T102C polymorphism of the 5-hydroxytryptamine type 2a-receptor gene: European Multicentre Association Study of Schizophrenia (EMASS) Group', *Lancet*, 347: 1294–6.

Williams J., Spurlock G., Holmans P. *et al.* (1998). 'A meta-analysis and transmission disequilibrium study of association between the dopamine D3 receptor gene and schizophrenia', *Molecular Psychiatry*, 3: 141–9.

Wright P., Donaldson P., Underhill J. *et al.* (1995). 'Schizophrenia: a HLA class I and II association study', *Psychiatric Genet*, 5 (suppl. 1): S35.

Zhong F., McCombs C. C., Olson J. M. *et al.* (1996). 'An autosomal screen for genes that predispose to celiac disease in the western counties of Ireland', *Nature Genet.*, 14: 329–33.

Chapter 2

The Catatonic Syndrome: A Review of Recent Clinical Experience

GEORGIOS PETRIDES AND MAX FINK

INTRODUCTION

Catatonia is a distinct motor syndrome, first described in 1874 by the German psychiatrist Karl Ludwig Kahlbaum in a monograph titled 'Die Katatonie oder das Spannungsirresein' ('Catatonia or tension insanity') (Kahlbaum, 1973). Kahlbaum viewed catatonia using the clinical method of classifying mental illness by symptoms, signs, and course of the disorder; he conceptualized catatonia as a motor syndrome characterized by lack of motion and speech, alternating with periods of excessive, purposeless motor activity, rigidity, negativism, verbigeration, automatic obedience, posturing, grimacing, and stereotypies. He described the syndrome to have a periodic course and, in some cases, a lethal outcome.

Kraepelin adopted the ideas and methods of Kahlbaum in developing a concept of mental diseases. He categorized psychoses into schizophrenia (dementia-praecox) and manic-depressive illness, and classified catatonia as a subtype of schizophrenia (Kraepelin, 1913). The Kraepelinian stance was adopted by many modern classificatory schemes, including DSM–III (American Psychiatric Association, 1980), DSM–III-R (American Psychiatric Association, 1987) and ICD–9 (World Health Organization, 1977).

A different approach to catatonia is to view it as a syndrome. A syndrome is an aggregate of characteristic symptoms and signs associated with a morbid process; it is distinguished from a disease by the absence of specification of an aetiology. The catatonic syndrome is defined as the presence of two or more signs from a defined cluster of signs in a person with a mental disorder. It occurs in patients with affective disorders (Taylor and Abrams, 1973, 1977, and 1978; Abrams and Taylor, 1976; Abrams *et al.*, 1979; Bräunig *et al.*, 1998), neurological illnesses (Gelenberg, 1976 and 1977; Gelenberg and Mandel, 1977; Fricchione *et al.*, 1983 and 1990), and schizophrenia. Surveys of patients newly admitted to academic in-patient psychiatric services find that 6–9 per cent of patients meet the criteria for catatonia; these patients suffer from diverse psychiatric syndromes more often than they suffer from schizophrenia (Rosebush *et al.*, 1990; Pataki *et al.*, 1992; Ungvari *et al.*, 1994a and b; Bush *et al.*, 1996a).

Our consideration of catatonia encompasses three questions. Should catatonia be viewed as a syndrome of diverse aetiology or as a specific pathology in schizophrenia? May the nosological status of catatonia be influenced by its response to treatment options? And, is the neuroleptic malignant syndrome (NMS) better characterized as a type of catatonia or as a specific, independent syndrome? In this chapter, we present our views on these three issues; our attitudes are based, in large part, on our experiences at the University Hospital at Stony Brook, New York.

Catatonia As a Subtype of Schizophrenia

Kraeplin (1913) dichotomized psychoses into manic-depressive illness and schizophrenia (dementia-praecox). This simple classification could not satisfactorily account for conditions such as delusional unipolar depression, schizoaffective disorder, and substance-induced psychoses. The limitation of the Kraepelinian system was most apparent when catatonic symptoms were present; catatonia was recognized only as a form of schizophrenia, and the presence of catatonic symptoms was considered sufficient and binding for that diagnosis.

Wernicke, Bleuler, Kleist, and Leonhard sought to define further disease categories for better correspondence with clinically observable symptoms and their course and outcome. Leonhard (1979), in particular, described a sophisticated and complex classification system that considered catatonia as a schizophrenia subtype with a specific heredity, familial clustering, and prognosis.

His classification subdivided psychoses into five categories: unipolar phasic psychosis, bipolar phasic psychosis, cycloid psychosis, the unsystematic schizophrenias, and the systematic schizophrenias.

In Leonhard's system, catatonia was typically classified under the systematic and unsystematic schizophrenias. The various forms described under the general category of simple systematic schizophrenia were parakinetic catatonia, affected catatonia, proskinetic catatonia, negativistic catatonia, and sluggish catatonia. The unsystematic schizophrenias included a form of periodic catatonia characterized by an episodic course with symptom-free intervals between episodes; the syndrome was associated with both hypo- and hyper-kinetic states, and with affective symptoms. Leonhard wrote 'systematic and unsystematic schizophrenias are totally unrelated, and only for historical reasons are called schizophrenias.' He considered that the unsystematic schizophrenias have a different course and prognosis. He suggested that periodic catatonia was more closely related to cycloid psychoses—what we now generally consider as periodic affective disorders.

Using Leonhard's classification of catatonia, German researchers conducted elegant studies and showed that periodic catatonia differed genetically from the other systematic catatonias. Periodic (unsystematic) catatonia demonstrated a strong familial pattern of transmission while systematic catatonias were low in heritability (Stöber *et al.*, 1995; Beckmann *et al.*, 1996). A suggestion was also made that 'it is unlikely that a major psychosis gene, contributing (to periodic catatonia), is at a locus on the sex chromosomes' (Franzek *et al.*, 1995). Although Leonhard tried to dissociate periodic catatonia from the Kraepelinian dementia praecox, its classification under schizophrenia did not help his cause.

The Anglo-American approach to catatonia was influenced by Kraepelin. Catatonia was strictly defined as a subtype of schizophrenia in DSM-II, DSM-III, and DSM-III-R. This classification was crude, and did not even allow for the finer distinctions made by Leonhard. Such a conceptualization (or lack of it) had an enormous effect on management strategies for patients with catatonic symptoms; the implication was that the treatment of catatonia should be that of schizophrenia (that is based on neuroleptic medications), and that the prognosis was also that of schizophrenia. This approach fostered the impression that catatonia is a rare form of mental illness. Further, this approach offered little incentive for the recognition of catatonia because it encouraged the mistaken belief that the prognosis was (by association with schizophrenia) also poor. Finally, this approach drew attention away from the unique response of catatonia to tranquillizing drugs and electroconvulsive therapy (ECT).

Catatonia as a Syndrome

The traditional German and Anglo-American stances notwithstanding, catatonic symptoms are now recognized to also occur in non-schizophrenic psychiatric disorders as well as in systemic illnesses. The view that catatonic symptoms arise in diverse conditions is not new. Kahlbaum (1973) wrote that 'all the main clinical forms of the various mental conditions may be present [during the course of catatonia]; i.e., forms of melancholy, mania, stupor..., confusion, and insanity' (p. 29). DSM-IV (American Psychiatric Association, 1994) reflects this recognition; for example, it includes a category for catatonia secondary to a general medical condition (295.93), and permits the use of a modifier for catatonia in mood disorders.

Beyond the acceptance of catatonic symptoms as non-specific symptoms or epiphenomena in medical and psychiatric states is the conceptualization of catatonia as a unique syndrome. In this section, we review the evidence that catatonic symptoms arise in diverse backgrounds, and consider the position that catatonia merits consideration as a separate syndrome.

Catatonia: A Broad Spectrum of Origin

Morrison (1973, 1975) reviewed the Iowa State Hospital charts of 250 patients diagnosed with excited, retarded, or mixed DSM-II catatonic schizophrenia; 10–15 per cent of these patients fulfilled research criteria for the diagnosis of an affective disorder. Abrams and Taylor (1976) identified catatonic symptoms in 14–20 per cent of patients who met the research criteria for mania. In a prospective study of patients with one or more catatonic symptoms, the same authors found that 62 per cent of patients were manic, 16 per cent had organic brain disease, 9 per cent were depressed, and only 7 per cent met criteria for schizophrenia.

Our experience was similar. A retrospective review of 20

catatonic schizophrenics diagnosed at the University Hospital at Stony Brook between 1985 and 1990 found that 7 (35 per cent) patients met criteria for bipolar disorder, with 6 patients meeting criteria for mania (Pataki *et al.*, 1992). In a prospective study at the same hospital, we reported that 21 (91 per cent) of 23 catatonic patients met criteria for diagnoses other than schizophrenia (Bush *et al.*, 1996a).

In their survey of catatonic patients in a university hospital, (Rosebush *et al.*, 1990) used a check-list for catatonic symptoms and found that just 2 of 12 catatonics met criteria for schizophrenia. (Bräunig *et al.*, 1998), studying consecutive in-patients diagnosed with bipolar disorder (manic or mixed type) using the structured clinical interview for DSM-III-R (SCID), found that 19 (31 per cent) of 61 patients had catatonic symptoms. The catatonic patients had more mixed episodes, more severe manic symptoms, more severe psychopathology, longer periods of hospitalization, and a more severe course than did the manic patients without catatonia.

Catatonia has thus been associated with many psychiatric and systemic disorders (Table 2.1). This accumulated experience supports the view that catatonic signs, like delusions and hallucinations, are not pathognomonic of schizophrenia. Indeed, some patients who present with a catatonic picture but with no other identifiable psychopathology fit a class of 'catatonia not otherwise specified'. Such patients manifest an abrupt onset of catatonic symptoms, respond to treatment fully and promptly, allow no other psychopathology to be identified, and proceed to a normal life course.

Table 2.1: Conditions Associated with Catatonia (DSM-IV codes indicated in parentheses)

Depression	296.2x; 296.3x; 296.5x; 296.89
Mania	296.0x; 296.4x
Mixed affective disorder	296.6x
Schizophrenia	295.xx; specifically, 295.2x
Dissociative disorder	300.15
Delirium	291.0; 292.81; 293.0
Neuroleptic malignant syndrome	333.92
Catatonic disorder due to general medical condition	293.89

In the spirit of these observations, Fink and Taylor (1991) advocated the separation of catatonia from schizophrenia in DSM-IV, and suggested the creation of a distinct category. This experience was brought to the attention of the DSM-IV committee members who did decide to break with the tradition of DSM-II and DSM-III. The result was the inclusion of a new class, that of *Catatonic Disorder Due to a General Medical Condition (293.89)*. And, in recognition of the reports that catatonia is commonly observed in patients with affective disorders as well as in those with systemic conditions, when catatonic signs appeared in such patients the modifier 'with catatonia' was recommended (Table 2.1).

In ICD-10 (World Health Organization, 1992), catatonia is classified as a subtype of schizophrenia (F20.2) and as an organic disorder F06.1). ICD-10 also recognizes that stupor may occur as part of a depressive (F32.3), manic (F30.2) or dissociative (F44.2) disorder; stupor is clinically indistinguishable from what the North American literature calls catatonia.

Catatonia: Syndromes in Literature

Several syndromes of catatonia described in literature take into account possible triggering factors, clinical presentations, and course; these are briefly discussed.

Lethal catatonia, also known as malignant catatonia or pernicious catatonia, was described by Stauder (1934) as an acute clinical disorder characterized by fever, autonomic instability, and hyperactivity or stupor; the characterization resembled the descriptions of catatonia by Kahlbaum. The disorder was considered to be 'lethal' because it was associated with an increased risk of a fatal outcome. Arnold and Stepan (1952) identified 34 cases of lethal catatonia; 18 of these patients died. It was observed that the survivors had received ECT within the first five days of the illness. Similar findings were reported by Mann *et al.* (1986 and 1990) and by Philbrick and Rummans (1994). The latter authors reviewed the results of 13 cases reported in the literature between 1986 and 1991, and 5 cases from their records at the Mayo Clinic. ECT was effective in both series.

Catatonic excitement, also known as catatonic furor, delirious mania or manic delirium, is characterized by excitement, purposeless agitation, and autonomic instability. It is usually seen during the course of bipolar illness. In the absence of a good clinical history, it can be difficult to differentiate from pernicious catatonia.

Catatonic stupor typically presents with complete immobility and mutism. If untreated, medical complications of prolonged immobility may develop; these include inanition, pulmonary embolism, and bladder infections. The complications may lead to death; thus, catatonic stupor may also be lethal. Instances of stupor, immobility, mutism, and rigidity have also been described as benign stupors (Hoch, 1921). Other terms that have been used include akinetic mutism and coma vigil; these characterize patients who are unresponsive, although their eyes remain open and they appear to be awake.

Recurrent or *periodic catatonia* is the condition in which signs of catatonia appear periodically. The *neuroleptic malignant syndrome* (NMS) is the syndrome of fever and rigidity which develops after the recent administration of neuroleptic agents. The *toxic serotonin syndrome*, which may occur in patients who have received serotonin reuptake inhibitors, may also exhibit catatonic features (Fink, 1996a). *Non-convulsive status epilepticus* (NCSE) describes catatonic patients who exhibit abnormal EEG activity.

The treatment of catatonic syndromes has generally been supportive and symptomatic. It may be noted that the various descriptive designations carry little merit beyond announcing the multiplicity of presentations and the possible lethality of the syndrome; no specific aetiology is assumed. NMS, however, has been viewed as a specific psychopathological state. It is characterized by rigidity, fever, autonomic instability, and marked changes in mental status. It is classified as a distinct syndrome by DSM-IV (333.92) (American Psychiatric Association, 1994). Clinically, no features distinguish NMS from other catatonic states, particularly from the malignant form of catatonia. Treatments effective in catatonia are also effective in NMS; ECT, which is especially effective in catatonia, may be life-saving in NMS (Davis *et al.*, 1991). Many argue that NMS is a form of malignant catatonia induced by neuroleptic medications (White and Robins, 1991; White, 1992; Fink, 1996b); in this context, in studies of catatonia at the University Hospital at Stony Brook, we encountered NMS when we searched for catatonia, and catatonia when we searched for NMS (Koch *et al.*, 1995 and 1999).

Experience at the University Hospital at Stony Brook

We gained much experience with catatonia during the last decade at the University Hospital at Stony Brook. Our interest was stimulated by a 36-year-old woman, suffering from lupus cerebritis, who presented with mutism, posturing, rigidity, negativism, and autonomic instability in the absence of a prior history of psychiatric disturbance. The catatonic syndrome did not respond to neuroleptic and anticonvulsant medications, nor to specific anti-lupus pharmacotherapy, but dissolved dramatically with ECT (Fricchione *et al.*, 1990). While the catatonic syndrome could only be classified under schizophrenia in DSM-III-R, the case did not meet the DSM-III-R criteria for schizophrenia; this prompted a retrospective examination of the University Hospital experience from 1985 to 1990 (Pataki *et al.*, 1992). The records of 20 patients diagnosed with DSM-III (295.2) catatonic schizophrenia were identified; on review, 7 (35 per cent) patients were found to meet criteria for bipolar disorder, with 6 meeting criteria for mania.

Studies of Acute and Chronic Catatonia

In a subsequent prospective study, we developed a standardized 14-item screening instrument and a 23-item rating scale to identify and assess patients with catatonia (Bush *et al.*, 1996b). The instruments included the signs and symptoms that are most frequently reported in descriptions of catatonia. We applied the screening instrument to 215 consecutive admissions to our acute care unit over a 6-month period; patients in whom two or more catatonic symptoms were identified underwent a full evaluation using the 23-item rating scale. Fifteen patients (7 per cent) met criteria for catatonia, and all presented with at least 3 symptoms (average=6.6). Our study group comprised these 15 patients along with 13 other catatonic patients who were referred just before or after the official screening period of the study. Of the 28 patients, 15 (54 per cent) met criteria for affective disorders, (nine had mania, two had mixed affective disorder, three had major depression, and one had schizoaffective depression), 6 (21 per cent) were diagnosed with systemic disorders (three had NMS, one had a seizure disorder after closed head injury, one had an anticholinergic delirium, and one had steroid-induced delirium). A further two patients (3 per cent) were diagnosed with schizophrenia, and one with atypical psychosis. These data support the view that catatonia is not uncommon among psychiatric patients, and that it is most often seen in disorders other than schizophrenia. In this case series, the most common catatonic symptom was mutism, followed by immobility, staring, and posturing. These findings suggest that catatonia may be present in mild or subtle forms, without dramatic and uncommon symptoms such as waxy flexibility, stereotypies, or echophenomena.

In 5 of the 28 patients, catatonia remitted spontaneously within 49 hours of admission and before the initiation of treatment. Twenty-one patients received a lorazepam trial. These patients were first challenged with intravenous lorazepam, administered in two doses of 1 mg each, spaced 5 mins apart. Catatonic symptomatology was rated during the challenge. Sixteen patients (76 per cent) improved during the challenge; their catatonic symptoms were subsequently observed to respond to oral lorazepam in doses of up to 8 mg/day. Thus, a positive response to lorazepam challenge predicted a good response to oral lorazepam. Correspondingly, when the lorazepam challenge failed to relieve the catatonic syndrome, larger doses of lorazepam administered over many days also failed to provide relief. In such instances, ECT proved to be an effective treatment. Four patients received ECT and each recovered. In three of the ECT-treated patients, catatonic symptoms disappeared after 3 treatments; one patient however needed 11 treatments (Bush *et al.*, 1996a).

To examine the application of the catatonia rating scale in patients who were not acutely ill, we studied patients diagnosed with catatonic schizophrenia in a long-stay hospital, the Pilgrim Psychiatric Center at Long Island, New York. Forty-two chronically hospitalized patients were rated with the Stony Brook catatonia rating scale and with standardized rating scales for parkinsonism, tardive dyskinesia, and akathisia. The catatonia rating scale successfully distinguished catatonia from other motor symptoms; rigidity was one catatonic sign which overlapped with other motor syndromes. The features of chronic catatonia did not differ from those of the acute syndrome (Bush *et al.*, 1997).

The Consistency of Catatonic Symptoms Across Episodes

One criterion for the diagnostic validity of the catatonic syndrome is the consistency of symptoms across episodes (Robins and Guze, 1970). We described five patients who presented with a second catatonic episode after an interval of 4.5–20 (mean = 10.7) months. These patients were rated on the 23-item catatonia rating scale on both occasions. They were observed to have 7–15 (mean = 9.6) catatonic symptoms during the first episode and 4–14 (mean = 9.6) catatonic symptoms during the second episode. In the five patients, 13–21 symptoms (mean = 16.6) showed a presence/absence agreement between the two episodes (Francis *et al.*, 1997).

ECT—Lorazepam Synergism in Catatonia

ECT and benzodiazepines are traditionally considered to be antagonistic, and their concurrent use is not recommended (American Psychiatric Association, 1990); nevertheless, we found a synergism between the two treatments in the management of the catatonic syndrome (Petrides *et al.*, 1997). We used lorazepam and ECT sequentially and concurrently in five prospectively identified cases of catatonia. The syndromes included acute, chronic, and episodic catatonia in patients with histories of depressive and (in several instances) psychotic symptoms. In each case, the combination of lorazepam with ECT was superior to monotherapy. In one patient, we were able to successfully discontinue maintenance ECT after adding lorazepam to the prescription despite the inefficacy of this medicine prior to ECT. The improved treatment response with ECT and lorazepam contrasts with reports suggesting unfavourable clinical results when benzodiazepines are combined with ECT (particularly unilateral treatment) for the management of depression (Kellner *et al.*, 1991; Cohen and Lawton, 1992).

The apparent synergism between lorazepam and ECT has implications for the pathophysiology of catatonia; it supports the view that GABA antagonism and dopamine receptor upregulation underlie the mechanism of action of benzodiazepines in catatonia (Rosebush and Mazurek, 1991) through a complex interaction between dopaminergic and GABA-ergic systems in the basal ganglia (Northoff, 1995). Electroconvulsive Shocks (ECS) increase diazepam binding sites in the cerebral cortex (Gulati *et al.*, 1986) and increase GABA concentrations in different areas of the brain (Bowdler *et al.*, 1982; Sanacora *et al.*, 1998).

An alternate explanation for the synergism is that ECT and benzodiazepines are both anticonvulsants that raise the seizure threshold. Seizure activity and/or kindling phenomena have been suggested as pathophysiological mechanisms in catatonia (Menza, 1989) as well as in manic states that are known to be associated with catatonia (Post *et al.*, 1986). This explanation encourages the study of brain electrical activity in catatonia. Available data suggest that in patients with catatonia a characteristic low voltage, fast frequency pattern is common; this is replaced by the more usual rhythmic alpha frequency after effective treatment (Hill, 1963).

Lorazepam in the Prophylaxis of Catatonia

While benzodiazepines and ECT are effective in acute catatonia, their usefulness in the prophylaxis of chronic, recurrent catatonia has not been established. We studied lorazepam prophylaxis in four patients with recurrent catatonia. Steady doses (1.5–6.5 mg/day) of lorazepam were used for up to five years with favourable results. The patients did not require escalating doses (indicating that tolerance to the benefits of the medication did not develop) nor did they report side effects (Petrides, 1997).

The most notable case in our experience (Bright-Long and Fink, 1993) was that of a 58-year-old woman with pseudodementia who, since age 49, had been diagnosed with dementia of presumably Alzheimer's type. This woman was referred to us for further evaluation. She appeared confused and perplexed. Her speech was mumbling and incoherent. Other symptoms included posturing, wandering, and incontinence. She was unable to care for herself or for her family. In view of a history of prior episodes of major depression, the diagnosis of pseudodementia was considered. Pharmacotherapy trials with tricyclic antidepressants, neuroleptics, lithium, and combinations thereof failed. ECT was administered to a total of 11 treatments; there was dramatic response—she became verbal, regained her ability to recognize her family members, and ultimately returned to her premorbid level of functioning for the first time in nine years.

Despite maintenance pharmacotherapy, she rapidly relapsed into pseudodementia. Maintenance ECT was prescribed at a frequency of 1–2 treatments every 6–8 weeks; these treatments were prompted by relapses, usually characterized by perplexity, mutism, posturing, stereotypic movements,, and negativism. Following such ECT treatments, the symptoms would remit, but would recur 6–8 weeks later. Lithium was thought to prolong symptom-free periods, but tricyclic antidepressants added no benefit. Maintenance ECT and lithium were therefore continued for 9 years when, on re-evaluation, it was thought that her catatonic syndrome might respond better to lorazepam. Oral lorazepam (0.5 mg thrice daily) was prescribed for prophylaxis. She did not relapse at her usual 6–8 week period, and her symptoms did not return for the next three years. She has not required further ECT.

Catatonia and the Neuroleptic Malignant Syndrome

When we screened patients for catatonia, we occasionally encountered patients with NMS, and when we studied patients with NMS, we found that they had many symptoms of catatonia. In our screening study (Bush *et al.*, 1996b), as reported earlier, 3 (20 per cent) of 15 prospectively identified catatonic patients also met criteria for NMS. In another study (Koch *et al.*, 1999), we reviewed the records of all patients treated for NMS at the University Hospital. Sixteen patients met the DSM-IV criteria for NMS; of these patients, 11 also met the more stringent NMS research criteria (Caroff and Mann, 1993). One patient exhibited catatonia before the onset of NMS; the other 15 patients met criteria for catatonia after the onset of NMS symptoms, scoring an average of 6.1 on the catatonia rating scale. There was a strong positive correlation between the severity of NMS and the severity of catatonia.

We examined the treatment of these patients (Francis *et al.*, 1999) Not surprisingly, all 16 patients had received benzodiazepines (mainly lorazepam) before the prompt resolution of NMS symptoms. None had received dopamine agonists or other NMS-specific medicines. These data support our view that NMS and catatonia are phenomenologically similar, that they respond to the same pharmacological treatments (benzodiazepines), and that they may therefore represent the same nosological entity (Fink, 1996a).

INCIDENCE

Having reached this point in our discussion of catatonia, we take up an issue which in conventional texts would have been examined rather earlier. This issue concerns the incidence of catatonia, and views related thereto.

Some authors consider that the incidence of catatonia has substantially decreased, and that catatonia may even be an extinct entity (Mahendra, 1981). One explanation for the presumed decrease in its incidence suggests that the introduction of neuroleptic medications altered the natural course of schizophrenia in which catatonia appears as a late syndrome. This explanation is unlikely to be valid because most historical as well as contemporary descriptions of catatonia refer to young patients in the very early stages of illness.

Rosebush *et al.* (1990) reported that 12 (9 per cent) of 140 patients admitted to a university psychiatric facility manifested catatonic signs; Ungvari *et al.* (1994a and b) reported an incidence of 8 per cent (18 of 212 patients); and, we (Bush *et al.*, 1996a) reported an incidence of 7 per cent (15 of 215 patients). In these reports, schizophrenia was diagnosed in only a minority of the catatonic patients. With the background of these studies, we suggest that alternate explanations for the apparent decrease in the incidence of catatonia are that clinicians are not trained to identify catatonic symptoms, that clinicians do not pay attention to catatonic symptoms as they consider these to be features of schizophrenia that will not alter their treatment approach, or that clinicians consciously or unconsciously ignore catatonic symptoms that occur in non-schizophrenic patients. The use of catatonia screening and rating instruments should help in the proper identification, prompt treatment, and better classification of catatonia.

TREATMENT

During the 1930s, an important discovery was that barbiturates effectively relieved catatonia. Previously, many catatonic patients had died, but with the use of barbiturates, more than half of such patients recovered quickly. For decades, intravenous amylobarbital (0.5–1 g) was widely used. Later, barbiturate therapy gave way to treatment with far safer drugs, the benzodiazepines. Presently, both diazepam and lorazepam are considered standard treatments. For the acutely ill patients, lorazepam (1–2 mg) or diazepam (10–20 mg) may be administered intravenously. The effect of intravenous lorazepam is very rapid, and the success or failure of such a challenge predicts the success or failure of larger oral doses over many days (Bush *et al.*, 1996a). Intramuscular or oral benzodiazepine treatment is also effective, but necessitates higher doses such as 8–16 mg/day for lorazepam and 40–80 mg/day for diazepam.

ECT is very effective in catatonic patients, even in those who fail to improve with benzodiazepines. Catatonic symptoms respond to ECT faster and more dramatically than do depressive or psychotic symptoms. It is fortunate that the first patients treated by Meduna (who introduced convulsive therapy) and Cerletti and Bini (who introduced electricity for the induction of seizures) were patients with catatonic symptoms (Fink, 1984). Severe, life-threatening forms of catatonia also respond to ECT. In our study, four patients who did not respond to lorazepam treatment were successfully treated with ECT (Bush *et al.*, 1996a). Indeed, we know of almost no cases of catatonia that were not relieved by adequate courses of ECT, administered using treatment methods that are considered to maximize effectiveness.

The use of benzodiazepines during a course of ECT is traditionally avoided and discouraged as these medications are considered to interfere with the efficacy of the treatment. In catatonia, however, both treatments are effective separately as well as together; in the latter situation, they may be therapeutically synergistic (Petrides *et al.*, 1997).

The separation of the catatonic syndrome from schizophrenia carries important therapeutic implications. ECT is seldom considered as a first-line treatment for schizophrenia, and benzodiazepines at best enjoy the status of an adjunctive treatment for this disorder; however, ECT and benzodiazepines are both effective treatments for catatonia. While neuroleptic drugs are standard treatments for schizophrenia, they may not relieve catatonia; in fact, these drugs may worsen catatonic symptoms or precipitate NMS or malignant catatonia. Thus, the management of catatonic patients as if they are examples of schizophrenia is both unwarranted and unsafe.

SUMMARY

Recent data contradict the traditional view that catatonia comprises a group of symptoms that is seen exclusively during the course of schizophrenia. Surveys and clinical reports describe catatonia as a non-specific syndrome that appears in many psychiatric and systemic illnesses. The syndromic view is simpler than the complex European classification of catatonia under specific schizophrenia subtypes. The syndromic view also offers useful treatment algorithms for a potentially lethal condition. Catatonia occurs in about 7–9 per cent of acutely ill psychiatric patients. Screening instruments and rating scales facilitate the diagnosis of catatonia. The phenomenology of chronic and acute forms of catatonia is similar. Recurrent episodes of catatonia in the same patient manifest the same symptoms. Catatonia and NMS share the same symptomatology and respond to the same treatments. Available evidence supports the view that NMS is a subtype of the catatonic syndrome.

Catatonia is readily treated with benzodiazepines and/or ECT regardless of the associated illness. These two treatments are therapeutically effective during acute catatonic episodes, and prophylactically effective in recurrent catatonia; their concurrent use may be therapeutically synergistic in catatonic patients.

REFERENCES

Abrams R. and Taylor M. A. (1976). 'Catatonia, a prospective clinical study', *Arch. Gen. Psychiatry*, 33: 579–81.

Abrams R., Taylor M. A., and Stolurow K. A. (1979). 'Catatonia and mania: patterns of cerebral dysfunction', *Biol. Psychiatry*, 14: 111–17.

American Psychiatric Association (1980). *Diagnostic and Statistical Manual of Mental Disorders*, 3rd ed., Washington: American Psychiatric Association.

——— (1987). *Diagnostic and Statistical Manual of Mental Disorders*, 3rd ed., revised, Washington: American Psychiatric Association.

——— (1990). *Electroconvulsive Therapy: Recommendations for Treatment, Training and Privileging*, Washington: American Psychiatric Association.

——— (1994). *Diagnostic and Statistical manual of Mental Disorders*, 4th ed., Washington: American Psychiatric Association.

Arnold O. H. and Stepan H. (1952). 'Untersuchungen zur Frage der akuten tödlichen Katatonie', *Wr Z f Nervenheilkunde*, 4: 235–87.

Beckmann H., Franzek E., and Stöber G. (1996). 'Genetic heterogeneity in catatonic schizophrenia: A family study', *Am. J. Med. Genetics*, 67: 289–300.

Bowdler J. M., Green A. R., and Minchin M. C. W. (1982). 'Regional GABA concentration and [3H]-diazepam binding in rat brain following repeated electroconvulsive shock', *J. Neur. Transmission*, 56: 3–12.

Bräunig P., Krüger S., and Shugar G. (1998). 'Prevalence and clinical significance of catatonic symptoms in mania', *Compr. Psychiatry*, 39: 35–46.

Bright-Long L. and Fink M. (1993) 'Reversible dementia and affective disorder: The Rip-van-Winkle syndrome', *Convulsive Ther.*, 9: 209–16.

Bush G., Fink M., Petrides G. *et al.* (1996a). 'Catatonia. II: Treatment with lorazepam and electroconvulsive therapy', *Acta. Psychiatr. Scand.*, 93: 137–43.

——— (1996b). 'Catationia. I: Rating scale and standardized examination', *Acta. Psychiatr. Scand.*, 93: 129–36.

Bush G., Petrides G. and Francis A. (1997). 'Catatonia and other motor syndromes in a chronically hospitalized psychiatric population', *Schizophr. Res.*, 27: 83–92.

Caroff S. N. and Mann S. C. (1993). 'Neuroleptic malignant syndrome', *Med. Clin. N. America*, 77: 185–202.

Cohen S. I. and Lawton C. (1992). 'Do benzodiazepines interfere with the action of electroconvulsive therapy?', *Br. J. Psychiatry*, 160: 545–6.

Davis J. M., Janicak P. G., Sakkas P. *et al.* (1991). 'Electroconvulsive therapy in the treatment of the neuroleptic malignant syndrome', *Convulsive Ther.*, 7: 111–20.

Fink M. (1984). 'Meduna and the origins of convulsive therapy', *Am. J. Psychiatry*, 141: 1034–41.

——— (1996a). 'Toxic serotonin syndrome or neuroleptic malignant syndrome?', *Pharmacopsychiatry*, 29: 159–61.

——— (1996b). 'Neuroleptic malignant syndrome and catatonia: One entity or two?', *Biol. Psychiatry*, 39: 1–4.

Fink M. and Taylor M. A. (1991). 'Catatonia: A separate category for DSM-IV? *Integrative Psychiatry*, 7: 2–10.

Francis A., Divadeenam K., Bush G. *et al.* (1997). 'Consistency of symptoms in recurrrent catatonia', *Compr. Psychiatry*, 38: 56–60.

Francis A., Petrides G., Chandragiri S. *et al.* (1999). 'Lorazepam in the treatment of neuroleptic malignant syndrome', *J. Clin. Psychiatry* (submitted).

Franzek E., Schmidtke A., Beckmann H., and Stöber G. (1995). 'Evidence against unusual sex concordance and pseudoautosomal inheritance in the catatonic subtype of schizophrenia', *Psychiatry Res.*, 59: 17–24.

Fricchione G. L., Cassem N. H., Hooberman D. *et al.* (1983). 'Intravenous lorazepam in neuroleptic-induced catatonia', *J. Clin. Psychopharm.*, 3: 338–42.

Fricchione G. L., Kaufman L. D., Gruber B. L. *et al.* (1990). 'Electroconvulsive therapy and cyclophosphamide in combination for severe neuropsychiatric lupus with catatonia', *Am. J. Medicine*, 88: 442–3.

Gelenberg A. J. (1976). 'The catatonic syndrome', *Lancet*, 2: 1339–41.

——— (1977). 'Catatonic reactions to high-potency neuroleptic drugs', *Arch. Gen. Psychiatry*, 34: 947–50.

Gelenberg A. J. and Mandel M. R. (1977). 'Catatonic reactions to high potency neuroleptic drugs', *Arch. Gen. Psychiatry*, 34: 947–50.

Gulati A., Srimal R. C., and Shawan B. N. (1986). Upregulation of brain benzodiazepine receptors by electroconvulsive shocks', *Pharm. Res. Commun.*, 18: 581–9.

Hill D. (1963). 'Epilepsy: clinical aspects', in JAV Bates *et al.* (eds), *Electroencephalography: A Symposium on its Various Aspects*, New York: Macmillan Co., 286–7; 404–6.

Hoch A. (1921). *Benign Stupors*, New York: Macmillan Co.

Kahlbaum K. L. (1973). *Catatonia*, Baltimore: Johns Hopkins University Press.

Kellner C. H., Nixon D. W., and Bernstein H. J. (1991). 'ECT drug interactions: a review', *Psychopharmacol. Bull.* 27: 595–609.

Koch M. A., Petrides G., and Francis A. J. (1995). 'Catatonia from neuroleptics and NMS: Two entities?', *APA New Research Abstracts*, NR 227: 117.

Koch M., Chandragiri S., Rizvi S. *et al.* (1999). 'Catatonic signs in neuroleptic malignant syndrome', *Comprehensive Psychiatry* (in press).

Kraepelin E. (1913). *Psychiatrie*, 8th ed., Loipzig: Johann Ambrosius Barth.

Leonhard K. (1979). *The Classification of Endogenous Psychoses*, 5th ed., New York: Irvington Publishers.

Mahendra B. (1981). 'Where have all the catatonics gone?', *Psychol. Med.*, 11: 669–71.

Mann S. C., Caroff S. N., Bleier H. R. *et al.* (1986). 'Lethal catatonia', *Am. J. Psychiatry*, 143: 1374–81.

——— (1990). 'Electroconvulsive therapy of the lethal catatonia syndrome', *Convulsive Ther.* 6: 239–47.

Menza M. A. (1989). 'Benzodiazepines and catatonia: An overview', *Biol. Psychiatry*, 26: 842–6.

Morrison J. R. (1973). 'Catatonia: retarded and excited types', *Arch. Gen. Psychiatry*, 28: 39–41.

——— (1975). 'Catatonia: Diagnosis and treatment, *Hosp. Community Psychiatry*', 26: 91–4.

Northoff G. (1995). 'Effects of benzodiazepines in catatonia–a pathophysiological model', in H. Beckman and K. J. Neumarker (eds), *Endogenous Psychosis*, Ullstein, Mosby.

Pataki J., Zervas I. M., and Jandorf L. (1992). 'Catatonia in a university in-patient service (1985–90), *Convulsive Ther.*, 8: 163–73.

Petrides G. (1997). 'Lorazepam for prophylaxis in recurrent catatonia', *ACNP Scientific Abstracts*, PO 296.

Petrides G., Divadeenam K., Bush G. *et al.* (1997). 'Synergism of lorazepam and ECT in the treatment of catatonia', *Biol. Psychiatry*, 42: 375–81.

Philbrick K. L. and Rummans T. A. (1994). 'Malignant catatonia', *J. Neuropsychiatry Clin. Neurosciences*, 6: 1–13.

Post R. M., Putnam F., Uhde T. W. *et al.* (1986). 'Electroconvulsive therapy as an anticonvulsant: Implications for its mechanism of action in affective illness', *Ann. NY Acad. Sci.*, 462: 376–88.

Robins E. and Guze S. B. (1970). 'Establishment of diagnostic validity in psychiatric illness: its application to schizophrenia', *Am. J. Psychiatry*, 126: 983–7.

Rosebush P. I. and Mazurek M. F. (1991). 'Lorazepam and catatonic immobility', *J. Clin. Psychiatry*, 52: 187–8.

Rosebush P. I., Hildebrand A. M., Furlong B. G. *et al.* (1990). 'Catatonic syndrome in a general psychiatric population: Frequency, clinical presentation, and response to lorazepam', *J. Clin. Psychiatry*, 51: 357–62.

Sanacora G., Mason G. F., Rothman D. L. *et al.* (1998). 'ECT effects on cortical GABA levels as determined by 1H-MRS', *ACNP Scientific Abstracts*, PO 200.

Stauder K. H. (1934). 'Die tödliche Katatonie', *Archiv. für. Psychiatrie und Nervenkrankheiten*, 102: 614–34.

Stöber G., Franzek E., Lesch K. P. *et al.* (1995). 'Periodic catatonia: a schizophrenic subtype with major gene effect and anticipation', *Eur. Arch. Psychiatry Clin. Neurosci.*, 245: 135–41.

Taylor M. A. and Abrams R. (1976). 'The phenomenology of mania: a new look at some old patients', *Arch. Gen. Psychiatry*, 29: 520–22.

——— (1977). 'Catatonia: prevalence and importance in the manic phase of manic-depressive illness', *Arch. Gen. Psychiatry*, 34: 1223–5.

——— (1978). 'The prevalence of schizophrenia: a reassessment using modern diagnostic criteria', *Am. J. Psychiatry*, 135: 945–8.

Ungvari G. S., Leung H. C. M. and Lee T. S. (1994a). 'Benzodiazepines and the psychopathology of catatonia', *Pharmacopsychiatry*, 27: 242–5.

Ungvari G. S., Leung C. M., Wong M. K. *et al.* (1994b). 'Benzodiazepines in the treatment of catatonic syndrome', *Acta. Psychiatr. Scand.*, 89: 285–8.

White D. A. C. (1992). 'Catatonia and the neuroleptic malignant syndrome—a single entity?', *Br. J. Psychiatry*, 161: 558–60.

White D. A. C. and Robins A. H. (1991). 'Catatonia: Harbinger of the neuroleptic malignant syndrome', *Br. J. Psychiatry*, 158: 419–21.

World Health Organization (1977). *International Classification of Diseases*, 9th rev., Geneva: World Health Organization.

World Health Organization (1992). *International Classification of Diseases*, 10th rev., Geneva: World Health Organization.

Chapter 3

Attention, Memory and Language Disturbances in Schizophrenia: Characteristics and Implications

CAMERON S. CARTER AND DEANNA M. BARCH

INTRODUCTION

While the investigation of cognitive dysfunction in schizophrenia dates back to Kraeplin (1919/1971), during recent years there has been a sharp increase in interest in this aspect of the illness. Two considerations appear to be responsible. The first is clinical, and reflects an increased awareness of the disabilities occasioned by these deficits, and of our inability to effectively treat them (Green, 1998). The second is methodological, and reflects the ascendency of cognitive neuroscience as a major, new, integrative neuroscientific discipline, the tools and constructs of which are readily applied to clinical research (Spitzer, 1993; Posner and Abdullev, 1996).

Cognitive impairment is a very relevant clinical aspect of schizophrenia. Several recent investigators (Connor and Herman, 1993; Green 1996; Klapow *et al.*, 1997; Davidson and McGlashan, 1997) have suggested that in schizophrenic patients cognitive impairment is strongly associated with functional disability. In fact, in such patients cognitive impairment appears to be a stronger predictor of poor social and occupational functioning than the positive symptoms (such as delusions and hallucinations) which are traditional targets of therapeutic efforts. This observation has been drawn from a very discouraging body of literature on the impact of antipsychotic medications on cognitive deficits: while the typical neuroleptics clearly have no positive impact upon cognition, existing data on atypical antipsychotics are mixed and suggest limited benefit at best (Goldberg *et al.*, 1990; Green *et al.*, 1997; Green, 1998). There has been a consequent surge of interest in the exploration of the relationship between cognitive dysfunction and disability in schizophrenia. Realization has dawned that beyond positive and negative symptoms, cognitive deficits and associated illness disabilities are highly appropriate targets for therapeutic development.

Cognitive neuroscience is a new and rapidly developing discipline in which assessment methods from the field of cognitive psychology are integrated with assessment methods from physiological sciences. Examples of experimental paradigms are functional neuroimaging in humans and single cell recording in primates, conducted while the subjects are engaged in particular behaviours. Cognitive neuroscience is presently one of the most active areas in neuroscience, and has provided a wealth of knowledge about neural mechanisms underlying normal cognition. The discipline has also provided psychopathology researchers with a new and powerful set of tools. As a result, the pathophysiology of cognitive disturbances in schizophrenia has become much better understood. Prerequisites for applying these tools, however, are knowledge of the kinds of cognitive deficits which are common in schizophrenia, and expertise in the choice of cognitive methods for studies using techniques such as functional neuroimaging.

This chapter will review several key issues related to recent developments in the understanding of cognitive dysfunction in schizophrenia. First, impairments in certain important cognitive systems will be discussed in detail. Next, possible neurobiological substrates of these impairments will be examined. Subsequently, the literature relating cognitive dysfunction to other aspects of symptomatology will be briefly considered. Finally, a short discussion will be presented on the implications of these findings for the development of effective treatments for this disabling aspect of the illness.

Attention, Memory and Language Disturbances in Schizophrenia

Scope

Cognitive dysfunction in schizophrenia can be studied using a variety of approaches. This review emphasizes only research which is amenable to analysis and interpretation using tools and constructs of experimental cognitive psychology. Such an approach has dominated the empirical study of human cognition for four decades. It promotes the use of a common taxonomy of cognition, and provides a theoretical clarity which is grounded in a vast body of empirical literature. It permits a mechanistic approach to the investigation of cognitive dysfunction in schizophrenia: task design is theoretically based, and tasks are administered in a systematic, hypothesis-driven manner. Most importantly, it allows an integration of human and non-human neuroscientific studies.

Disturbances have been observed at a number of levels of information processing in schizophrenia, including those which are clearly perceptual or pre-attentive (Saccuzzo and Braff, 1981; Green *et al.*, 1994; Carter *et al.*, 1996a). This review examines disturbances of controlled cognitive processes with specific reference to those involving attention, memory, and language production; that is, processes which have an important functional and clinical relevance in schizophrenia. Wherever appropriate, however, attention is paid to automatic processes that may contribute to disturbances of cognitive control in schizophrenic patients.

Attention in Schizophrenia

Attention refers to a number of processes which ultimately determine the degree to which information is processed and responded to, and the degree to which it is not. Taxonomies of attention generally classify these processes into a few broad categories (Posner and Petersen, 1990; LaBerge, 1995). Such theoretical frameworks are now becoming increasingly constrained by our knowledge of brain function. Thus, while these taxonomies emphasize mechanisms by which both perceptual and response-related processes may be modulated by attention (Posner and Petersen, 1990), they also consider the interactive nature and parallel organization of the neural circuitry that implements attentional processes (Cohen *et al.*, 1990).

Within these widely accepted theoretical frameworks, executive processes which modulate attention in a task-appropriate manner are distinguished from attentional processes which modulate stimulus processing and response selection through local changes in activity in information processing pathways. Vigilance is distinguished from preparatory and selective aspects of attention (LaBerge, 1995). These and other aspects of attention have been extensively studied in schizophrenia. A specific profile of attention has emerged: certain aspects of attention have been found to be intact while others have been found to be impaired.

The Continuous Performance Task (CPT; Rosvold *et al.*, 1956) is a cognitive paradigm that has frequently been used to investigate attention in schizophrenia. In this task, subjects concentrate on a sequence of stimuli that appear on a computer monitor and respond when a pre-specified target stimulus occurs. Schizophrenic patients are reliably impaired on this task, especially when it is more difficult to discriminate target from non-target stimuli (Nuechterlein and Dawson, 1984), or when a memory load is added. Many variants of the CPT have been employed to study attentional processes in schizophrenia; certain of these are briefly discussed.

Vigilance is the ability to maintain an attentive state over time. Conclusions about vigilance in schizophrenic patients have been drawn from an examination of their performances on the CPT. Essentially, impairment is distributed across the time course of the task, and does not worsen as the task prolongs (Green, 1998). Vigilance is thus unimpaired in schizophrenia.

Preparatory attention is the ability to take advantage of a cue or warning to improve the detection of a stimulus (LaBerge, 1995). Preparatory attention can be studied using, for example, a spatial cuing task (Posner, 1980; Posner and Cohen, 1984). Here, subjects watch a monitor for the occurrence of a simple stimulus (the probe). At a variable interval before the appearance of this probe, a cue warns the subject about the location at which the probe is likely to appear; this cue is either an arrow or a brief brightening of a box. Expectedly, normal subjects respond more quickly when a cue correctly predicts the location of the probe; such a cue is called a valid cue.

Many studies have used variants of the spatial cuing task to examine preparatory attention in schizophrenia (Posner *et al.*, 1988; Strauss *et al.*, 1991 and 1992; Carter *et al.*, 1992; Nestor *et al.*, 1992; Bustillo *et al.*, 1997). The results have been rather mixed; however, a fairly consistent finding is that patients *are* able to improve their performance with a valid cue. It therefore appears that preparatory attention is intact in schizophrenia.

This conclusion has been confirmed using the Global/Local Task (Carter *et al.*, 1996a). In this task, subjects are shown a complex visual stimulus consisting of a large letter made up of many copies of a smaller letter. They are asked to decide which of two target letters, one of which is always present, has appeared. The target may be either at the small letter (local) level or at the large letter (global) level. When patients are cued that in a given block of trials 80 per cent of the targets will appear at a particular level, they significantly improve their performance for targets at that level, and their performance resembles that of normal subjects.

Selective attention is the ability to process goal-relevant information and ignore goal-irrelevant material. A disturbance in selective attention results in distractibility. The Stroop task, one of the most widely used procedures in cognitive science (Stroop, 1935; Macleod, 1991), is the classical paradigm used to investigate selective attention. In the Stroop task, subjects are presented with words that are written in different colours. The words may be colour-related (e.g., RED, BLUE) or colour-unrelated (e.g., HORSE, ABCDE). The colour-related words may be colour-congruent (e.g., RED written in a red shade) or colour-incongruent (e.g., RED written in a blue shade). Subjects are instructed to ignore the meaning of the words, and to name only the colours of the words. In this task, colour-related words affect subjects performances. The colour-incongruent words predispose subjects to slower responses and to errors (they read the word instead of naming the colour); this effect is known as *interference*. Colour-congruent words predispose to faster responses; this effect is known as *facilitation*. The occurrence of interference and facilitation is thought to reflect the fact that reading a word is an automatic response; in other words there is a prepotent response tendency to read a stimulus if it is a word.

The original version of the Stroop task used cards, and many Stroop card studies were performed in schizophrenic patients over the years. Virtually all of these studies were confounded by a failure to take into account the general impairments (such as an overall slow response to all types of stimulus) which patients show while performing the task (Perlstein *et al.*, 1998); nevertheless, it was generally concluded that patients are more distractable than controls.

Recent studies have used a computerized version of the Stroop task. Single stimuli are presented, and response time and response accuracy are both monitored on-line. Such studies have provided reliable evidence of impaired selective attention in schizophrenia. In comparison with controls, patients show more interference in response to colour-incongruent stimuli, and more facilitation in response to colour-congruent stimuli (Carter *et al.*, 1992; Taylor *et al.*, 1996; Perlstein *et al.*, 1998; Cohen *et al.*, 1999).

Increased distractibility in schizophrenia has also been observed using other tasks. By way of example, in the antisaccade task subject must overcome the prepotent response to make a saccade to the location of onset of visual stimulus, and must make a saccade to a location in the opposite visual field, instead. Schizophrenic patients make significantly more errors on this task than controls: they direct saccades towards the target (which is the distracting stimulus in this context) rather than in the opposite direction (Crawford *et al.*, 1995).

In conclusion, these results suggest that while aspects of attention such as vigilance and preparation are intact, the use of task-irrelevant distractors reliably impairs the active selection of task-relevant information in schizophrenic patients (Table 3.1).

Table 3.1: Attention in Schizophrenia

Aspect of attention	Task	Finding
Vigilance	Continuous performance task	No impairment; errors do not worsen as the task prolongs
Preparatory attention	Spatial cuing task; Global/Local task	No impairment; performance improves with cuing
Selective attention	(a) Stroop task	Impairment is present; increased interference and increased facilitation are seen
	(b) Antisaccade task	Impairment is present

Memory in Schizophrenia

Memory, like attention, refers to a broad group of cognitive functions. In most models of memory, short-term memory is distinguished from long-term memory; this distinction may reflect the involvement of independent neural systems. The concept of short-term memory has been elaborated into a working memory system comprised of storage buffers and a central executive. The former handles transitory information while the latter manipulates the functioning of the system. Information from working memory may or may not become encoded into long-term memory. Models of long-term memory have largely been based on studies of amnestic individuals with medial temporal lobe damage associated with a resultant inability to acquire new memories. In these models, declarative memory which is consciously acquired is distinguished from non-declarative memory which is unconsciously acquired (e.g., Squire and Zola-Morgan, 1988; Squire, 1992).

Working memory is hypothesized to consist of a set of buffers for the storage or maintenance of information, and functions on a time scale of a few seconds. For example, a 7-digit phone number retrieved from a directory is usually held in mind only for as long as it takes to dial it; the number may not be recalled later if the line was busy. Working memory has been extensively studied in schizophrenia and has been shown to be reliably impaired in this disorder. Schizophrenic patients show impairment in spatial working memory (Park and Holzman, 1992; Keefe *et al.*, 1995; Carter *et al.*, 1996b; Stone *et al.*, 1998) as well as verbal working memory (Servan-Schreiber *et al.*, 1996). Deficits of verbal working memory are most evident when patients are challenged with a high information load (Carter *et al.*, 1998), when they have to deal with distraction (Keefe *et al.*, 1995), and when they are required to manipulate rather than maintain information in working memory (Gold *et al.*, 1997).

As already discussed, classical models of working memory invoke a system characterized by short-term storage buffers in which information is maintained, and a central executive which updates and operates upon the information in the short-term store. It is unclear whether working memory disturbances in schizophrenia reflect deficits in maintenance processes (Park and Holzman, 1992), executive processes (Barch and Carter, 1998), or both (Carter *et al.*, 1996b). Since schizophrenic patients are often impaired in tests (e.g., the Stroop task) of executive but not maintenance processes, and since these impairments correlate strongly with global working memory impairment (Barch and Carter, 1998), it is likely that the impairments lie in executive processes in working memory rather than solely in the buffer systems. This conclusion is also supported by the finding that schizophrenic patients generally perform well on simple span tasks which are considered to be standard measures of the integrity of the buffer systems (Clare *et al.*, 1993; Gold *et al.*, 1997). The determination of the exact mechanisms underlying working memory impairments in schizophrenia is an active area of investigation, and may have important implications for our understanding of the neurobiology of cognitive disability in this disorder.

Declarative or explicit memory involves the conscious acquisition of memories for facts and events. The integrity of declarative memory in schizophrenia is controversial because it is difficult to assess memory functions in the presence of deficits in attention and working memory. Patients are known to show impairments on standard learning and memory tests such as list learning (Goldberg *et al.*, 1990; Tamlyn *et al.*, 1992; Schmand *et al.*, 1992; Schwartz *et al.*, 1992; Clare *et al.*, 1993); however, an impairment in attention allocation and executive processes could easily account for these deficits. It has frequently been reported that patients with schizophrenia show impaired recall but intact recognition on such tasks, and that they are able to improve their recall performance into the normal range when provided with cues such as the category of items (Schwartz *et al.*, 1992; Beatty *et al.*, 1993). In addition, studies have found that recall is improved when strategies such as semantic chunking are provided to improve encoding (Koh, 1978). These data strongly suggest that patients have difficulties not with the storage of memories *per se*, but with the executive processes associated with the encoding and retrieval of items.

A recent set of studies which attempted to show a specific deficit in declarative memory in schizophrenia did not satisfactorily control for deficits in executive processes in working memory, which could in turn result in findings of impaired long-term memory performance. The task used to control for the integrity of the working memory system required subjects to remember short strings of letters (a subspan task), a procedure which evaluates the buffer systems but not the executive component of working memory (Tamlyn *et al.*, 1992). As mentioned earlier, working memory impairment for verbal material is most evident in schizophrenia in the presence of distraction, or when subjects are required to engage executive processes to manipulate the content of the buffers (Gold *et al.*, 1997; Barch and Carter, 1998). Thus, the studies by Tamlyn *et al.* (1992) did not rule out the possibility that the declarative memory deficits observed in patients with schizophrenia were actually due to deficits in attention or executive functions. Further work is required to clarify this issue.

Non-declarative or implicit memory refers to a range of knowledge and abilities (including motor, perceptual, and cognitive skills) which are acquired through events or mechanisms that are not explicitly or consciously recollected. Many studies have shown that schizophrenic patients acquire procedural knowledge as effectively as controls; for example, patients acquire simple motor skills and patterns at the same rate and to the same degree as normal subjects (Goldberg *et al.*, 1990; Schwartz *et al.*, 1992; Clare *et al.*, 1993).

Semantic knowledge is another example of a skill that is implicitly acquired; thus, implicit memory in schizophrenia can also be studied by examining semantic processing. A mixed body of literature suggests that semantic priming is abnormal in schizophrenia. Semantic priming is an aspect of memory thought to reflect in part non-declarative processes (Tulving and Schachter, 1990; Squire, 1992). In studies on semantic priming, subjects are required to respond to a letter string by making a lexical decision such as whether the stimulus is a valid word or not; in some paradigms, the subjects are required to pronounce the words verbally. The target stimulus, to which the subject is required to respond, is immediately preceded by a priming stimulus, to which no response is necessary. It has been found that subjects respond faster to targets which are valid words if the priming stimulus is also a valid word. Subjects also respond faster if the target is semantically related to the priming stimulus. These accelerations of response illustrate a phenomenon known as the semantic priming effect.

An original report by Maher and colleagues (Manshreck *et al.*, 1988) suggested that schizophrenic patients showed increased semantic priming effects, measured as faster response times to making a lexical decision when the target was preceded by a related word. Thus, patients were better able to conclude that a letter string such as DOCTOR is a valid word when it was preceded by the letter string NURSE. This finding was suggested to reflect increased spreading activation in networks representing semantic knowledge in schizophrenia.

There have been some published replications of this finding (Kwapil *et al.*, 1990; Spitzer, 1993; Henik *et al.*, 1995) but also a number of non-replications (Vinogradov *et al.*, 1992; Henik *et al.*, 1992; Barch *et al.*, 1996), leading to the suggestion that increased semantic priming effects might not be a reliable finding in schizophrenia. It is noteworthy that all studies which reported this finding addressed medicated patients, suggesting that the finding might in fact be a medication effect rather than a reliable aspect of the psychopathology of schizophrenia (Barch *et al.*, 1996). Based on these results, it is likely that some aspects of non-declarative memory (procedural learning and priming effects) are preserved in schizophrenia.

In conclusion, working memory and declarative memory are both impaired in schizophrenic patients, probably as a result of deficits in executive processing; non-declarative memory is, however, intact (Table 3.2). Memory functioning in schizophrenia has been summarized in Table 3.2.

Table 3.2: Memory Functioning in Schizophrenia

Aspect of memory	Finding
Working memory:	
Buffer storage	Intact
Executive processing	Impaired
Declarative memory:	
Encoding	Impaired
Storage	Intact
Retrieval	Impaired
Non-declarative memory:	
Procedural learning	Intact
Priming effects	Intact

Language Processing in Schizophrenia

As with attention and memory, language processing involves a broad range of cognitive functions. In general, processes involved in language production are distinguished from those involved in language comprehension. Disturbed language production has historically been one of the hallmark clinical symptoms of schizophrenia, phenomenologically classified as loosening of association or formal thought disorder. However, despite a long-time interest in disturbed language production, there has been little consensus on the components which are disturbed in schizophrenia.

Psycholinguistic approaches have recently been used to compartmentalize the processes operating during language production. For example, Levelt (1989) classified language production into the following components:

1. Forming and maintaining a discourse plan.
2. Grammatically and phonologically encoding information to be expressed.
3. Monitoring both one's own and other's speech.
4. Editing speech for errors.
5. Articulation.

Patients with schizophrenia occasionally make grammatical and phonological errors in their speech (Barch and Berenbaum, 1996), but such disturbances are relatively infrequent (Andreasen, 1979). While patients do appear to be reliably impaired in at least some higher level components of language production, the exact source of these deficits is still unclear. Consider *reference*, for example; this is the process of referring to information that has been either previously mentioned in speech, or is outside of but relevant to the speech context. The ability to produce clear references is consistently impaired in schizophrenia (Harvey, 1983; Harvey and Brault, 1986; Docherty *et al.*, 1988; Docherty *et al.*, 1996a and b); in a model such as that of Levelt (1989), these referential impairments could arise from difficulties in forming and maintaining a discourse plan, monitoring speech, or even editing speech for errors.

The production of clear references is linked to working memory function. Studies on healthy adults (e.g., Pratt *et al.*, 1989) show that there is a positive correlation between the use of clear references and performance on verbal working memory tasks. An explanation for this finding is that verbal working memory is used to maintain representations of prior discourse; these representations facilitate appropriate reference use. Studies on patients with schizophrenia (e.g., Docherty *et al.*, 1996a and b) show that the production of unclear references is linked to deficits on tasks which measure working memory function and executive processes. An explanation for these findings is that the production of unclear references reflects an inability to maintain prior discourse information in working memory as well as an inability to use that information to guide and edit ongoing language production.

Much data suggests that verbal working memory plays an important role in language comprehension. Just and Carpenter (1992) argued that syntactic, semantic, and referential aspects of earlier sentence comprehension are maintained and manipulated in working memory to facilitate later sentence comprehension. In schizophrenia, there is a relatively consistent evidence that patients are impaired in at least some aspects of sentence comprehension (Morice and McNicol, 1985; Condray *et al.*, 1995). These deficits become apparent in event-related potential studies that examine the N400 component during language comprehension. The N400 is thought to index the degree to which a target word is predicted by its preceding context; less predictable words elicit larger N400's (Kutas and Hillyard, 1980). Studies have shown that schizophrenic patients, unlike healthy controls, consistently produce a N400 to predicted words (Koyama *et al.*, 1991; Niznikiewicz *et al.*, 1997). This suggests that in such patients the previous sentence context does not appropriately influence later sentence comprehension; impaired verbal working memory may be responsible for such a comprehension deficit.

Although these results demonstrate that schizophrenic patients have language comprehension deficits, the precise mechanism underlying the deficits is unclear. It is unlikely that the deficits are due to disturbances in semantic decoding of single words, or due to disturbances in comprehension of simple syntactic structures because patients do not show disturbances in these areas (Morice and McNicol, 1985). Instead, the deficits are more likely to be due to either difficulty in maintaining the prior sentence context, or due to disturbances in executive functions that (in normal persons) allow the prior context to facilitate later language comprehension through an integration of current and prior sentence information.

In conclusion, schizophrenic patients exhibit deficits in both production and comprehension of language. However, these deficits probably originate from impairments in aspects of working memory and executive functions.

EXECUTIVE IMPAIRMENT AND IMPAIRMENT IN HIGHER COGNITION IN SCHIZOPHRENIA

Executive processes have been referred to as a potential common thread which links deficits in attention, memory, and language processing in schizophrenia. These executive processes may also form the basis for a general set of disturbances that extend across the domains of higher cognition. The term 'executive process' itself needs clarification since it has been used in relation to a number of domains of cognition as well as a wide range of tasks in cognitive psychology and neuropsychology.

Executive processes describe a broad range of operations that are involved in initiating and maintaining controlled information processing and co-ordinated mental activity. Executive processes include goal or context representation and maintenance, attention allocation and stimulus-response mapping, and performance monitoring (Shallice, 1988; Cohen *et al.*, 1990; Carter *et al.*, 1998). Deficits in executive processes have been frequently reported in schizophrenia using a range of methodologies from neuropsychology and experimental cognitive psychology. Such deficits have served as the basis of a number of general theories of cognitive dysfunction in schizophrenia; these have been well discussed elsewhere (Calloway and Naghdi, 1982; Braff, 1993; Cohen and Servan-Schreiber, 1992; Posner and Abdullaev, 1996; Barch and Carter, 1998; Andreasen *et al.*, 1998).

The specific abnormalities within the executive system are yet to be defined in schizophrenia. Well-articulated theories emphasize impaired context representation and maintenance (Shakov, 1962; Cohen and Servan-Schreiber, 1992), impaired attention allocation (Braff, 1993), and impaired performance monitoring (Feinberg, 1978; Malenka *et al.*, 1982; Frith and Done, 1989; Gray *et al.*, 1990). Disruption of one or more of these processes could account for cognitive disturbances in areas such as selective attention, working memory, encoding and recall in declarative memory, as well as language production and comprehension.

To date, no single theory of impaired executive control has garnered overwhelming empirical support over other theories that explain cognitive disability in schizophrenia. Thus, further research is needed to clarify whether a disruption of one specific aspect of executive functions in schizophrenia is sufficient to account for the range of higher cognitive deficits observed, or whether several different executive deficits exist, with each contributing to different aspects of cognitive disability. It is precisely in this endeavour that the tools and constructs of cognitive neuroscience may help enhance the current understanding of the nature of cognitive deficits in schizophrenia. The different components of executive processes described earlier are being linked to discrete elements of a distributed neural network in the brain. This will allow the development of functional-anatomical hypotheses about the neural substrates of cognitive deficits in schizophrenia.

In conclusion, impairments in executive processes probably explain the observed deficits in aspects of attention, memory, and language processing in schizophrenia; however, the relative roles of different executive functions remains to be defined.

Neurobiological Substrates of Cognitive Disability in Schizophrenia

In recent years, more attention has been paid to the neurobiological substrates of cognitive functioning in schizophrenia than to the neurobiological substrates of any other aspect of the illness. One explanation is that cognitive functioning in schizophrenia can be very reliably and objectively measured while assessment of other aspects of the illness (such as delusions and hallucinations) relies upon the patients' self-report and clinical inference. Another explanation is that the use of cognitive activation during functional brain imaging procedures such as positron emission tomography (PET) and functional magnetic resonance imaging (fMRI) brings pathophysiology research in schizophrenia into direct contact with mainstream cognitive neuroscience, thus providing unprecedented opportunities for empirical research into the neurobiology of cognition.

The neural network involved in executive processes includes the dorsolateral prefrontal cortex (DLPFC) and the anterior cingulate cortex (ACC). In general, results to date suggest that schizophrenic patients have impairments in this neural network. These findings suggest hypothetical mechanisms through which disturbances at the neural level may result in disturbed cognition and disorganized behaviour in schizophrenia. Besides in the DLPFC and the ACC, functional imaging studies in schizophrenia have identified disturbances in temporo-limbic regions including the hippocampus (Tamminga *et al.*, 1992; Nordahl *et al.*, 1996), the superior temporal gyrus (Frith *et al.*, 1995; Dolan *et al.*, 1995; Ganguli *et al.*, 1997; O'Leary *et al.*, 1996), and the striatum and cerebellum (Buchsbaum, 1990; Andreasen *et al.*, 1992). Just as this review focused on the disturbances of higher cognitive functions in schizophrenia because of their clinical significance, so too will it focus on the physiological disturbances in circuits underlying executive functions in order to place these disturbances in their neurobiological context.

Regional cerebral blood flow to the frontal lobes of the brain is increased during certain neuropsychological tasks. In a pioneering study, Ingvar and Franzen (1974) showed that this response was attenuated in schizophrenic patients; these findings were suggested to imply *functional hypofrontality*. Subsequently, many but not all investigations reported reduced blood flow or metabolism in the DLPFC in schizophrenia (Berman *et al.*, 1986; Buchsbaum 1990; Andreasen *et al.*, 1992).

Functional hypofrontality is most reliably observed when patients are performing working memory and other tasks which engage cognitive systems that are known to elicit neural activity in this region of the brain (Goldman-Rakic, 1987 and 1991; Carter *et at.*, 1998). Functional hypofrontality is less reliably demonstrable when patients are studied at rest (Gur and Gur, 1995).

What does hypofrontality reflect? While a definitive answer is as yet unavailable, two possibilities exist: hypofrontality may indicate impaired maintenance of information in working memory, or it may indicate impaired executive processes related to representing context or task demand information, that is, information that must be represented or maintained in order that a given task be performed as instructed. Two observations about the pattern of cognitive dysfunction in schizophrenia provide pertinent clues. First, schizophrenic patients show impairments across a range of tasks involving executive control, many of which do not place high maintenance loads on working memory (Barch and Carter, 1998). Second, during working memory tasks schizophrenic patients often show impairments with even very short delays, when the demand for maintenance in memory is minimal (Carter *et al.*, 1996b; Keefe *et al.*, 1995). Such observations suggest that the DLPFC dysfunction in schizophrenia is more likely to reflect impairment of executive processes such as context or task representation. However, these observations do not rule out the possibility that maintenance (memory) processes associated with the DLPFC are also impaired.

While much of the interest in functional hypofrontality in schizophrenia has centered on the DLPFC, hypoactivity in ACC has also been frequently observed in functional brain imaging research. Tamminga and colleagues (1992) reported reduced resting ACC and hippocampal metabolism in a large group of unmedicated schizophrenic patients. Buchsbaum and colleagues (Seigel *et al.*, 1993; Haznedar *et al.*, 1997) described cingulate hypometabolism in the resting state in a large unmedicated sample. Liddle *et al.* (1992) found that resting regional cerebral blood flow in the ACC correlated specifically with the level of behavioural disorganization in patients with schizophrenia. The term 'resting' here is used to describe subjects who were not required to perform any task at the time the data were obtained.

A number of studies have examined ACC functioning in schizophrenia during cognitive activation. Andreasen *et al.* (1992) studied unmedicated schizophrenic patients using single photon emission computerized tomography (SPECT); assessments were conducted while the subjects performed the Tower of London task, a test of executive function. Patients were found to show decreased ACC activity. Reduced ACC activation was also reported during two other classical measures of executive processes: an auditory-verbal supraspan memory task (Ganguli *et al.*, 1997) and a verbal fluency task (Dolan *et al.* 1995).

The Stroop task elicits response competition, requires the strategic allocation of attention, but places very low demands on maintenance processes in working memory: schizophrenic patients were found to show reduced ACC activation during this task as well (Carter *et al.*, 1997a).

What does ACC hypofunction reflect? Recent work using event-related fMRI has suggested that the ACC plays an evaluative role during the executive control of cognition. It detects conditions, such as a competition between simultaneously activated but incompatible response tendencies, which may induce poor task performance. This detection occurs 'on-line' and may provide a signal to other components of the executive system, thus indicating the need for an increased control through processes such as improved attention allocation (Carter *et al.*, 1998). ACC hypofunction in schizophrenia may therefore indicate an impairment in performance monitoring, which is a critical element of executive functioning.

In conclusion, schizophrenic patients show hypoactivity in both the DLPFC and the ACC. Hypoactivity of the former is associated with impairment of context and task representation. Hypoactivity of the latter is associated with impairment of on-line performance monitoring during cognitive processing. The DLPFC and the ACC may therefore represent the neuroanatomical substrates of these executive functions.

The Relationship Between Cognitive Dysfunction and Symptoms in Schizophrenia

The complex literature on the relationship between cognitive deficits and symptoms in schizophrenia has been extensively reviewed (Walker and Lewine, 1988; Strauss, 1993; Green, 1998). Since frontal cortical dysfunction has been associated with the presence of negative symptoms, one would expect that these symptoms would be associated with cognitive disability. While there is some support for the association between negative symptoms and spatial working memory (Keefe *et al.*, 1995; Carter *et al.*, 1996b), the literature is in general inconclusive. Some investigators have therefore suggested that cognitive dysfunction might reflect a separate domain of the illness, distinct from the conventionally described clinical symptoms.

Difficulties in demonstrating associations between negative symptoms and cognitive deficits might in part reflect the practical difficulty of distinguishing drug induced Parkinsonism from 'true' negative symptoms of frontal lobe origin. But, because disorganization is also a part of the frontal lobe syndrome, another reason for the paucity of literature linking frontal lobe symptoms with cognitive deficits is that many studies (particularly the older ones) used a two-factor model of schizophrenia, dividing symptoms into positive and negative syndromes; recent research has suggested that the factor structure of schizophrenia is actually more complex, and probably includes a disorganization factor as well (Liddle and Barnes, 1990; Andreasen *et al.*, 1995; Arndt *et al.*, 1995).

In studies that have used a three-factor approach to symptomatology in schizophrenia, both medicated and unmedicated patients show occasional relationships between negative symptoms on the one hand, and deficits in selective attention and verbal working memory on the other; in contrast, robust relationships are evident between these cognitive deficits and the syndrome of disorganization (Barch *et al.*, 1998; Cohen *et al.*, 1999). This is consistent with previous hypotheses describing the relationship between disorganization and attentional disturbances (Liddle and Morris, 1991). Interestingly, nearly a century ago Bleuler (1911–50) suggested that disturbances in the control of attention were responsible for the associational disturbances that distinguished the schizophrenias from other major psychoses.

Targeting Cognitive Disability in Treatment

The first step towards developing effective treatments for cognitive disability in schizophrenia is to continue the paradigm shift which is already under way. The traditional emphasis on positive and negative symptoms as treatment outcome measures needs to be expanded to include measures of cognitive function, especially measures of attention, memory, and language processing.

The second step is to utilize the burgeoning information on the likely pathophysiological substrates of the cognitive disability. As discussed earlier, functional neuroimaging studies suggest that disturbances in the DLPFC and ACC circuitry produce executive impairments, leading to deficits in attention, memory, and language processing. Disturbances in the DLPFC and ACC circuitry have also been described in postmortem studies of the brains of schizophrenic patients. Further, reductions in markers of glutamate function and (GABA-ergic) inhibitory interneuron function, and reductions in afferent dopaminergic modulatory input have been reported in the DLPEC and the ACC (Benes, 1995; Akbarian *et al.*, 1996; Meador-Woodruff *et al.*, 1997; Woo *et al.*, 1998). Pharmacological approaches will therefore need to target the function of the DLPFC and ACC circuits. Such approaches may open a whole new avenue of opportunity for disability reduction in schizophrenia.

Preliminary studies that used glycine, cycloserine and d-serine (Heresco Levy *et al.*, 1996; Leiderman *et al.*, 1996; Goff *et al.*, 1996; Tsai *et al.*, 1998) to enhance glutamate function support the feasibility of these approaches; new agents which enhance glutamate effects through more specific mechanisms are currently under development. Transient benefits on cognitive function were observed after stimulant challenge (Goldberg *et al.*, 1991; Carter *et al.*, 1997b; Barch *et al.*, 1997); in one study, these benefits extended beyond effects on working memory to include improvement in measures of the organization of language production (Carter *et al.*, 1997b; Barch *et al.*, 1997). Agents which enhance phasic dopamine in the cortex may also attenuate cognitive deficits. Strategies for the pharmacological modulation of local inhibitory function are also under development.

It may be noted here that neuroleptic drugs do not benefit cognition; in fact, certain neuroleptic and co-administered anticholinergic drugs have even been reported to have an adverse impact. Available data on atypical antipsychotic drugs are mixed and suggest limited benefit at best (Goldberg *et al.*, 1990; Green *et al.*, 1997; Green, 1998). More data are required from carefully controlled studies that use appropriate and sophisticated measures to assess the effect of the atypical agents on cognitive functions.

Finally, cognitive rehabilitation measures may stimulate neuroplastic responses in the DLPFC and the ACC. Cognitive rehabilitation may therefore assist in the attenuation of cognitive disability in schizophrenia. Preliminary data using procedures adapted from cognitive rehabilitation approaches to patients with closed head injury support the possible efficacy of this treatment method (Hogarty and Flesher , 1998). A recent study examined patients with chronic schizophrenia who had been randomized to receive computer-based attention training or a control procedure; after eighteen sessions of treatment, CPT assessments demonstrated significantly greater improvement in experimental as compared with control patients (Medalia *et al.*, 1998).

In Conclusion

A growing body of data describes the clinical importance of cognitive disability in schizophrenia. The deficits observed cut across a number of domains of cognitive functioning, including selective attention, working memory, and language processing. These deficits probably result from disturbances in executive processes, such as goal or context representation and maintenance, strategy formation, and performance monitoring. Evidence from functional neuroimaging studies suggests that these higher cognitive deficits are related to physiological dysfunction in circuits underlying executive functions in the brain, such as the DLPFC and the ACC. At the local circuit level, disturbances may be present in glutamatergic and GABA-ergic neurotransmission, and in the modulation of these by dopamine. The development of novel therapies targeting these disturbances at the local circuit level in medial and dorsolateral prefrontal cortices promises to begin a new phase in the therapeutics of schizophrenia.

References

Akbarian S., Sucher N. J., Bradley D. *et al.* (1996). 'Selective alterations in gene expression for NMDA receptor subunits in prefrontal cortex of schizophrenics', *J. Neurosci.*, 16: 19–30.

Andreasen N. C. (1979). 'Thought, language, and communication disorders: II. Diagnostic significance', *Arch. Gen. Psychiatry*, 36: 1325–30.

Andreasen N. C., Rezai K., Alliger R. *et al.* (1992). 'Hypofrontality in neuroleptic-naive patients and in patients with chronic schizophrenia: assessment with xenon 133 single photon emission computed tomography and the Tower of London', *Arch. Gen. Psychiatry*, 49: 943–58.

Andreasen N. C., Arndt S., Alliger R. *et al.* (1995). 'A longitudinal study of symptom dimensions in schizophrenia: prediction and patterns of change', *Arch. Gen. Psychiatry*, 52: 341–52.

Andreasen N. C., Paradiso S and O'Leary D. S. (1998). '"Cognitive dysmetria" as an integrative theory of schizophrenia: A dysfunction in cortical-subcortical-cerebellar circuitry', *Schizophr. Bull.*, 24: 203–18.

Arndt S., Andreasen N. C., Flaum M. *et al.* (1995). 'Symptoms of schizophrenia: methods, meanings, and mechanisms', *Arch. Gen. Psychiatry*, 52: 352–60.

Baddeley A. (1986). *Working Memory*, Oxford: Oxford University Press.

Barch D. M. and Berenbaum H. (1996). 'Language production and thought disorder in schizophrenia', *J. Abnorm. Psychol.*, 105: 81–8.

Barch D. M. and Carter C. S. (1998). 'Selective attention in schizophrenia: Relationship to verbal working memory', *Schizophr. Res.*, 33: 53–61.

Barch D. M., Cohen J. D., Servan-Schreiber D. *et al.* (1996). 'Semantic priming in schizophrenia: and examination of spreading activation using word pronunciation and multiple SOA's', *J. Abnorm. Psychol.*, 105: 592–601.

Barch D. M., Carter C. S., Braver T. S. *et al.* (1997). 'The effect of d-amphetamine on working memory and language deficits in schizophrenia', *Schizophr. Res.*, 24: 129.

Barch D. M., Carter C. S., Hachten P. C. *et al.* (1998). 'The "benefits" of distractibility: The mechanisms underlying increased Stroop effects in schizophrenia', *Schizophr. Bull.* (in press).

Beatty W., Jocic Z., Monson N. *et al.* (1993). 'Memory and frontal lobe dysfunction in schizophrenia and schizoaffective disorder', *J. Nerv. Ment. Dis.*, 181: 448–53.

Benes F. M. (1995). 'Is there a neuroanatomic basis for schizophrenia?', *Neuroscientist*, 1: 112–20.

Berman K., Zec R. and Weinberger D. (1986). 'Physiological dysfunction of dorsolateral prefrontal cortex in schizophrenia: II. Role of neuroleptic treatment, attention and mental effort', *Arch. Gen. Psychiatry*, 43: 126–35.

Bleuler E. (1911). *Dementia Praecox or The Group of Schizophrenias*, Translated by J. Zinkin, New York; International Universities Press, 1950.

Braff D. (1993). 'Information processing and attention dysfunction in schizophrenia', *Schizophr. Bull.*, 19: 233–59.

Buchsbaum M. (1990). 'The frontal lobes, basal ganglia and temporal lobes as sites for schizophrenia', *Schizophr. Bull.*, 16: 379–89.

Bustillo J. R., Thaker G., Buchanan R. W. *et al.* (1997). 'Visual information-processing impairments in deficit and non-deficit schizophrenia', *Am. J. Psychiatry*, 154: 647–54.

Calloway E. and Naghdi S. (1982). 'An information processing model for schizophrenia', *Arch. Gen. Psychiatry*, 39: 339–47.

Carter C. S., Robertson L. C. and Nordahl T. E. (1992). 'Abnormal processing of irrelevant information in chronic schizophrenia: selective enhancement of Stroop facilitation', *Psychiatry Res.*, 41: 137–46.

Carter C. S., Robertson L. C., Chaderjian M. R. *et al.* (1994). 'Attentional asymmetry in schizophrenia: the role of illness subtype and symptomatology', *Prog. Neuropsychopharm. Biol. Psychiatry*, 18: 661–83.

Carter C. S., Robertson L. C., Nordahl T. E. *et al.* (1996a). 'Attentional and perceptual asymmetries in schizophrenia: further evidence for a left hemisphere deficit', *Psychiatry Res.*, 62: 111–19.

Carter C. S., Robertson L. C., Nordahl T. E. *et al.* (1996b). 'Spatial working memory deficits and their relationship to negative symptoms in unmedicated schizophrenia patients', *Biol. Psychiatry*, 40: 930–2.

Carter C. S., Mintun M., Nichols T. *et al.* (1997a). 'Anterior cingulate gyrus dysfunction and selective attention dysfunction in schizophrenia: An ^{15}O–H_2O PET study during Stroop Task performance', *Am. J. Psychiatry*, 154: 1670–5.
Carter C. S., Barch D., Jonathan D. *et al.* (1997b). 'CNS catecholamines and cognitive dysfunction in schizophrenia', *Schizophr. Res.*, 24: 211A.
Carter C. S., Braver T. S., Barch D. M. *et al.* (1998). 'Anterior cingulate cortex, error detection, and the on-line monitoring of performance', *Science*, 280: 747–9.
Clare L., McKenna P. J., Mortimer A. M. *et al.* (1993). 'Memory in schizophrenia: what is impaired and what is preserved', *Neuropsychologia*, 31: 1225–41.
Cohen J. D. and Servan-Schreiber D. (1992). 'Context, cortex, and dopamine: A connectionist approach to behaviour and biology in schizophrenia', *Psychol. Rev.*, 99: 45–77.
Cohen J. D., Dunbar K. and McClelland J. L. (1990). 'On the control of automatic processes: A parallel distributed processing model of the Stroop effect', *Psychol. Rev.*, 97: 332–61.
Cohen J. D., Barch D. M., Carter C. S. *et al.* (1999). 'Schizophrenic deficits in the processing of context: Converging evidence from three theoretically motivated cognitive tasks', *J. Abnorm. Psychology* (in press).
Condray R., Steinhauer S. R. and Goldstein G. (1992). 'Language comprehension in schizophrenics and their brothers', *Biol. Psychiatry*, 32: 790–802.
Condray R., van Kammen D. P., Steinhauer S. R. *et al.* (1995). 'Language comprehension in schizophrenia: trait or state indicator?', *Biol. Psychiatry*, 38: 287–96.
Connor R. O. and Herman H. (1993). 'Assessment of contributions to disability in people with schizophrenia during rehabilitation', *Aust. N. Z. J. Psychiatry*, 27: 595–600.
Crawford T. J., Haeger B., Kennard C. *et al.* (1995). 'Saccadic abnormalities in psychotic patients: 1. Neuroleptic-free psychotic patients', *Psychol. Med.*, 25: 461–71.
Davidson L. and McGlashan T. H. (1997). 'The varied outcomes of schizophrenia', *Can. J. Psychiatry*, 42: 34–43.
Docherty N., Schnur M. and Harvey P. D. (1988). 'Reference performance and positive and negative thought disorder: A follow-up study of manics and schizophrenics', *J. Abnorm. Psychol.*, 97: 437–42.
Docherty N. M., Hawkins K. A., Sledge W. H. *et al.* (1996a). 'Working memory, attention, and communication disturbances in schizophrenia', *J. Abnorm. Psychol.*, 105: 212–19.
Docherty N. M., DeRosa M. and Andreasen N. C. (1996b). 'Communication disturbances in schizophrenia and mania', *Arch. Gen. Psychiatry*, 53: 358–64.

Dolan R., Frith C. D., Friston K. J. *et al.* (1995). 'Dopaminergic modulation of impaired cognitive activation in the ACC in schizophrenia', *Nature*, 378: 180–3.

Feinberg I. (1978). 'Efference copy and corollary discharge: implications for thinking and its disorders', *Schizophr. Bull.*, 4: 636–40.

Frith C. D. and Done D. J. (1989). 'Experiences of alien control in schizophrenia reflect a disorder in the central monitoring of action', *Psychol. Med.*, 19: 359–63.

Frith C. D., Friston K. J., Herold S. *et al.* (1995). 'Regional brain activity in chronic schizophrenia patients during the performance of a verbal fluency task', *Br. J. Psychiatry*, 167: 343–9.

Ganguli R., Carter C. S., Mintun M. *et al.* (1997). 'Abnormal cortical physiology in schizophrenia: A PET blood flow study during rest and supraspan memory performance', *Biol. Psychiatry*, 41: 33–42.

Goff D. C., Tsai G., Manoach D. S. *et al.* (1996) 'D-cycloserine added to clozapine for patients with schizophrenia', *Am. J. Psychiatry*, 153: 1628–30.

Gold J. M., Carpenter C., Randolph C. *et al.* (1997). 'Auditory working memory and Wisconsin card sorting test performance in schizophrenia', *Archives of General Psychiatry*, 54: 159–65.

Goldberg T. E., Saint-Cyr J. and Weinberger D. R. (1990). 'Assessment of procedural learning and problem solving in schizophrenic patients using Tower of Hanoi type tasks', *Neuropsychiatry and Clin. Neurosci.*, 2: 165–73.

Goldberg T. E., Bigelow L. B., Weinberger D. R. *et al.* (1991). 'Cognitive and behavioral effects of the coadministration of dextroamphetamine and haloperidol in schizophrenia', *Am. J. Psychiatry*, 148: 78–84.

Goldberg T. E., Greenberg R. D., Griffin S. J. *et al.* 1993). 'The effect of clozapine on cognition and psychiatric symptoms in patients with schizophrenia', *British Journal of Psychiatry*, 162: 43–8.

Goldman-Rakic P. S. (1987). 'Circuitry of primate prefrontal cortex and regulation of behaviour by representational memory', in Plum F (ed.) *Handbook of Physiology: The Nervous system*, Bethesda: American Physiological Society, 5: 373–417.

——— (1991). 'Prefrontal cortical dysfunction in schizophrenia: The relevance of working memory', in Carroll BJ, Barrett JE (eds) *Psychopathology and the Brain*, New York: Raven Press, 1–23.

Gray J., Feldon J., Rawlins J. *et al.* (1990). 'The neuropsychology of schizophrenia', *Behavioral and Brain Sciences*, 14: 1–84.

Green M. F. (1996). 'What are the functional consequences of neurocognitive deficits in schizophrenia?', *Am J. Psychiatry*, 153: 321–30.

——— (1998). *Schizophrenia from a neurocognitive perspective: Probing the impenetrable darkness*, Boston, MA: Allyn and Bacon.

Green M. F., Nuechterlein K. H. and Mintz J. (1994). 'Backward masking in schizophrenia and mania: specifying a mechanism', *Arch. Gen. Psychiatry*, 51: 939–44.

Green M. F., Marshall Jr. B. D., Wirshing W. C. *et al.* (1997). 'Does risperdone improve verbal working memory in treatment-resistant schizophrenia?', *Am. J. Psychiatry*, 154: 799–804.

Gur R. C. and Gur R. E. (1995). 'Hypofrontality in schizophrenia: RIP', *Lancet*, 345: 1383–4.

Harvey P. D. (1983). 'Speech competence in manic and schizophrenic psychoses: The association between clinically rated thought disorder and cohension and reference performance', *J. Abnor. Psychol.*, 92: 368–77.

Harvey P. D. and Brault J. (1986). 'Speech performance in mania and schizophrenia: The association of positive and negative thought disorder and reference failure', *J. Communic. Disord.*, 19: 161–73.

Haznedar M. M., Buchsbaum M. S., Luu C *et al.* (1997). 'Decreased anterior cingulate gyrus metabolic rate in schizophrenia', *Am J. Psychiatry*, 154: 682–4.

Henik A. Priel B. and Umansky R. (1992). 'Attention and automaticity in semantic processing of schizophrenic patients', *Neuropsychiatry Neuropsychol. Behav. Neurol.*, 5: 161–9.

Henik A., Nissimov E., Priel B. *et al.* (1995). 'Effects of cognitive load on semantic priming in patients with schizophrenia', *J. Abnorm. Psychol.*, 104: 576–84.

Heresco-Levy U., Silipo G. and Javitt D. C. (1996). 'Glycinergic augmentation of NMDA receptor-mediated neurotransmission in the treatment of schizophrenia', *Psychopharmacol. Bull.*, 32: 731–40.

Hogarty G. E. and Flesher S. (1998). 'Practice principles of cognitive enhancement therapy for schizophrenia', *Schizophr. Bull.* (in press).

Ingvar D. H. and Franzen G. (1974). 'Distribution of cerebral activity in chronic schizophrenia', *lancet*, 2: 1484–6.

Just M. A. and Carpenter P. A. (1992). 'A capacity theory of comprehension: Individual differences in working memory', *Psychol. Rev.*, 99: 122–49.

Keefe R. S. E., Roitman S. E. L., Harvey P. D. *et al.* (1995) 'A pen-and-paper human analogue of a monkey prefrontal cortex activation task: Spatial working memory in patients with schizophrenia', *Schizophr. Res.*, 17: 25–33.

Klapow J. C., Evans J., Patterson T. L. *et al.* (1997). 'Direct assessment of functional status in older patients with schizophrenia', *Am. J. Psychiatry*, 154: 1022–4.

Koh S. D. (1978). 'Remembering of verbal materials by schizophrenic young adults', in Schwartz S (ed.), *Language and Cognition in Schizophrenia*, New Jersey: Lawrence Erlbaum, 55–99.

Koyama M., Nageishi Y., Shimokochi M. *et al.* (1991). 'The N400 component of event-related potentials in schizophrenic patients: A preliminary study', *Electroencephalogr. Clin. Neurophysiol.*, 78: 124–32.

Kraeplin E. (1971). *Dementia praecox and paraphrenia*, Edinburgh: Churchill Livingston (original work published 1919; translated by Barclay RM).

Kutas M. and Hillyard S. A. (1980). 'Reading senseless sentences: brain potentials reflect semantic incongruity', *Science*, 207: 203–5.

Kwapil T. R., Hegley D. C., Chapman L. J. *et al.* (1990). 'Facilitation of word recognition by semantic priming in schizophrenia', *J. Abnorm. Psychol.*, 3: 215–21.

LaBerge D. (1995). *Attentional Processing*, Cambridge: Harvard University Press.

Leiderman E., Zylberman I., Zukin S. R. *et al.* (1996). 'Preliminary investigation of high-dose oral glycine on serum levels and negative symptoms in schizophrenia: an open-label trial', *Biol. Psychiatry*, 39: 213–15.

Levelt W. J. M. (1989). *Speaking: From Intention to Articulation*, Cambridge: MIT Press.

Liddle P. F. and Barnes T. R. E. (1990). 'Syndromes of chronic schizophrenia', *Br. J. Psychiatry*, 157: 558–61.

Liddle P. F. and Morris D. L. (1991). 'Schizophrenic syndromes and frontal lobe performance', *Br. J. Psychiatry*, 158: 340–45.

Liddle P. F., Friston K. J., Frith C. D. *et al.* (1992) 'Patterns of cerebral blood flow in schizophrenia', *Br. J. Psychiatry*, 160: 179–86.

Macleod C. M. (1991). 'Half a century of research on the Stroop effect: an integrative review', *Psychol. Bull.*, 109: 163–203.

Malenka R. C., Angel R. W., Hampton B. *et al.* (1982). 'Impaired central error-correcting behavior in schizophrenia', *Arch. Gen. Psychiatry*, 39: 101–7.

Manschreck T. C., Maher B. A., Milavetz J. J. *et al.* (1988). 'Semantic priming in thought disordered schizophrenic patients', *Schizophr. Res.*, 1: 61–6.

Meador-Woodruff J. H., Haroutunian V., Pochik P. *et al.* (1997). 'Dopamine receptor transcript expression in striatum and prefrontal and occipital cortex: Focal abnormalities in orbitofrontal cortex in schizophrenia', *Arch. Gen. Psychiatry*, 54: 1089–95.

Medalia A., Aluma M., Tyron W., Merriam A. E. Effectiveness of attention training in schizophrenia. Schizophr Bull (1998); 24: 147–152.

Morice R. and McNicol D. (1985). 'The comprehension and production of complex syntax in schizophrenia', *Cortex*, 21: 567–80.

Nestor P. G., Faux S. F., McCarley R. W. *et al.* (1992). 'Attentional cues in chronic schizophrenia: abnormal disengagement of attention', *J. Abnorm. Psychol.*, 101: 682–9.

Niznikiewicz M. A., O'Donnel B. F., Nestor P. G. *et al.* (1997). 'ERP assessment of visual and auditory language processing in schizophrenia', *J. Abnorm. Psychol.*, 106: 85–94.

Nordahl T. E., Kusubov N., Carter C. *et al.* (1996). ' Temporal lobe metabolic differences in medication-free outpatients with schizophrenia via the PET-600', *Neuropsychopharmacol.*, 15: 541–54.

Nuechterlein K. H. and Dawson M. E. (1984). 'Information processing and attentional dysfunction in the developmental course of schizophrenia', *Schizophr. Bull.*, 10: 160–203.

O'Leary D. S., Andreasen N. C., Hurtig R. T. *et al.* (1996). 'Auditory attentional deficits in schizophrenia: a positron emission tomography study', *Arch. Gen. Psychiatry*, 53: 633–41.

Park S. and Holzman P. S. (1992). 'Schizophrenics show spatial working memory deficits', *Arch. Gen. Psychiatry*, 49: 975–82.

Perlstein W. M., Carter C. S., Barch D. M. *et al.* (1998). 'The Stroop task and attention deficits in schizophrenia: a critical evaluation of card and single-trial stroop methodologies', *Neuropsychol.*, 12: 414–25.

Posner M. I. (1980). 'Orienting of attention: The VII Sir Frederic Bartlett Lecture', *Q. J. Exp. Psychol.*, 32: 3–25.

Posner M. I. and Abdullaev Y. G. (1996). 'What to image? Anatomy, circuitry and plasticity of human brain function', in Toga AW, Mazziota JC (eds), *Brain Mapping: The Methods*, Academic press: New York, 408–19.

Posner M. I. and Cohen Y. (1984). 'Components of visual orienting', in Bouma H. Bouwhuis D. G. (eds) *Attention and Performence*, Hillsdale: Erlbaum, 531–56.

Posner M. I. and Dahaene S. (1995). 'Attentional networks', *Trends Neurosci.*, 17: 75–9.

Posner M. I. and Petersen S. E. (1990). 'The attention system of the human brain', *Ann. Rev. Neurosci.*, 13: 25–42.

Posner M. I., Early T. S., Reiman E. *et al.* (1988). 'Asymmetries of attentional control in schizophrenia', *Arch. Gen. Psychiatry*, 45: 814–21.

Pratt M. W., Boyes C., Robins S. *et al.* (1989). 'Telling tales: Aging, working memory, and the narrative cohesion of story retellings', *Devel. Psychol.*, 4; 628–35.

Rosvold K. E., Mirsky A. F., Sarason I. *et al.* (1956). 'A continuous performance test of brain damage', *J. Consult. Clin. Psychol.*, 20: 343–50.

Saccuzzo D. P. and Braff D. L. (1981). 'Early information processing deficits in schizophrenia', *Arch. Gen. Psychiatry*, 38: 175–9.

Schmand B., Beand N. and Kuipers T. (1992). 'Procedural learning of cognitive and motor skills in psychotic patients', *Schizophr. Res.*, 8: 157–70.

Schwartz B. L., Rosse R. B. and Deutsch S. I. (1992). 'Towards a neuropsychology of memory in schizophrenia', *Psychopharmacol. Bull.*, 28: 341–51.

Seigel B. V., Buchsbaum M. S., Bunney W. *et al.* (1993). 'Cortico-striatal-thalamic circuits and brain glucose metabolism in 70 unmedicated schizophrenic patients', *Am J. Psychiatry*, 150: 1325–36.

Servan-Schreiber D., Cohen J. D. and Steingard S. (1996). 'Schizophrenic deficits in the processing of context: A test of neural network simulations of cognitive functioning in schizophrenia', *Arch. Gen. Psychiatry*, 53: 1105–12.

Shakov D. (1962). 'Segmental set: A theory of the formal psychological deficit in schizophrenia', *Arch. Gen. Psychiatry*, 6: 1–17.

Shallice T. (1988). *From Neuropsychology to Mental Structure*, Cambridge: Cambridge University Press.

Spitzer M. (1993). 'The psychopathology, neuropsychology and neurobiology of associative and working memory in schizophrenia', *Eur. Arch. Psychiatry Clin. Neurosci.*, 243: 57–70.

Squire L. (1992). 'Declarative and non-declarative memory Multiple brain systems supporting learning and memory', *J. Cog. Neurosci.*, 4: 232–43.

Squire L. and Zola–Morgan S. (1988). 'Declarative and non-declarative memory: multiple brain systems supporting learning and memory', *Trends Neurosci.*, 11: 170–5.

Stone M., Gabrieli J. D., Stebbins G. T. *et al.* (1998). 'Working and strategic memory deficits in schizophrenia', *Neuropsychol.*, 12: 278–88.

Strauss M. E. (1993). 'Relations of symptoms to cognitive deficits in schizophrenia', *Schizophr. Bull.*, 19: 215–31.

Strauss M. E., Novakovic T., Tien A. *et al.* (1991). 'Disengagment of attention in schizophrenia', *Psychiatry Res.*, 37: 139–46.

Strauss M. E., Alphs L. and Boekamp J. (1992). 'Disengagment of attention in chronic schizophrenia', *Psychiatry Res.*, 43: 87–92.

Stroop J. R. (1935). 'Studies of interference in serial verbal reactions', *J. Exp. Psychol.*, 18: 643–62.

Tamlyn D., McKenna P., Mortimer A. *et al.* (1992). 'Memory impairment in schizophrenia: its extent, affiliations and neuropsychological character', *Psychol. Med.*, 22: 101–15.

Tamminga C. A., Thaker G. K., Buchanan R. *et al.* (1992). 'Limbic system abnormalities identified in schizophrenia with fluorodeoxyglucose and neocortical alterations with the deficit syndrome', *Arch. Gen. Psychiatry*, 49: 522–30.

Taylor S., Kornblum S. and Tandon R. (1996). 'Facilitation and interference of selective attention in schizophrenia', *J. Psychiatr. Res.*, 30: 251–9.

Tsai G., Yang P., Chung L. *et al*. (1998). 'D-serine added to antipsychotics for the treatment of schizophrenia', *Biol. Psychiatry*, 44: 1081–9.

Tulving E. and Schachter D. (1990). 'Priming and human memory systems', *Science*, 247: 301–6.

Vinogradov S., Ober B. A. and Shenaut G. K. (1992). 'Semantic priming of word pronunciation and lexical decision in schizophrenia', *Schizoph. Res.*, 8: 171–81.

Walker E. and Lewine R. J. (1988). 'Negative symptom distinction in schizophrenia: validity and etiological relevance', *Schizophr. Res.*, 1: 315–28.

Woo Tu, Whitehead R. E., Melchitzky D. S. *et al*. (1998). 'A subclass of prefrontal gamma-aminobutyric acid axon terminals are selectively altered in schizophrenia', *Proc. Natl. Acad. Sci. USA*, 95: 5341–6.

Chapter 4

MRI Hyperintensities and the Vascular Origins of Late Life Depression

HAROLD A. SACKEIM, SARAH H. LISANBY, MITCHELL S. NOBLER, RONALD L. VAN HEERTUM, ROBERT L. DELAPAZ AND BRETT MENSH

ENCEPHALOMALACIA IN MAJOR DEPRESSION

In comparison with healthy controls, high rates of abnormality have consistently been observed in magnetic resonance imaging (MRI) evaluations of elderly patients with major depressive disorder (MDD) (Krishnan *et al.*, 1988 and 1997; Coffey *et al.*, 1990; Zubenko *et al.*, 1990; Rabins *et al.*, 1991; Lesser *et al.*, 1991; Coffey *et al.*, 1993; Fujikawa *et al.*, 1993; Krishnan, 1993; Hickie *et al.*, 1995; Greenwald *et al.*, 1996; Iidaka *et al.*, 1996; Lesser *et al.*, 1996). These abnormalities appear as areas of increased signal intensity in balanced, T_2-weighted, and fluid-attenuated inversion recovery (FLAIR) images. The abnormalities can be classified into three types. As seen in Fig. 4.1, *periventricular hyperintensities* (PVH) are a halo or rim adjacent to ventricles; in severe forms, these invade the surrounding deep white matter. *Deep white matter hyperintensities* (DWMH) are single, patchy, or confluent foci, which may be observed in subcortical white matter, with or without PVH. Hyperintensities (HIs) may also be found in *deep gray structures*,

Acknowledgements: Preparation of this chapter was supported in part by Grants MH35636, MH55646, and MH01244 from the National Institute of Mental Health, Bethesda, MD.

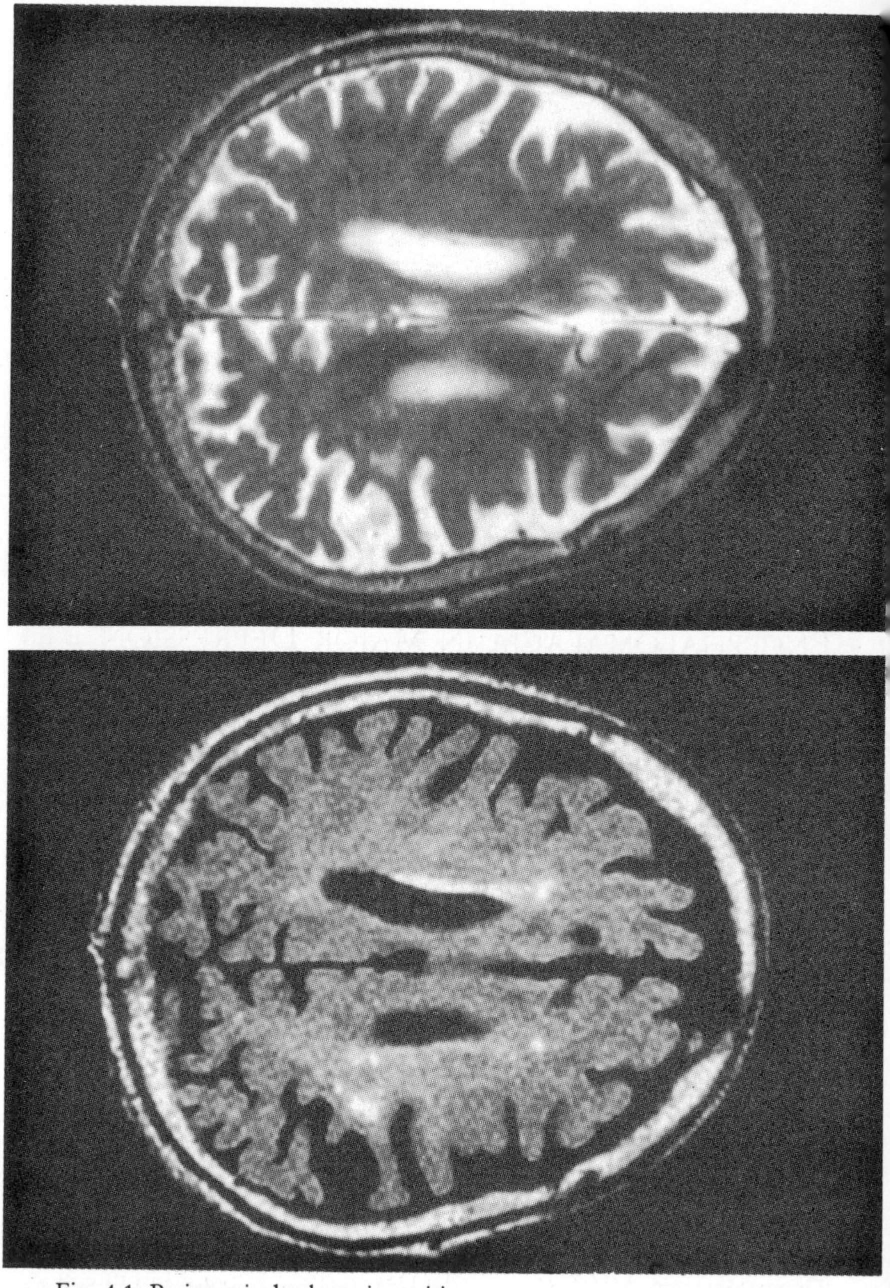

Fig. 4.1: Periventricular hyperintensities.

particularly the basal ganglia, thalamus, and pons. Computed tomography (CT) lucencies (hypodensities) have also been reported in MDD (Coffey *et al*., 1988; Kohlmeyer, 1988; Zubenko *et al*., 1990), but with lower prevalence due to reduced imaging sensitivity (Barnes and Enzmann, 1981; Awad *et al*., 1986a). These abnormalities have been referred to as leukoencephalopathy (Krishnan *et al*., 1988), leuko-araiosis (Hachinski *et al*., 1987), subcortical arteriosclerotic encephalopathy (Solomon *et al*., 1987), encephalomalacia (Awad *et al*., 1986b), and unidentified bright object (UBOs; Swayze *et al*., 1990). Since the HIs in MDD are not restricted to white matter and since their aetiology is not established, the term encephalomalacia is used in this review.

In one of the largest prospective MRI series (Coffey *et al*., 1989 and 1990), all 51 elderly (age >60 years) depressed patients referred for electroconvulsive therapy (ECT) were found to have HIs. Over half the HIs were rated as moderate to severe. In 51 per cent of these patients, lesions of subcortical gray nuclei were also observed. These rates of abnormality greatly exceeded those found in a healthy control sample. Basal ganglia abnormalities best discriminated between depressed and control groups (*see* Fig. 4.2).

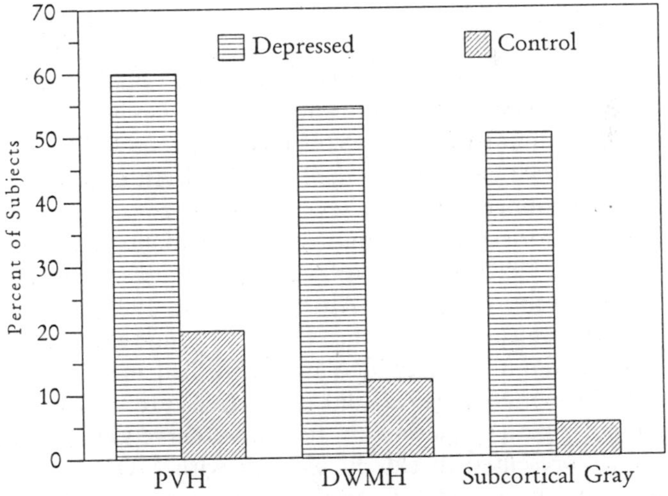

Fig. 4.2: Ratio of MRI hyperinensity in a sample of severely depressed in-patients and matched controls (after Coffey *et al.* 1990). (PVH=periventricular hyperintensity: DWMH=deep white matter hyperintensity).

Depressed samples studied to date have often included patients with comorbid medical illnesses, and have not adequately controlled for cerebrovascular disease (CVD) risk factors, medication, or drug abuse. Nonetheless, in the reports by Coffey *et al.* (1989 and 1990), the rate of encephalomalacia in MDD patients greatly exceeded that of normal controls even when MDD patients with pre-existing neurological conditions were excluded. In a replication study (Coffey *et al.*, 1993), MDD patients had marked increases in the frequency of PVH, DWMH, and basal ganglia and thalamic HIs relative to controls matched for CVD risk factors. After adjusting for age, MDD patients were over five times more likely than controls to exhibit PVH (age-adjusted odds ratio = 5.32). In other studies, when excluding the characteristic halo or caps at the ventricles, only 10–30 per cent of elderly, healthy controls had MRI white matter abnormalities (typically mild in severity); rates of subcortical gray matter abnormalities were also low (Brandt-Zawadski *et al.*, 1985; Gerard and Weisberg, 1986; Kertesz *et al.*, 1988; Fazekas, 1989; Rao *et al.*, 1989; Mirsen *et al.*, 1991; Boone *et al.*, 1992; Matsubayashi *et al.*, 1992; Christiansen *et al.*, 1994; Breteler *et al.*, 1994a; Golomb *et al.*, 1995).

The rate or severity of encephalomalacia in geriatric depression may equal or exceed that in Alzheimer's disease (Rezek *et al.*, 1986; Erkinjuntti *et al.*, 1987 and 1994; Aharon-Peretz *et al.*, 1988; Filley *et al.*, 1989; Leys *et al.*, 1990; Diaz *et al.*, 1991; Lopez *et al.*, 1992; Brilliant *et al.*, 1995) and may be comparable to that in multi-infarct dementia (Erkinjuntti *et al.*, 1987; Hershey *et al.*, 1987; Aharon-Peretz *et al.*, 1988; Zubenko *et al.*, 1990; Almkvist *et al.*, 1992). In considerably younger samples, several groups have reported that MRI HIs are more common among bipolar patients than controls (Dupont *et al.*, 1990 and 1995a; Swayze *et al.*, 1990; Figiel *et al.*, 1991a; Strakowski *et al.*, 1993; Altschuler *et al.*, 1995; Botteron *et al.*, 1995). In contrast, Aylward *et al.* (1994) found that older (age > 38 years) and not younger bipolar patients had an excess of HIs. Similarly, Brown *et al.* (1992) did not detect an excess of HIs in young bipolar patients, although they did observe that severe HIs were over-represented in elderly patients with MDD.

Few studies have directly compared rates of encephalomalacia between elderly depressed patients and those with another neuropsychiatric illness. Zubenko *et al.* (1990) used MRI or CT assessments in 67 elderly patients with MDD, 61 patients with

Alzheimer's disease and multi-infarct dementia, and 44 healthy controls. As compared with controls, both the clinical groups had markedly greater prevalences of cortical atrophy, cortical infarction, gray matter lacunae, and subcortical white matter HIs (MRI) or lucencies (CT). The MDD and dementia groups differed only in cortical atrophy scores, with less abnormality observed in MDD. The MDD group had slightly more subcortical white matter abnormalities than the dementia group despite the inclusion of many multi-infarct patients in the latter category.

Rabins *et al.* (1991) performed MRI in 21 elderly in-patients with MDD, 16 patients with Alzheimer's disease, and 14 normal controls. The MDD patients differed from controls in basal ganglia HIs and DWMH, and tended to differ in PVH. Alzheimer's disease patients differed from controls in DWMH, and only tended to differ in basal ganglia HIs and PVH. A similar but larger study was conducted by O'Brien *et al.* (1996); DWMH and PVH were examined in 60 patients with MDD, 61 patients with Alzheimer's disease, and 39 control participants. After controlling for vascular risk factors and blood pressure, DWMH were found to be more severe in the MDD group, while PVH were more severe in the Alzheimer's group. Ebmeier *et al.* (1997) compared 13 patients with early-onset MDD, 11 patients with late-onset MDD, and 20 patients with Alzheimer's disease. There were no significant differences among the groups in the ratings of DWMH or PVH, although severity ratings tended to be higher in the late-relative to the early-onset MDD patients.

Encephalomalacia and Depression: Clinical Correlates

Information is beginning to accumulate on the clinical and historical features of depressive illness with associated encephalomalacia. For example, Coffey *et al.* (1988, 1989, 1990, 1991 and 1993) suggested that medication-resistant patients with late-onset MDD (onset >60 years) are at an increased risk for encephalomalacia. The patients were consecutive referrals to an ECT service and were unusual in two respects: 80 per cent had late-onset depression, and 86 per cent were said to be medication-resistant (Coffey *et al.*, 1988). However, the criteria for medication resistance were not consistent with accepted standards (Keller *et al.*, 1986; Sackeim *et al*., 1990a; Prudic *et al*., 1996;), and included medication-intolerant patients. In the sections that follow, encephalomalacia is examined in various clinical contexts.

Age at Onset

A substantial number of studies have found an association between encephalomalacia and age at onset of illness. Lesser *et al*. (1991) reported an excess of large DWMH in patients with late-onset psychotic depression as compared with normal controls. Figiel *et al*. (1991b) found that a higher rate of caudate HI and large DWMH distinguished late-onset from early-onset MDD in a small sample of patients with unipolar depression. In relatively small samples of elderly MDD patients and controls with a similar frequency of CVD risk factors, Krishnan *et al*. (1993) found that late-onset illness was associated with smaller volumes of the caudate and lenticular nuclei, and greater frequency and severity of DWMH. In a subsequent study, Krishnan *et al*. (1997) studied 32 elderly MDD Patients with encephalomalacia and 57 MDD patients without encephalomalacia. Controlling for age, the group characterized by MRI abnormalities had later age at onset, and tended to have a lower rate of positive family history of mood disorder.

Fujiwaka *et al*. (1993 and 1994) found a higher rate of 'silent cerebral infarctions' in late-compared to early-onset MDD. Patients with these large HIs also had a lower rate of family history of mood disorder. Hickie *et al*. (1995) found that late age at onset and negative family history of mood disorder were associated with more severe DWMH. Lesser *et al*. (1996) found that independent of current age, patients with late-onset (>35 years) MDD had larger areas of white matter HIs than patients with early-onset recurrent MDD. Salloway *et al*. (1996) compared 15 patients with late-onset (>60 years) MDD to 15 patients with early-onset MDD using semi-automated measures of DWMH and PVH area. A marked difference was observed, with the late-onset group having twice as much of subcortical HIs as the early-onset group. O'Brein *et al*. (1996) reported that severe DWMH were most common in in-patients with late-onset MDD. Dahabra *et al*. (1998) compared small groups of early- and late-onset elderly patients who had recovered from an episode of MDD. White matter HIs were more common in the late-onset group, as was ventricular enlargement.

Thus, a large number of independent investigations have found higher prevalence and/or greater severity of encephalomalacia in late- relative to early-onset depression. Few studies have yielded negative results (Dupont *et al.*, 1995a; Greenwald *et al.*, 1996; Iidaka *et al.*, 1996; Ebmeier *et al.*, 1997). There is also a suggestion, less consistently observed, that MDD patients with these MRI abnormalities are less likely to have a positive family history of mood disorder.

In an unpublished pilot study, we performed MRI in 30 consecutive in-patients participating in ECT research, with heavy T_2-weighting (Phillips 1.5T, TR 3500, TE 80 in the transaxial plane, 6.5 mm width, 1.5 mm gap, covering total cerebrum). T_1-weighted scans (TR 700, TE 34, coronal plane) were also obtained. A heavily T_2-weighted sequence was chosen for greater sensitivity to subtle water content abnormalities. The scans were blindly rated for DWMH and PVH using the visual anchors developed by Coffey *et al.* (1990) HIs in the basal ganglia, thalamus, and pons (or brain stem) and diffuse increases in background white matter signal intensity were also scored. The total sample (age $= 56.0 \pm 14.8$ years; 50 per cent female) had a high rate of encephalomalacia: 70 per cent had evidence of PVH and 70 per cent had DWMH. The frequency of HIs was 53.3 per cent in white matter underlying the cerebral cortex, 43.3 per cent in the basal ganglia, 43.3 per cent in the thalamus, and 50 per cent in the brainstem. A diffuse increase in background signal in the centrum semiovale was noted in 80 per cent of subjects. The absence of matched controls limited interpretation; nonetheless, the high rate of HIs in subcortical gray matter structures was striking. Coffey *et al.* (1990 and 1993) found that only 5 per cent of normal controls had basal ganglia or thalamic HIs. Therefore, our findings may be particularly consequential since neurological illness and insult were rigorously excluded.

Other findings in our study were that abnormalities in the deep gray structures covaried with ratings of white matter HIs, for example, basal ganglia abnormality covaried with PVH ($p < .02$). There were no sex difference. Age was associated with an increased likelihood of encephalomalacia (PVH: $p < .005$; basal ganglia: $p < .05$). We also observed high rates of diffuse T_2 signal increase in the centrum semiovale; this could suggest a generalized abnormality of the white matter, and such findings have been associated with white matter pallor or edema at autopsy.

To focus on an elderly sample, we examined the findings in 21 patients (age >50 years), and divided this group into early- (<50 years) and late-onset (>50 years) categories. As seen in Fig. 4.3, late-onset patients (n=12, age=64.2±7.5 years) tended to differ from early-onset patients (n=9, age=63.2±11.1 years) in rates of basal ganglia and thalamic HIs, and differed significantly in DWMH ($p<.05$). This preliminary study thus confirmed a high rate of white matter and subcortical gray matter MRI signal abnormalities in severely depressed in-patients, and demonstrated an association between specific abnormalities and age at onset of mood disorder.

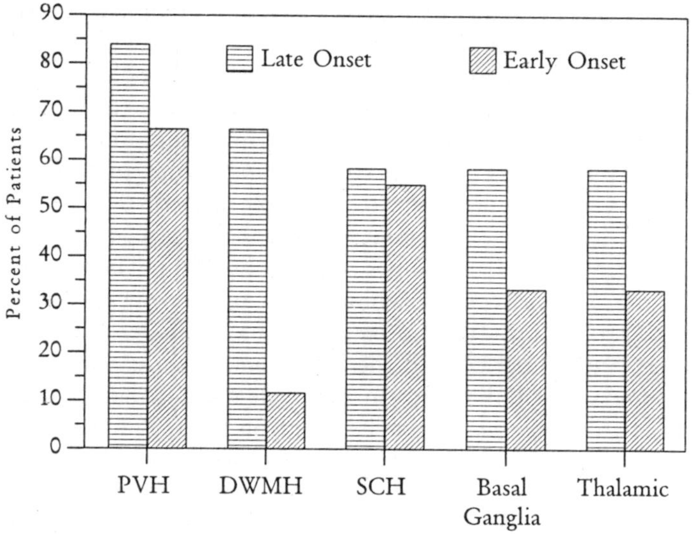

Fig. 4.3: A pilot study of MRI hyperintensities at the New York State Psychiatric Institute. Compared to elderly patients with early-onset Major Depression, patients with late-onset illness had a significantly higher rate of hyperintensity in the basal ganglia and thalamus, and tended to have a higher rate in the deep white matter. (SCH=subcortical hyperintensity).

Severity and Nature of Depressive Symptoms

With the exception of the study of Lesser *et al.* (1994), the MRI research has in general focused on in-patients with severe symptoms, often those who had been referred for ECT. Generalizability to the far more common cases of out-patient MDD therefore remains to be established, particularly since symptom severity has not shown association with encephalomalacia. There is no consistent indication of a difference in the rates or severity of encephalomalacia in psychotic and nonpsychotic depression. Indeed, Krishnan *et al.* (1997) reported that patients with encephalomalacia were less likely to have psychotic symptoms, but more likely to present with anhedonia. Phenomenological differences as a function of encephalomalacia have rarely been examined.

Treatment Response and Long-Term Outcome

The relationship of encephalomalacia to short-term treatment outcome is little studied. Even less is known about the predictive value of encephalomalacia for long-term clinical course. Coffey *et al.* (1989 and 1990) suggested that patients with encephalomalacia show positive response to ECT; however, ratings of improvement were obtained retrospectively and globally. In contrast, Hickie *et al.* (1995) reported that the greater severity of DWMH predicted poorer outcome with either heterogeneous pharmacological regimens or ECT. In a retrospective study, Fujikawa *et al.* (1996) reported that MDD patients with severe, silent cerebral infarction (in both perforating and cortical areas) had longer hospital stay and poorer response to antidepressant pharmacotherapy than MDD patients without infarction. In a study of 44 MDD patients aged 65–85 years, Simpson *et al.* (1997) found that globally-assessed short-term clinical outcome was poorer in patients with DWMH and HIs in the basal ganglia or pons. To date, there has been no prospective evaluation of the prognostic significance of these structural abnormalities using a standardized pharmacological protocol. The available evidence is consistent, however, in suggesting that encephalomalacia is associated with poorer short-term response to antidepressant treatments.

In a sample of 37 patients followed-up for an average of 14 months, Hickie *et al.* (1997) provided the first evidence that DWMH in MDD may predict poor long-term outcome. DWMH, late age of onset, and CVD risk factors were linked to chronic depression and cognitive decline, with a subgroup of patients developing a vascular dementia. The link between poor outcome and encephalomalacia was supported by another recent study:

O'Brien *et al.* (1998) followed-up 60 MDD patients aged over 55 years for an average of 32 months. The outcome measure was time to relapse into depression, or the occurrence of cognitive decline. Patients with severe white matter HIs at baseline had a median survival time of only 136 days, in contrast to 315 days in those without severe HIs. In the light of the recurrent and often chronic nature of MDD, and given the evidence that depressive symptoms in the elderly may be prodromal to dementing conditions, further investigation of the prognostic significance of encephalomalacia is clearly needed.

Adverse Effects

There is some evidence that elderly MDD patients with basal ganglia HIs may be prone to develop delirium when treated with antidepressant medications (Figiel *et al.*, 1989) or ECT (Figiel *et al.*, 1990a and b). However, these reports were based on small samples, did not examine the specificity of the basal ganglia HIs, and did not examine the relationship between other types of encephalomalacia and adverse effects. The link between basal ganglia HIs and ECT-induced delirium is compatible with the clinical observation that patients with basal ganglia disorders such as Parkinson's disease are more prone to prolonged confusional states when treated with ECT (Kellner *et al.*, 1994; Fall *et al.*, 1995).

Fujikawa *et al.* (1996) retrospectively assessed the role of silent cerebral infarction on response to and adverse effects with pharmacotherapy in MDD patients aged over 50 years. Patients with silent infarction had a higher incidence of treatment-related CNS adverse effects than those without infarction. The frequency of adverse effects increased with the severity of infarction.

Cognition and Neurological Signs

In normal subjects, it is unclear whether the limited encephalomalacia observed is associated with cognitive impairment (George *et al.*, 1986; Steingart *et at.* 1987; Rao *et al.*, 1989; Mirsen *et al.*, 1991; Schmidt *et al.*, 1993). There may be threshold effects for cognitive impairments associated with HI volume (Boone *et al.*, 1992). Nonetheless, in normal and neurological samples there is a concentration of replicated findings associating encephalomalacia with deficits in attention and motor speed (Gupta *et al.*, 1988; Junque *et al.*, 1990; van Swieten *et al.*, 1991a; Almkvist *et al.*, 1992; Matsubayashi *et al.*, 1992; Schmidt *et al.*, 1993; Ylikoski *et al.*, 1993; Abe *et al.*, 1994; Breteler *et al.*, 1994b; Fukui *et al.*, 1994; Baloh *et al.*, 1995; Longstreth *et al.*, 1996). These are hallmark areas of abnormality in geriatric depression (Sackeim and Steif, 1988; Zakzanis *et al.*, 1998). In nonpsychiatric patient samples, the most common neurological abnormalities associated with encephalomalacia are gait disturbances (George *et al.*, 1986; Steingart *et al.*, 1987; Hendrie *et al.*, 1989; Baloh *et al.*, 1995), tendency to fall (Masdeu *et al.*, 1989; Baloh *et al.*, 1995), extensor plantar reflex (Steingart *et al.*, 1987; Cadelo *et al.*, 1991), and primitive reflexes (Steingart *et al.*, 1987; Junque *et al.*, 1990; Cadelo *et al.*, 1991).

Despite these findings in normal and neurological samples, there has been limited investigation of the neuropsychological correlates of encephalomalacia in MDD. Ebmeier *et al.* (1997) found that severity of DWMH was inversely related to global cognitive function (Mini-Mental State scores) in elderly patients with MDD. In the most comprehensive study to date, Lesser *et al.* (1996) contrasted 60 late-onset (>50 years) MDD patients , 35 early-onset (<35 years) MDD patients, and 165 normal controls. All subjects were at least 50 years of age. The late-onset group had greater DWMH than either of the other groups. Cognitive deficits were most marked in the late-onset group, and pertained to non-verbal intelligence, non-verbal memory, constructional ability, executive function, and speed of processing. Patients with more severe DWMH had significantly poorer scores on tests of executive function.

Simpson *et al.* (1997) conducted neuropsychological assessments following the treatment of an elderly MDD sample. HIs in the pons were associated with reduced psychomotor speed; basal ganglia HIs were linked to impaired category productivity; and, PVH were associated with recall deficits. Since the severity of encephalomalacia in this study was also associated with clinical outcome, the findings regarding the neuropsychological correlates may have been confounded with the clinical state. Jenkins *et al.* (1998) used the California Verbal Learning Test to compare 12 elderly MDD patients with moderate to severe PVH and 12 matched MDD patients without encephalomalacia. The patients with PVH showed poorer performance as compared with control patients on a number of learning and memory indices, with the pattern of deficits resembling that in subcortical degenerative disorders (Huntington's and Parkinson's diseases). Clearly, there is a need for comprehensive neuropsychological and neurological evaluations of elderly MDD patients in relation to the structural and functional imaging deficits.

AETIOLOGY OF ENCEPHALOMALACIA

Neuropathology: Links with Cerebrovascular Disease

The pathogenesis of the MRI abnormalities in MDD is unknown. In other samples, these abnormalities have usually been attributed to ischaemic CVD, with the HIs reflecting increased water content in perivascular space, axon and myelin loss, astrocyte proliferation (gliosis), and/or frank infarction (Caplan and Schoene, 1978; Awad *et al.*, 1986c; Janota *et al.*, 1989; van Swieten *et al.*, 1991b; Chimowitz *et al.*, 1992; Boiten *et al.*, 1993; Pantoni and Garcia, 1995). Typically, the HIs occur in watershed areas supplied by small arterioles that branch off long penetrating medullary and lenticulostriate arteries. These areas receive limited collateral supply and are particularly vulnerable to vascular insult (De Reuck, 1971). In all the populations studied, including MDD patients and normal controls, age has been the most critical correlate (Awad *et al.*, 1987; Schmidt *et al.*, 1992; Christiansen *et al.*, 1994; Manolio *et al.*, 1994; Jorgensen *et al.*, 1995; Lesser *et al.*, 1996). To a lesser extent, these abnormalities are also associated with hypertension, diabetes, coronary heart disease, or other vascular risk factors (Gerard and Weisberg, 1986; Awad *et al.*, 1986a and 1987; Fazekas *et al.*, 1988; Krishnan *et al.*, 1988; Lechner *et al.*, 1988; Coffey *et al.*, 1989; Cadelo *et al.*, 1991; Breteler *et al.*, 1994a; Lindgren *et al.*, 1994; Manolio *et al.*, 1994; Howard *et al.*, 1995; Henon *et al.*, 1996; Longstreth *et al.*, 1996).

In a CT scan study of patients with Alzheimer's disease, frank CVD at 1-year follow-up was observed only in patients with baseline white matter lucencies (Lopez *et al.*, 1992). In 215 patients with lacunar infarction, a prospective 3-year follow-up indicated that baseline encephalomalacia predicted subsequent stroke, new-onset dementia, and death (Miyao *et al.*, 1992). Several other recent studies indicate that encephalomalacia predicts subsequent stroke, myocardial infarction, and vascular death (van Swieten *et al.*, 1992; Inzitari *et al.*, 1995; Tarvonen-Schroder *et al.*, 1995). Boiten *et al.* (1993) found a considerably higher rate of encephalomalacia in patients with asymptomatic lacunar infarcts than in patients with symptomatic lacunar infarcts (odds ratio = 10.7). These groups differed in the location and implicated vascular territories of the infarcts, with the suggestion offered that ischaemia due to arteriosclerosis leads to encephalomalacia and silent lacunar infarcts, while microatheromatosis more commonly produces symptomatic lacunar infarcts. Tohgi *et al.* (1991) reported greater 24-hour variability in blood pressure among patients with HIs, suggesting periodic ischaemic compromise.

Induction of similar T_2-weighted abnormalities in animals is now done by MCA occlusion (Gill *et al.*, 1995). Awad *et al.* (1993) reported the first prospective *de novo* appearance of DWMH in humans. Despite full anticoagulation, 4 of 8 patients undergoing therapeutic ICA occlusion (detachable balloon technique) developed ipsilateral subcortical HIs. This large array of findings supports a vascular aetiology of encephalomalacia. The Awad *et al.* (1986c) suggestion of *état criblé* is also compatible; pulsation in ectatic or tortuous blood vessels that are rigidified by sclerosis may mechanically increase water-filled perivascular space, or occasion the same results with parenchymal atrophy due to ischaemic substrate supply. Some types of PVH may be due to CSF leakage into the surrounding tissue (Hachinski *et al.*, 1987). Caps at the horns of the lateral ventricles are common in normals, may not be age-related, and may be due to interstitial flow into ventricles, combined with low myelin content and ependymitis granularis (Fazekas *et al.*, 1993). Therefore, including 'caps' in encephalomalacia ratings can lead to high false positive rates.

There has been considerable histopathological investigation of HIs, but not in MDD. The findings generally support a vascular aetiology, as areas of MRI HIs in neurological and normal samples commonly show arteriolar hyalinization, ectasia, enlarged perivascular (Virchow-Robin) space, gliosis, spongiosis, and/or lacunar infarcts (Awad *et al.*, 1986c; George *et al.*, 1986; Kirkpatrick and Hayman, 1987; Braffman *et al.*, 1988; Marshall *et al.*, 1988; Janota *et al.*, 1989; Grafton *et al.*, 1991; Tabaton *et al.*, 1991; Chimowitz *et al.*, 1992; Munoz *et al.*, 1993). Van Swieten *et al.* (1991b) found that DWMH were invariably accompanied by demyelination and gliosis, and less consistently with increased perivascular space. The demyelination was strongly associated with increased wall thickness of small arterioles. Van Swieten *et al.* therefore concluded that arteriosclerosis in small arterioles (<150 um) is the primary cause of DWMH, leading to demyelination, and then cell loss with progression. Munoz *et al.* (1993) suggested that some pathological changes could also be due to microaneurysms at the points of arteriole bifurcation, resulting in leakage of serum proteins (edema). Fazekas *et al.* (1993) observed that the size and appearance of MRI-defined PVH and DWMH were strongly associated with the extent of ischaemic tissue damage. Moody *et al.* (1995) recently reported the novel findings that venous collagenosis is strongly associated with encephalomalacia. They found marked thickening of periventricular post-capillary venules and collecting veins that provide drainage of the centrum semiovale, and suggested that disordered venous drainage results in distal chronic ischaemia and brain edema.

The initial magnetic resonance spectroscopy studies have been inconsistent, but there are suggestions of altered metabolite concentrations (reduced aspartate and creatine, elevated lactate) in the HIs, indicating disturbed metabolic processes (Sappey-Marinier *et al.*, 1992; Confort-Gouny *et al.*, 1993; Oppenheimer *et al.*, 1995). In the elderly depressed, autopsy refusal and the relatively low mortality rate limit prospective neuropathological investigation. However, the hypothesis that encephalomalacia in MDD is due to impaired blood flow (vascular insufficiency) in subcortical watershed areas can be tested with *in vivo* perfusion imaging. Positron Emission Tomography (PET) and Single Photon Emission Computed Tomography (SPECT) studies in stroke samples have consistently shown correspondence between the identified areas of hypoperfusion and the structural abnormalities identified by CT, MRI, or neuropathology. The spatial extent of the perfusion deficit is typically larger than the areas of tissue necrosis defined by pathology or structural imaging (Baron *et al.*, 1986; Perani *et al.*, 1988; Seiderer *et al.*, 1989; Sette *et al.*, 1989), and remote functional changes (diaschisis) may be observed (Pappata *et al.*, 1990; Andrews, 1991). This indicates that effects of punctate lesions, smaller in size than the spatial resolution of state-of-the-art PET (~4 mm FWHM), should be observable due to their association with a larger area of functional deficit. The conventional view is that punctate ischaemic lesions, having exceeded a cerebral blood flow (CBF) threshold for infarction, are often surrounded by a penumbra of above threshold but nonetheless compromised CBF (Tamura *et al.*, 1981; Gill *et al.*, 1995).

Pathophysiology of Encephalomalacia

No study has quantified regional cerebral blood flow (rCBF) or regional cerebral metabolic rate (rCMR) by co-registering functional and structural images, and quantifying perfusion and metabolism in the areas of asymptomatic, MRI-defined HIs. Our group is currently engaged in such research. In recent years, at least 20 studies have examined more general perfusion or metabolic abnormalities in subjects with encephalomalacia. These studies are briefly examined.

One study used the ^{133}Xe lateral projection technique to quantify cortical CBF in normal subjects categorized by MRI HIs (Fazekas *et al.*, 1988; Fazekas, 1989). Reduced global CBF, particularly in the slow compartment (white matter), was seen in asymptomatic subjects with DWMH. In the same subjects, using visual inspection of PET images, reductions in cerebral metabolic rate for glucose (CMR_{glu}) were not observed in cortical areas neighbouring MRI HIs. Kobayashi *et al.* (1991) found that DWMH were associated with reduced global cortical gray matter CBF in 246 neurologically healthy adults, as did Isaka *et al.* (1993) in 47 asymptomatic elderly. Using stable xenon CT, Kobari *et al.* (1990) found that cerebral atrophy ratings, age, and subcortical white matter CBF were each associated with CT lucencies in normal subjects. Also using stable xenon CT, Kawamura *et al.* (1991) found reduced CBF to be related to encephalomalacia in multi-infarct dementia, with low CBF in the putamen and thalamus being predictive of CT subcortical frontal lucencies.

Herholz *et al.* (1990), using PET, found that severe DWMH were associated with diffuse cortical CBF reductions in patients with internal carotid arteriosclerotic disease. Meguro *et al.* (1990) used the ^{15}O-PET steady-state method to quantify rCBF, regional cerebral metabolic rate for oxygen ($rCMRO_2$), regional oxygen extraction fraction (rOEF), and regional cerebral blood volume (rCBV) in 28 asymptomatic individuals with CVD risk factors. More severe PVH were associated with global reductions in gray matter CBF and in the CBF/CBV ratio, with the latter parameter being free of partial volume effects. In contrast, OEF tended to increase with severe PVH, while there was only a trend for reduced global $CMRO_2$ with increasing PVH. These effects were consistent across gray matter regions and suggested a compensatory mismatch between metabolism and CBF ('misery perfusion'): as CBF declined, OEF increased to maintain metabolic rate. De Reuck *et al.* (1992), also using the ^{15}O-PET steady-state method, reported similar findings: white matter CT lucencies were associated with lowered CBF in frontal and parietal gray and white matter, in both demented and normal subjects; particularly in the frontal white matter, encephalomalacia was associated with increased OEF, and with greater reductions in rCBF than in $rCMRO_2$.

Yao *et al.* (1992) confirmed the pattern of decreased perfusion and increased OEF in individuals with marked encephalomalacia. Matsushita *et al.* (1994) used intracerebral cannulation (AV O_2 difference) and stepwise manipulated blood pressure in 51 hypertensive patients with lacunar infarcts. Whole brain cerebrovascular resistance was greater and CBF autoregulation was impaired in patients with severe PVH, while $CMRO_2$ was preserved. Similarly, Hatazawa *et al.* (1997) compared 8 normal subjects without encephalomalacia and 15 asymptomatic individuals with white matter HIs, using $H_2{}^{15}O$, $C^{15}O$, and $^{15}O_2$ PET. White matter HIs were associated with reduced CBF and increased OEF in the cerebral white matter and basal ganglia, without effects in the thalamus.

Waldemar *et al.* (1994) studied 18 patients with Alzheimer's disease using both ^{133}Xe and HMPAO SPECT. They found that severity of PVH, severity of DWMH, and volume of DWMH were significantly and negatively correlated with global CBF, CBF in various cortical regions, and CBF in central white matter. There were particularly strong (inverse) correlations between DWMH volume and CBF in central white matter ($r=-0.56$) and the hippocampus ($r=-0.72$). The diffuse nature of the association between DWMH and CBF deficits suggested that deafferentation of cortical regions by subcortical HIs (diaschisis) did not play a role in producing the characteristic temporoparietal CBF and CMR deficits in Alzheimer's disease (Sackeim *et al.*, 1993). Rather, the HIs appeared to be associated with a more global ischaemic process.

In the only similar study on MDD, Lesser *et al.* (1994) reported a trend for patients with large areas of white matter HI to have the greatest deficits in whole brain CBF. Of note, in this elderly sample (age $>$ 60 years) whole brain CBF was markedly diminished across the MDD group, and the subgroup with HIs had the largest deficit.

Oppenheimer *et al.* (1995), using gadolinium-DPTA perfusion imaging with fMRI, found evidence that areas of asymptomatic HI often show marked deficits in rCBV. They hypothesized that this abnormality results from decompensation in these delimited areas, where vasodilation is not able to compensate for reduced rCBF; there is a consequent reduction in rCBV and, ultimately, necrosis. A negative study was, however, reported by Claus *et al.* (1996), who examined encephalomalacia in a sample of 60 community elders studied with HMPAO SPECT: individuals with and without white matter HIs did not differ in CBF indices. In contrast, Miyazawa *et al.* (1997) assessed CBF in the centrum semiovale in 135 normal subjects who differed in severity of DWMH. Severity of white matter HIs was associated with age and hypertension. There was a strong inverse relation between the severity of DWMH and CBF, even when controlled for age.

Promoting vasodilation through the use of a hypercapnic challenge may be a particularly useful method to investigate the pathophysiology of encephalomalacia. Brown *et al.* (1990) used stable xenon CT and showed that in comparison with controls, CVD patients with encephalomalacia had diminished white matter CBF response to acetazolamide. In 28 asymptomatic subjects, Isaka *et al.* (1993) found that the extent of PVH was marginally (inversely) related to global gray matter resting CBF ($r = -0.36$), but strongly (inversely) related to global CBF after hypercapnic challenge with acetazolamide ($r = -0.78$) as well as to the CBF change between rest and hypercapnia ($r = -0.57$). This study linked PVH in asymptomatic individuals to a diffuse reduction in cerebrovascular dilatory capacity (i.e., hemodynamic reserve), suggesting that small vessel disease may characterize not only the territories of the subcortical HIs, but may be widespread in the cortical gray matter. In a study using HMPAO SPECT in patients with unilateral carotid occlusive disease, severity of DWMH and PVH was linked to perfusion deficits at rest, with the associations being magnified following acetazolamide (hypercapnic) challenge (Isaka *et al.*, 1997).

Thus, virtually all of these 20 studies conducted in diverse populations (with only one in MDD) found relationships between white matter abnormalities and measures of perfusion. While CBF deficits in white matter were common, diffuse cortical gray matter deficits were also observed. The findings consistently linked encephalomalacia to low CBF and increased OEF, suggesting that the relationships between the structural and functional deficits are more marked for perfusion than metabolism measures. This has been observed in work assessing both CBF and $CMRO_2$ or CMR_{glu}.

It is not known if a similar uncoupling occurs in geriatric depression. Indeed, it is almost invariably assumed that rCBF deficits in mood disorders reflect disturbed patterns of neuronal activity rather than a constrained vascular substrate. We hypothesize that this assumption is false in geriatric or late-onset depression, and that deficits are greater for global CBF than for global CMR. Further, the findings linking encephalomalacia to reduced CBF response to hypercapnia suggest that limited vasodilatory capacity may be an important correlate, and that structure/function relationships become magnified with hypercapnic (vasodilatory) challenge.

Longitudinal Perspective

Across populations, the cross-sectional studies have all indicated that the likelihood and severity of encephalomalacia increase with age. In addition, the possibility that encephalomalacia and perfusion deficits in MDD are progressive is suggested by the associations with CVD risk factors; by the follow-up results in neurologic samples which indicate increased rates of future CVD, functional compromise, and death as a function of baseline encephalomalacia; by the histopathological findings in areas containing HIs; and, by the hypothesis of an underlying ischaemic CVD. Several groups are conducting MRI studies examining change in encephalomalacia at long-term follow-up in patients with MDD. However, the only data reported to date were limited to an examination of MDD patients before, and 6 months after ECT (Coffey *et al.*, 1991). Blind ratings showed strong test-retest stability in HI evaluations, with the only change being a worsening of encephalomalacia in 4 patients; however, the follow-up interval was probably too short to observe more frequent MRI changes. In this context, perfusion imaging may provide more sensitive measures of progressive effects than MRI. If ischaemia in deep structures leads to encephalomalacia, it should exist prior to MRI evidence of structural deficits, and its quantification should be more sensitive to progressive change.

Perfusion and Metabolic Abnormalities in Major Depression

Our research and other studies described in this section have shown that many elderly patients with MDD have marked abnormalities in CBF. We used the ^{133}Xenon inhalation technique to quantify rCBF in medication-free, elderly depressed samples without a history of neurological illness or insult. Patients were studied prior to, during, and following ECT. A pretreatment comparison of resting studies in 41 patients with 40 matched controls revealed a global flow reduction of ~15 per cent in cortical CBF (Sackeim *et al.*, 1990a). This deficit was comparable to that seen in many forms of frank CVD, and was found to be equivalent to that in matched patients with Alzheimer's disease (Sackeim *et al.*, 1993). We applied a new method, the Scaled Subprofile Model (SSM) (Moeller *et al.*, 1987; Moeller and Strother, 1991; Alexander and Moeller, 1994), which is designed to reveal abnormal regional topographies (covariance patterns). We observed that the depressed group had marked abnormality in a specific cortical pattern, independent of the global CBF deficit (Sackeim *et al.*, 1990a and 1993). The abnormality in this pattern increased with both patients' age and symptom severity. Such CBF deficits need not reflect static or progressive CVD, but could be due to functional metabolic abnormalities associated with the depressed state. However, other related data sets suggest involvement of a CVD process.

First, in a recently completed study, we used hypercapnic challenge with the ^{133}Xenon inhalation method. Since CO_2 is a potent vasodilator, occlusive or ischaemic CVD is often revealed by hypercapnic hyporeactivity (Yamamoto *et al.*, 1980; Levine *et al.*, 1986; Tatemichi *et al.*, 1988; Vorstrup, 1988). In 25 MDD in-patients, 11 (44 per cent) showed global cortical hypercapnic hyporeactivity, indicating inadequate vasodilatory capacity. Hyporeactivity was associated with markedly reduced global CBF in the resting baseline state, with late onset of depression, with the presence of hypertension, and with poor clinical response to ECT. In a second group of 17 elderly MDD out-patients, we found that 29.4 per cent had global CBF hypercapnic hyporeactivity.

Second, in a large sample, we found that the specific rCBF abnormalities at resting baseline did not resolve with clinical recovery aftèr ECT but were stable (Nobler *et al.*, 1994). When assessed acutely (1 hour) and in the short-term (1 week) after ECT, there were further rCBF reductions, with responders showing the most marked decreases both globally and in a grouping of anterior cortical regions.

Third, in another pilot study, we treated 20 elderly out-patients with either nortriptyline or sertraline. Clinical response was similarly associated with reduced CBF in anterior cortical regions. Therefore, it would appear that the baseline deficits in resting rCBF observed in elderly patients with MDD contain a major trait (state-independent) component.

Our findings, suggesting marked global and topographic cortical deficits at baseline in elderly depressed patients, have been replicated in other studies of relatively elderly samples. Upadhyaya *et al.* (1990) assessed rCBF with HMPAO SPECT in 18 elderly (age >66 years) patients with MDD, 14 patients with Alzheimer's disease, and 12 normal controls. Global cortical CBF (normalized against cerebellum) was reduced in the MDD group, and deficits were most marked in frontal, temporal, and parietal regions. Kumar *et al.* (1993) reported that resting global CMR_{glu} was markedly reduced in a small sample (n=8) with late-life MDD, with the reduction being comparable to that in age-matched patients with Alzheimer's disease; the pattern of cortical regional abnormalities in the elderly MDD was also similar to our characterization (Sackeim *et al.*, 1990a and 1993).

Bench *et al.* (1993) conducted $C^{15}O_2$ PET studies at rest in 40 MDD patients (of whom half were medicated) and 23 controls. The sample was mixed in age, and the mean age was 57 years. The data analytic method, using Statistical Parametric Mapping (SPM), was insensitive to global effects, averaging over neural and non-neural (CSF) voxels, and the focus was on regional differences. The MDD group had CBF reductions in the dorsolateral prefrontal cortex, angular gyrus (inferior parietal lobule), and anterior cingulate gyrus. Curran *et al.* (1993) studied 20 medicated elderly MDD patients (mean age=70 years) with HMPAO SPECT. The quantification method (normalization against occipital cortex) also limited the capacity to observe global cortical effects. Depressed patients had reduced CBF in frontal, temporal, anterior cingulate, thalamus, and caudate regions. Of note, clinical outcome at 6–18 months was best in MDD patients with the least evidence of baseline CBF abnormalities. Lesser *et al.* (1994) compared 39 elderly, medication-free out-patients with mild to moderate MDD and 20 controls using both the ^{133}Xe technique for full CBF quantification and HMPAO SPECT to examine regional distribution. Whole brain CBF was 13.5 per cent less in MDD patients, although these patients were younger than controls. Late-onset patients had nonsignificantly lower global CBF than early-onset patients. There were marked deficits in frontal, temporal, and parietal regions.

There is now extensive literature on rCBF and rCMR baseline abnormalities in *younger* MDD samples as well. While the literature is not fully consistent (e.g., Drevets *et al.*, 1992; Biver *et al.*, 1994), there is a general agreement that MDD is accompanied by CBF and CMR reductions, most commonly in the prefrontal cortex (for reviews, *see* Sackeim and Prohovnik, 1993; Soares and Mann, 1997; Drevets, 1998). The findings of reduced global CBF and CMR, however, appear less commonly in younger than in older MDD samples. Indeed, Devous *et al.* (1993) reported differences between normal controls and MDD patients in the relationship between rCBF and age. The possibility of age-specificity was also underscored in a recent study that we reported on younger MDD, bipolar manic, and normal subjects (Rubin *et al.*, 1995). In line with the literature, the younger MDD patients had primarily anterior frontal cortical CBF deficits, without the global disturbance or the covarying reductions in the superior temporal and anterior parietal cortices that have been observed in older MDD patients. Consequently, there is reason to suspect that the magnitude of global CBF and CMR deficits increases among the depressed elderly.

At least 15 studies have reported inverse correlations between depressive symptom scores and frontal CBF or CMR (George *et al.*, 1994). In addition, studies in the context of Parkinson's disease, Huntington's chorea, and post-stroke have also implicated CBF/CMR deficits in the fronto-temporal cortex in secondary MDD (Mayberg *et al.*, 1990 and 1992; Ring *et al.*, 1994; Okada *et al.*, 1997). In primary mood disorder samples, subcortical disturbance has been less well studied, although there is some evidence of reduced functional activity in the basal ganglia and anterior cingulate (Baxter *et al.*, 1985; Buchsbaum *et al.*, 1986; Hagman *et al.*, 1990; Bench *et al.*, 1993).

There has yet to be a study using high resolution PET to characterize such perfusion or metabolic deficits in a large sample with late-onset MDD.

Effects of Treatment on Perfusion and Metabolic Abnormalities

Basic science research indicates that electroconvulsive shocks and most antidepressant medications have marked effects on capillary permeability, rCBF, and $rCMR_{glu}$; these indices are reduced in a regionally distributed manner (Gerber *et al.*, 1983; Caldecott-Hazard *et al.*, 1988). However, there is only limited information on the effects of antidepressant medication and clinical recovery on rCBF or rCMR in MDD, with virtually no information on geriatric depression (for review, *see* Drevets, 1998).

In a recent report, we identified seven brain imaging studies that reported results before and after treatment with antidepressants (Rubin *et al.*, 1994). Medication regimens and time-points of imaging were often heterogeneous within a study. The median sample size was 10 patients, suggesting a high risk of Type II error. Interpretations of changes related to clinical outcome must therefore be made with caution; nonetheless, the intuitive notion that baseline deficits reverse with successful antidepressant treatment was not supported in several instances. In one of the larger studies (n=20), Reischies *et al.* (1989) reported a trend for reduced CBF (^{133}Xe SPECT) in the prefrontal cortex following treatment with various antidepressant medications. Goodwin *et al.* (1993) used HMPAO SPECT to assess medication-free patients in depressed and euthymic states. Marked deficits in the frontal, temporal, and parietal cortices were observed during the depressed state, and there was no change during euthymia. Indeed, patients with more endogenous baseline symptoms later showed reduced CBF in the frontal regions. Clinical recovery was, however, associated with a bilateral increase in the anterior cingulate and putamen.

Baxter *et al.* (1985 and 1989) and Martinot *et al.* (1990) reported that a metabolic asymmetry in the dorsolateral prefrontal cortex reversed following antidepressant treatment, but both a global cortical reduction in CMR_{glu} and a pronounced reduction across the frontal cortex remained unaltered. Using the ^{133}Xe planar technique in a relatively elderly sample, Passero *et al.* (1995)

reported normalization in the left prefrontal CBF abnormalities, but no change in the right frontal deficits following 6 months of antidepressant treatment. In a recently completed study restricted to late-life MDD (onset >60 years), we used ^{133}Xe projection technique to compare responders and non-responders to nortriptyline or sertraline. Clinical response was associated with further reductions in frontal cortical CBF.

Surprisingly, there is more information on the effects of ECT on CBF and CMR than on the effects of antidepressant medications on these parameters. Both acutely and in the short-term, many studies report that ECT results in reductions of functional activity in anterior cortical regions (Silfverskiold *et al.*, 1986; Rosenberg *et al.*, 1988; Volkow *et al.*, 1988; for reviews, *see* Nobler and Sackeim, 1998 and Sackeim, 1999). Our work has indicated that greater reductions of this type, particularly in the anterior prefrontal regions, are associated with superior clinical outcome (Nobler *et al.*, 1994). Consequently, there is reason to suspect that some of the CBF/CMR abnormalities in MDD do not resolve with clinical response and reflect persistent deficits. In turn, this would suggest that functional imaging deficits at baseline partly reflect trait abnormalities, compatible with a CVD process. There is a clear need for high resolution imaging studies using prospective, standardized medication trials, concentrating on the patient population likely to manifest the most profound baseline deficits in CBF and CMR; that is, elderly patients with late-onset depression.

THEORETICAL INTEGRATION

The notion that CVD plays in important role in late-life MDD is not new (Gilarowsky, 1926; Post, 1962; Krishnan and McDonald, 1995). A recent suggestion has been that 'vascular depression' be included as an official subtype of MDD within the diagnostic nomenclature (Steffens and Krishnan, 1998). Considering these views and the literature that we have reviewed, we offer a comprehensive theory of the role of CVD in MDD. This theory is based on the evidence describing structural, vascular, and metabolic abnormalities in MDD, and includes specific, testable hypotheses. Our essential argument is that many elderly patients with MDD, particularly those with late-onset illness, have a diffuse vascular insufficiency syndrome which leads to both encephalomalacia and depression.

According to this argument and the available evidence, the HIs in subcortical gray and deep white matter result from an ischaemic process linked to arteriosclerosis and hypertension, and develop in watershed vascular territories which have high intrinsic vulnerability due to poor collateral supply (De Reuck, 1971). More generalized CBF deficits are also present. At first, such global deficits are more demonstrable in CBF than CMR because compensatory changes maintain the metabolic rate despite decreased perfusion; this phenomenon of 'misery perfusion' occurs in occlusive CVD (Sette *et al.*, 1989) and has been observed in PET studies of encephalomalacia (Meguro *et al.*, 1990; De Reuck *et al.*, 1992; Yao *et al.*, 1992). The compensatory changes initially involve increased CBV and OEF. With further CBF reduction, compensation is inadequate, and global CMR reductions are observed.

CO_2 or acetazolamide challenge provides a stronger test of vascular insufficiency than does the measurement of resting CBF; diminished CBF reactivity to hypercapnia indicates an inadequate hemodynamic reserve due to limited perfusion pressure, maximal vasodilation, or tissue infarction (Kanno *et al.*, 1988). Such vascular insufficiency would be expected in multi-infarct dementia but not in Alzheimer's disease, and compatible hypercapnic results have indeed been reported (Tachibana *et al.*, 1984). If tied to an underlying persistent CVD process, hyporeactivity to hypercapnia in late-onset MDD should not reverse with clinical response; rather, if the vascular insufficiency syndrome is progressive, global resting as well as hypercapnic CBF deficits should worsen at long-term follow-up. Consequently, it might be expected that encephalomalacia and the course of depression may both worsen with time; indeed, the presence of encephalomalacia has been suggested to predict poorer long-term prognosis (Hickie *et al.*, 1997; O'Brien *et al.*, 1998).

The mechanism whereby vascular insufficiency leads to MDD is unknown. A common hypothesis, based on the encephalomalacia findings, emphasizes deafferentation (Brown, 1993; Krishnan, 1993; Krishnan and McDonald, 1995; Alexopoulos *et al.*, 1997). Thus the pathophysiology of late-onset MDD may in many ways be similar to that of Binswanger's disease. Consider: MRI HIs are the key to the diagnosis of Binswanger's disease; the condition is associated with an excess of CVD risk factors, and is attributed to hypoperfusion in subcortical watershed areas; and, in the early stages, Binswanger's disease is characterized by blunted affect, poor concentration, slowness, and a diminished learning rate, all of which are commonly observed in MDD (Caplan and Schoene, 1978; Kinkel *et al.*, 1985; Roman, 1987; Gupta *et al.*, 1988; Boone *et al.*, 1992; Pantoni and Garcia, 1995). The dementia of Binswanger's disease is often thought to be due to a cortical disconnection syndrome resulting from the subcortical lesions. Whether or not MDD is associated with such a type of subcortical disconnection or deafferentation pathology may be contingent on the anatomic specificity to white matter tracts and gray matter nuclei involved.

Anatomic specificity in the relationship between location of abnormalities and risk for depression is suggested by the high rate of basal ganglia and thalamic HIs in MDD; some imaging studies in MDD have also observed reduced metabolism in the basal ganglia (Baxter *et al.*, 1985 and 1989; Buchsbaum *et al.*, 1986; Hagman *et al.*, 1990; Bench *et al.*, 1993) and reduced caudate volume (Krishnan *et al.*, 1992 and 1993). It is noteworthy that textbook diseases of the basal ganglia (Parkinson's disease, Huntington's disease) carry an elevated risk for the development of MDD (Cummings, 1993), and that depressed Parkinson's patients, like elderly patients with MDD, have prominent reductions in frontal CBF and CMR (Mayberg *et al.*, 1990; Ring *et al.*, 1994). There is also evidence from stroke patients that basal ganglia infarcts are more likely to be associated with depression than thalamic infarcts (Starkstein *et al.*, 1988).

Anatomical specificity is also suggested by the frontal location of the cortical CBF and CMR deficits in MDD; these may explain why the white matter HIs in MDD have a more frontal distribution than those in normal controls. Such an association of frontal abnormalities with depression is supported by several strands of evidence: post-stroke depression is more common with large anterior PVH than with large posterior PVH (Bokura *et al.*, 1994), depressive symptoms in patients with Alzheimer's disease are associated with HIs in frontal white matter (Lopez *et al.*, 1997), frontal predominance of DWMH exists in primary mood disorders (Figiel *et al.*, 1991a; Krishnan *et al.*, 1993; Aylward *et al.*, 1994; Dupont *et al.*, 1995b; Greenwald *et al.*, 1998) and T_1

relaxation values are increased specifically in frontal white matter in patients with depression (Dolan *et al.*, 1990).

In view of this evidence, precise detailing of the anatomic distribution of MRI abnormalities in MDD is necessary, and the location of such abnormalities should be examined in relation to abnormal patterns of subcortical and cortical rCBF and rCMR.

Returning to the theme of deafferentation, disruption of specific subcortical nuclei or their ascending pathways (e.g., the thalamo-corticostriatal tract) may result in persistent, topographically distributed CBF and CMR deficits that give rise to some depressive manifestations. For example, medical dorsal thalamic and medical pulvinar/lateral posterior thalamic nuclei modulate activity in the anterior and posterior portions (respectively) of the prefrontal-parietal network (Trojanowski and Jacobson, 1976; Mesulam *et al.*, 1983); in our research, abnormalities were evident in these areas in patients with MDD. Establishing such localization may suggest a final common pathway for various expressions of MDD, independent of aetiology. In this connection, the phenomenon of deafferentation resulting in distal metabolic suppression (wherein coupling between CBF and CMR is maintained) has been often observed with subcortical lacunar infarcts (Sette *et al.*, 1989; Pappata *et al.*, 1990).

Our theory therefore suggests that the global disturbances in CBF and CMR originate from diffuse vascular insufficiency, while the cortical topographic effects may at least partly reflect secondary metabolic dysregulation due to deafferentation. Combined assessment of encephalomalacia, rCBF under rest and hypercapnic challenge conditions, and resting $rCMR_{glu}$ would allow for rigorous tests of this and of alternative hypotheses. As in prior research on non-MDD samples, we expect that the severity of encephalomalacia in MDD, largely independent of location, will be linked to global CBF deficits in gray and white matter. These effects will strengthen with hypercapnic challenge, and will be less prominent in measures of global CMR.

An alternate interpretation of the research that we have reviewed is that the global cortical reductions in functional activity in elderly patients with MDD are not due to a generalized vascular insufficiency, but are instead metabolic in origin and reflect primary dysfunction in subcortical nuclei with widespread cortical projection. Indeed, in our own pilot work we found evidence that thalamic HIs in MDD are associated with reduced global cortical gray matter CBF (unpublished observation). Similarly, it is possible that lesions in the pons disrupt ascending monoamine systems with widespread subcortical and cortical projection (Krishnan, 1993). However, were such an alternate deafferentation account true, one would expect tight coupling between global CBF and CMR deficits, with both linked to specific anatomic distributions of encephalomalacia. Further, the CBF response to hypercapnia would be preserved, and the relationship between global CBF deficits and encephalomalacia would not be expected to strengthen with hypercapnia.

In contrast to our view regarding the global CBF deficits, we hypothesize that the regional cortical CBF profile reflects metabolic dysregulation. In support of this view, in our first report detailing the cortical topographic deficit we noted that its distribution did not conform to the major cerebral arteries, making a primary vascular origin unlikely, at least with regard to major vessel disease (Sackeim *et al.*, 1990b). An alternate view is that the cortical topographic deficit could reflect distributed dilatory incapacity in small vessels. However, were this the case, one would expect that manifestation of the CBF topographic deficit would accentuate under conditions promoting generalized vasodilatation. Regions with normal dilatory capacity would show normal CBF response to hypercapnia, and regions within the baseline topographic disturbance would show a blunted response. Instead, in our recently completed study of hypercapnia in MDD, we found no change in the degree of manifestation of abnormal MDD cortical topography between states of rest and hypercapnia; there was a high correlation of 0.71 in measurements of the specific topographic deficit between the two states. These data support the view that the regional deficit primarily reflects abnormal metabolic demand.

In short, there is now considerable evidence implicating abnormal cerebrovascular and metabolic processes in MDD. The evidence to date is compatible with our theory that a substantial proportion of the baseline CBF and CMR deficits in late-onset MDD reflect trait disturbances that fail to normalize with clinical recovery. Longitudinal examination of both the structural and functional deficits, relating progression to clinical course, is the research strategy that will best address key questions in this field.

Significance of Encephalomalacia

Progressive CVD is not likely to account for all cases of geriatric or, specifically, late-onset MDD. Further, in some patients it is likely that CVD manifestations are coincidental. It is also conceptually possible that some structural and functional abnormalities *result* from depressive illness or its treatment, rather than precede MDD expression. Nonetheless, the evidence implicating disturbed vascular processes in many patients with late-onset MDD is substantial. We believe that steps to evaluate the relevance of these deficits to the pathophysiology and aetiology of MDD should first address the relationship between the structural and functional abnormalities, and next examine whether these deficits are progressive in a subgroup of elderly patients with late-onset MDD.

At the clinical level, it has been suggested that encephalomalacia predicts poorer outcome and greater sensitivity to side effects with antidepressant treatment (Figiel *et al.*, 1989 and 1990a and b; Hickie *et al.*, 1995; Fujikawa *et al.*, 1996). These important claims have never been tested with a rigorous, standardized treatment protocol. It has also been suggested that patients with encephalomalacia have a poorer long-term prognosis (Hickie *et al.*, 1997; O'Brien *et al.*, 1998). However, a comprehensive prospective evaluation of the structural and functional deficits in relation to the course of MDD and neuropsychological impairment has yet to be conducted.

Establishing that a progressive CVD process contributes to late-onset MDD should have important implications for our understanding of the phenomenology, prevention, and treatment of the disorder. There is evidence that in some patients the course of affective illness may become more virulent with aging, showing shorter periods of euthymia between episodes, more abrupt onset of acute symptoms, and greater resistance to treatment (Murphy *et al.*, 1988; Goodwin and Jamison, 1989). Late-onset MDD may be particularly treatment-resistant (Alexopoulos *et al.*, 1996), although this is controversial (Little *et al.*, 1998). Treatment of MDD often involves the use of drugs with potential cardiovascular and cerebrovascular effects (e.g., tricyclic antidepressants). The effects of these drugs include hypotension or reduction in CBF (Preskorn *et al.*, 1982; Nobler *et al.*, 1994) and reduction in metabolism (Gerber *et al.*, 1983; Caldecott-Hazard *et al.*, 1988).

Such effects may aggravate a CVD process, and limit efficacy (Wehr and Goodwin, 1987; Georgotas *et al.*, 1989) or enhance side effects (Figiel *et al.*, 1989; Fujikawa *et al.*, 1996). Thus, there is the possibility that some treatments may be effective in suppressing the expression of the acute depressive episode but may, in the long run, contribute to disease progression. Finally, tying the functional and structural abnormalities in MDD to a CVD process may suggest alternative methods of treatment and new approaches to disease prevention.

REFERENCES

Abe K., Fujimura H., Toyooka K. *et al.* (1994). 'Involvement of the central nervous system in myotonic dystrophy', *J. Neurol. Sci.*, 127: 179–85.

Aharon-Peretz J., Cummings J. L. and Hill M. A. (1988). 'Vascular dementia and dementia of the Alzheimer type: cognition, ventricular size, and leuko-araiosis', *Arch. Neurol.*, 45: 719–21.

Alexander G. E. and Moeller J. R. (1994). 'Application of the scaled subprofile model to functional imaging in neuropsychiatric disorders: a principal components approach to modeling brain function in disease', *Human Brain Mapping*, 2: 79–94.

Alexopoulos G. S., Meyers B. S., Young R. C. *et al.* (1996). 'Recovery in geriatric depression', *Arch. Gen. Psychiatry*, 53: 305–12.

——— (1997). 'Vascular depression hypothesis', *Arch. Gen. Psychiatry*, 54: 915–22.

Almkvist O., Wahlund L. O., Andersson-Lundman G. *et al.* (1992). 'White-matter hyperintensity and neuropsychological functions in dementia and healthy aging', *Arch. Neurol.*, 49: 626–32.

Altshuler L. L., Curran J. G., Hauser P. *et al.* (1995). 'T2 hyperintensities in bipolar disorder: magnetic resonance imaging comparison and literature meta-analysis', *Am. J. Psychiatry*, 152: 1139–44.

Andrews R. J. (1991). 'Transhemispheric diaschisis: A review and comment', *Stroke*, 22: 942–9.

Awad I. A., Modic M., Little J. R. *et al.* (1986a). 'Focal parenchymal lesions in transient ischemic attacks: correlation of computed tomography and magnetic resonance imaging', *Stroke*, 17: 399–403.

Awad I. A., Johnson P. C., Spetzler R. F. *et al.* (1986b). 'Incidental subcortical lesions identified on magnetic resonance imaging in the elderly: II. Postmortem pathological correlations', *Stroke*, 17: 1090–7.

Awad I. A., Spetzler R. F., Hodak J. A. *et al.* (1986c). 'Incidental subcortical lesions identified on magnetic resonance imaging in the elderly:

I. Correlation with age and cerebrovascular risk factors', *Stroke*, 17: 1084–9.

——— (1987). 'Incidental lesions noted on magnetic resonance imaging of the brain: prevalence and clinical significance in various age groups', *Neurosurgery*, 20: 222–7.

Awad I. A., Masaryk T. and Magdinec M. (1993). 'Pathogenesis of subcortical hyperintense lesions on magnetic resonance imaging of the brain: Observations in patients undergoing controlled therapeutic internal carotid artery occlusion', *Stroke*, 24: 1339–46.

Aylward E. H., Roberts-Twillie J. V., Barta P. E. *et al.* (1994). 'Basal ganglia volumes and white matter hyperintensities in patients with bipolar disorder', *Am. J. Psychiatry*, 151: 687–93.

Baloh R. W., Yue Q., Socotch T. M. *et al.* (1995). 'White matter lesions and disequilibrium in older people: I. Case-control comparison', *Arch. Neurol.*, 52: 970–4.

Barnes D. M. and Enzmann D. R. (1981). 'The evaluation of white matter disease as seen on computed tomography', *Radiology*, 138: 379–83.

Baron J. C., D'Antona R., Pantano P. *et al.* (1986). 'Effects of thalamic stroke on energy metabolism of the cerebral cortex. A positron tomography study in man', *Brain*, 109: 1243–59.

Baxter L., Phelps M., Maziotta J. *et al.* (1985) 'Cerebral metabolic rates for glucose in mood disorders', *Arch. Gen. Psychiatry*, 42: 441–7.

Baxter L. R. Jr, Schwartz J. M., Phelps M. E. *et al.* (1989). 'Reduction of prefrontal cortex glucose metabolism common to three types of depression', *Arch. Gen. Psychiatry*, 46: 243–52.

Bench C. J., Friston K. J., Brown R. G. *et al.* (1993). 'Regional cerebral blood flow in depression measured by positron emission tomography: the relationship with clinical dimensions', *Psychol. Med.*, 23: 579–90.

Biver F., Goldman S., Delvenne V. *et al.* (1994). 'Frontal and parietal metabolic disturbances in unipolar depression', *Biological Psychiatry*, 36: 381–8.

Boiten J., Lodder J. and Kessels F. (1993). 'Two clinically distinct lacunar infarct entities? A hypothesis', *Stroke*, 24: 652–6.

Bokura H., Kobayashi S., Yamaguchi S. *et al.* (1994). 'Significance of periventricular hyper-intensity in T2-weighted MRI on memory dysfunction and depression after stroke', *Rinsho. Shinkeigaku*, 34: 438–42.

Boone K. B., Miller B. L., Lesser I. M. *et al.* (1992). 'Neuropsychological correlates of white-matter lesions in healthy elderly subject: A threshold effect', *Arch. Neurol.*, 49: 549–54.

Botteron K. N., Vannier M. W., Geller B. *et al.* (1995). 'Preliminary study of magnetic resonance imaging characteristics in 8 to 16 year-olds with mania', *J. Am. Acad. Child. Adolesc. Psychiatry*, 34: 742–9.

Braffman B. H., Zimmerman R. A., Trojanowski J. Q. *et al.* (1988). 'Brain MR: Pathologic correlation with gross histopathology: 2. Hyperintense white-matter foci in the elderly', *Am. J. Neuroradio.*, 19: 629–36.

Brandt-Zawadski M., Fein G., Van Dyke C. *et al.* (1985). 'MR imaging of the aging brain', *Am. J. Neuroradio.* 16: 675–82.

Breteler M. M., van Swieten J. C., Bots M. L. *et al.* (1994a). 'Cerebral white matter lesions, vascular risk factors, and cognitive function in a population-based study: the Rotterdam Study', *Neurology*, 44: 1246–52.

Breteler M. M. B., van Amerongen N. M., van Swieten J. C. *et al.* (1994b). 'Cognitive correlates of ventricular enlargement and cerebral white matter lesions on magnetic resonance imaging: the Rotterdam Study', *Stroke*, 25: 1109–15.

Brilliant M., Hughes L., Anderson D. *et al.* (1995). 'Rarefied white matter in patients with Alzheimer disease', *Alzheimer Dis. Assoc. Disord.*, 9: 39–46.

Brown F. W. (1993). 'The neurobiology of late-life psychosis', *Crit. Rev. Neurobiol.*, 7: 275–89.

Brown M. M., Pelz D. M. and Hachinski V. (1990). 'Xenon-enchanced CT measurement of cerebral blood flow in cerebrovascular disease', (abstr.), *J. Neurol. Neurosurg. Psychiatry*, 53: 815.

Brown F. W., Lewine R. J., Hudgins P. A. *et al.* (1992). 'White matter hyperintensity signals in psychiatric and nonpsychiatric subjects', *Am. J. Psychiatry*, 149: 620–5.

Buchsbaum M. S., Wu J., DeLisi L. E. *et al.* (1986). 'Frontal cortex and basal ganglia metabolic rates assessed by positron emission tomography with [18F]2-deoxyglucose in affective illness', *J. Affective Disord.*, 10: 137–52.

Cadelo M., Inzitari D., Pracucci G. *et al.* (1991). 'Predictors of leukoaraiosis in elderly neurological patients', *Cerebrovasc. Dis.*, 1: 345–51.

Caldecott-Hazard S., Mazziotta J. and Phelps M. (1988). 'Cerebral correlates of depressed behavior in rats, visualized using 14C-2-deoxyglucose autoradiography', *J. Neurosci.*, 8: 1951–61.

Caplan L. R. and Schoene W. C. (1978). 'Clinical features of subcortical arteriosclerotic encephalopathy (Binswanger disease), *Neurology*, 28: 1206–15.

Chimowitz M. I., Estes M. L., Furlan A. J. *et al.* (1992). 'Further observations on the pathology of subcortical lesions identified on magnetic resonance imaging', *Arch. Neurol.*, 49: 747–52.

Christiansen P., Larsson H. B., Thomsen C. *et al.* (1994). 'Age dependent white matter lesions and brain volume changes in healthy volunteers', *Acta. Radiol.*, 35: 117–22.

Claus J. J., Breteler M. M., Hasan D. *et al.* (1996). 'Vascular risk factors, atherosclerosis, cerebral white matter lesions and cerebral perfusion in a population-based study', *Eur. J. Nucl. Med.*, 23: 675–82.

Coffey C. E., Figiel G. S., Djang W. T. *et al.* (1988). 'Leukoencephalopathy in elderly depressed patients referred for ECT', *Biol. Psychiatry.*, 24: 143–61.

——— (1989). 'White matter hyperintensity on magnetic resonance imaging: clinical and neuroanatomic correlates in the depressed elderly', *J. Neuropsychiatry Clin. Neurosci.*, 1: 135–44.

——— (1990). 'Subcortical hyperintensity on magnetic resonance imaging: a comparison of normal and depressed elderly subjects', *Am. J. Psychiatry*, 147: 187–9.

Coffey C. E., Weiner R. D., Djang W. T. *et al.* (1991). 'Brain anatomic effects of electroconvulsive therapy: A prospective magnetic resonance imaging study', *Arch. Gen. Psychiatry*, 48: 1013–21.

Coffey C. E., Wilkinson W. E., Weiner R. D. *et al.* (1993). 'Quantitative cerebral anatomy in depression: A controlled magnetic resonance imaging study', *Arch. Gen. Psychiatry*, 50: 7–16.

Confort-Gouny S., Vion-Dury J., Nicoli F. *et al.* (1993). 'A multiparametric data analysis showing the potential of localized proton MR spectroscopy of the brain in the metabolic characterization of neurological diseases', *J. Neurol. Sci.*, 118: 123–33.

Cummings J. L. (1993). 'The neuroanatomy of depression', *J. Clin. Psychiatry*, 54 (Suppl. 11): 14–20.

Curran S. M., Murray C. M., Van Beck M. *et al.* (1993). 'A single photon emission computerised tomography study of regional brain function in elderly patients with major depression and with Alzheimer-type dementia', *Br. J. Psychiatry*, 163: 155–65.

Dahabra S., Ashton C. H., Bahrainian M. *et al.* (1998). 'Structural and functional abnormalities in elderly patients clinically recovered from early- and late-onset depression', *Biol. Psychiatry*, 44: 34–46.

De Reuck J. (1971). 'The human periventricular arterial blood supply and the anatomy of cerebral infarctions', *Eur. Neurol.*, 5: 321–34.

De Reuck J., Decoo D., Strijckmans K. *et al.* (1992). 'Does the severity of leukoaraiosis contribute to senile dementia?: A comparative computerized and positron emission tomographic study', *Eur. Neurol.*, 32: 199–205.

Devanand D. P., Sano M., Tang M. X. *et al.* (1996). 'Depressed mood and the incidence of Alzheimer's disease in the elderly living in the community', *Arch. Gen. Psychiatry*, 53: 175–82.

Devous M. D. Sr, Gullion C. M., Grannemann B. D. *et al.* (1993). 'Regional cerebral blood flow alterations in unipolar depression', *Psychiatry Res.*, 50: 233–56.

Diaz J. F., Merskey H., Hachinski V. C. *et al.* (1991). 'Improved recognition of leukoaraiosis and cognitive impairment in Alzheimer's disease', *Arch. Neurol.*, 48: 1022–5.

Dolan R. J., Poynton A. M., Bridges P. K. *et al.* (1990). 'Altered magnetic resonance white-matter T1 values in patients with affective disorder', *Br. J. Psychiatry*: 157: 107–10.

Drevets W. C. (1998). 'Functional neuroimaging studies of depression: the anatomy of melancholia', *Ann. Rev. Med.*, 49: 341–61.

Drevets W. C., Videen T. O., Price J. L. *et al.* (1992). 'A functional anatomical study of unipolar depression', *J. Neurosci.*, 12: 3628–41.

Dupont R. M., Jernigan T. L., Butters N. *et al.* (1990). 'Subcortical abnormalities detected in bipolar affective disorder using magnetic resonance imaging: Clinical and neuropsychological significance' (*see* comments), *Arch. Gen. Psychiatry*, 47: 55–9.

Dupont R. M., Butters N., Schafer K. *et al.* (1995a). Diagnostic specificity of focal white matter abnormalities in bipolar and unipolar mood disorder', *Biol. Psychiatry*, 38: 482–6.

Dupont R. M., Jernigan T. L., Heindel W. *et al.* (1995b). 'Magnetic resonance imaging and mood disorders: Localization of white matter and other subcortical abnormalities', *Arch. Gen. Psychiatry*, 52: 747–55.

Ebmeier K. P., Prentice N., Ryman A. *et al.* (1997). 'Temporal lobe abnormalities in dementia and depression: a study using high resolution single photon emission tomography and magnetic resonance imaging', *J. Neurol. Neurosurg. Psychiatry*, 63: 597–604.

Erkinjuntti T., Ketonen L., Sulkava R. *et al.* (1987). 'Do white matter changes on MRI and CT differentiate vascular dementia from Alzheimer's disease?', *J. Neurol. Neursurg. Psychiatry*, 50: 37–42.

Erkinjuntti T., Gao F., Lee D. H. *et al.* (1994). 'Lack of difference in brain hyperintensities between patients with early Alzheimer's disease and control subjects', *Arch. Neurol.*, 51: 260–8.

Fall P. A., Ekman R., Granerus A. K. *et al.* (1995). 'ECT in Parkinson's disease: Changes in motor symptoms, monoamine metabolites and neuropeptides', *J. Neural. Transm. Park. Dis. Dement. Sect.*, 10: 129–40.

Fazekas F. (1989). 'Magnetic resonance signal abnormalities in asymptomatic individuals: their incidence and functional correlates', *Eur. Neurol.*, 29: 164–8.

Fazekas F., Niederkorn K., Schmitd R. *et al.* (1988). 'White matter signal abnormalities in normal individuals: correlation with carotid ultrasonography, cerebral blood flow measurements, and cerebrovascular risk factors', *Stroke*, 19: 1285–8.

Fazekas F., Kleinert R., Offenbacher H. *et al.* (1993). 'Pathologic correlates of incidental MRI white matter signal hyperintensities', *Neurology*, 43: 1683–9.

Figiel G. S., Krishnan K. R., Breitner J. C. *et al.* (1989). 'Radiologic correlates of antidepressant-induced delirium: the possible significance of basal-ganglia lesions', *J. Neuropsychiatry Clin. Neurosci.*, 1: 188–90.

Figiel G. S., Coffey C. E., Djang W. T. *et al.* (1990a). 'Brain magnetic resonance imaging findings in ECT-induced delirium', *J. Neuropsychiatry Clin. Neurosci.*, 2: 53–8.

Figiel G. S., Krishnan K. R. and Doraiswamy P. M. (1990b). ' Subcortical structural changes in ECT-induced delirium', *J. Geriatr. Psychiatry Neurol.*, 3: 172–6.

Figiel G. S., Krishnan K. R., Rao V. P. *et al.* (1991a). 'Subcortical hyperintensities on brain magnetic resonance imaging: a comparison of normal and bipolar subjects', *J. Neuropsychiatry Clin. Neurosci.*, 3: 18–22.

Figiel G. S., Krishnan K. R., Doraiswamy P. M. *et al.* (1991b). 'Subcortical hyperintensities on brain magnetic resonance imaging: a comparison between late age onset and early-onset elderly depressed subjects', *Neurobiol. Aging*, 12: 245–7.

Filley C. M., Davis K. A., Schmitz S. P. *et al.* (1989). 'Neuropsychological performance and magnetic resonance imaging in Alzheimer's disease and normal aging', *Neuropsychiatry Neuropsychol. Behav. Neurol.*, 2: 81–92.

Fujikawa T., Yamawaki S. and Touhouda Y. (1993). 'Incidence of silent cerebral infarction in patients with major depression', *Stroke*, 24: 1631–4.

——— (1994). 'Background factors and clinical symptoms of major depression with silent cerebral infarction', *Stroke*, 25: 798–801.

Fujikawa T., Yokota N., Muraoka M. *et al.* (1996). 'Response of patients with major depression and silent cerebral infarction to antidepressant drug therapy, with emphasis on central nervous system adverse reactions', *Stroke*, 27: 2040–2.

Fukui T., Sugita K., Sato Y. *et al.* (1994). 'Cognitive functions in subjects with incidental cerebral hyperintensities', *Eur. Neurol.*, 34: 272–6.

George A. E., deLeon M. J., Kalvin A. *et al.* (1986). 'Leukoencephalopathy in normal and pathologic aging', *Am. J. Neuroradio.*, 17: 567–70.

George M. S., Ketter T. A. and Post R. M. (1994). 'Prefrontal cortex dysfunction in clinical depression', *Depression*, 2: 59–72.

Georgotas A., McCue R. E. and Cooper T. B. (1989). 'A placebo-controlled comparison of nortriptyline and phenelzine in maintenance therapy of elderly depressed patients', *Arch. Gen. Psychiatry*, 46: 783–6.

Gerard G. and Weisberg L. A. (1986). 'MRI periventricular lesions in adults', *Neurology*, 36: 998–1001.

Gerber J. C., Choki J., Brunswick D. J. *et al.* (1983). 'The effects of antidepressant drugs on regional cerebral glucose utilization in the rat', *Brain Res.*, 269: 319–25.

Gilarowsky D. (1926). 'Ueber die rolle der arteriosklerose in der genese psychischer erkankungen des voralters', *Allg. Z. Psychiatr.*, 84: 169–75.

Gill R., Sibson N. R., Hatfield R. H. *et al.* (1995). 'A comparison of the early development of ischaemic damage following permanent middle cerebral artery occlusion in rats as assessed using magnetic resonance imaging and histology', *J. Cereb. Blood Flow Metab.*, 15: 1–11.

Golomb J., Kluger A., Gianutsos, J. *et al.* (1995). 'Nonspecific leukoencephalopathy associated with aging', *Neuroimaging Clin. N. Am.* 5: 33–44.

Goodwin F. K. and Jamison K. R. (1989). *Manic-Depressive Illness*, New York: Oxford University Press.

Goodwin G. M., Austin M. P., Dougall N. *et al.* (1993). 'State changes in brain activity shown by the uptake of 99mTc-exametazime with single photon emission tomography in major depression before and after treatment', *J. Affect. Disord.*, 29: 243–53.

Grafton S. T., Sumi S. M., Stimac G. K. *et al.* (1991). 'Comparison of postmortem magnetic resonance imaging and neuropathologic findings in the cerebral white matter', *Arch. Neurol.*, 48: 293–8.

Greenwald B. S., Kramer-Ginsberg E., Krishnan R. R. *et al.* (1996). 'MRI signal hyperintensities in geriatric depression', *Am. J. Psychiatry*, 153: 1212–15.

Greenwald B. S., Kramer-Ginsberg E., Krishnan K. R. *et al.* (1998). 'Neuroanatomic localization of magnetic resonance imaging signal hyperintensities in geriatric depression', *Stroke*, 29: 613–17.

Gupta S. R., Naheedy M. H., Young J. C. *et al.* (1988). 'Periventricular white matter changes and dementia', *Arch. Neurol.*, 45: 637–41.

Hachinski V., Potter P. and Merskey H. (1987). 'Leuko-araiosis', *Arch. Neurol.*, 44: 21–3.

Hagman J. O., Buchsbaum M. S., Wu J. C. *et al.* (1990). 'Comparison of regional brain metabolism in bulimia nervosa and affective disorder assessed with positron emission tomography', *J. Affective Disord.*, 19: 153–62.

Hatazawa J., Shimosegawa E., Satoh T. *et al.* (1997), 'Subcortical hypoperfusion associated with asymptomatic white matter lesions on magnetic resonance imaging', *Stroke*, 28: 1944–7.

Hendrie H. C., Farlow M. R., Austrom Guerriero M. *et al.* (1989). 'Foci of increased T2 signal intensity on brain MR scans of healthy elderly subjects', *Am. J. Neuroradiol.*, 10: 703–7.

Henon H., Godefroy O., Lucas C. *et al.* (1996). 'Risk factors and leukoaraiosis in stroke patients', *Acta. Neurol. Scand.*, 94: 137–44.

Herholz K., Heindel W., Rackl A. *et al.* (1990). 'Regional cerebral blood flow in patients with leuko-araiosis and atherosclerotic carotid artery disease', *Arch. Neurol.*, 47: 392–6.

Hershey L. A., Modic M. T., Greenough P. G. *et al.* (1987). 'Magnetic resonance imaging in vascular dementia', *Neurology*, 37: 29–36.

Hickie I., Scott E., Mitchell P. *et al.* (1995). 'Subcortical hyperintensities on magnetic resonance imaging: Clinical correlates and prognostic significance in patient with severe depression', *Biol. Psychiatry*, 37: 151–60.

Hickie I., Scott E., Wilhelm K. *et al.* (1997). 'Subcortical hyperintensities on magnetic resonance imaging in patients with severe depression: a longitudinal evaluation', *Biol. Psychiatry*, 42: 367–74.

Howard R., Cox T., Almeida O. *et al.* (1995). 'White matter signal hyperintensities in the brains of patients with late paraphrenia and the normal, community-living elderly', *Biol. Psychiatry*, 38: 86–91.

Iidaka T., Nakajima T., Kawamoto K. *et al.* (1996), 'Signal hyperintensities on brain magnetic resonance imaging in elderly depressed patients', *Eur. Neurol.*, 36: 293–9.

Inzitari D., Di Carlo A., Mascalchi M. *et al.* (1995). 'The cardiovascular outcome of patients with motor impairment and extensive leukoaraiosis', *Arch. Neurol.*, 52: 687–91.

Isaka Y., Iiji O, Ashida K. *et al.* (1993). 'Cerebral blood flow in asymptomatic individuals: relationship with cerebrovascular risk factors and magnetic resonance imaging signal abnormalities', *Jpn. Circ. J.*, 57: 283–90.

Isaka Y., Nagano K., Narita M. *et al.* (1997). 'High signal intensity on T2-weighted magnetic resonance imaging and cerebral hemodynamic reserve in carotid occlusive disease', *Stroke*, 28: 354–7.

Janota I., Mirsen T. R., Hachinski V. C. *et al.* (1989). 'Neuropathologic correlates of leuko-araiosis', *Arch. Neurol.*, 46: 1124–8.

Jenkins M., Malloy P., Salloway S. *et al.* (1998). 'Memory processes in depressed geriatric patients with and without subcortical hyperintensities on MRI', *J. Neuroimaging*, 8: 20–6.

Jorgensen H. S., Nakayama H., Raaschou H. O. *et al.* (1995). 'Leukoaraiosis in stroke patients: The Copenhagen Stroke Study', *Stroke*, 26: 588–92.

Junque C., Pujot T., Vendrell P. *et al.* (1990). 'Leukoaraiosis on magnetic resonance imaging and speed of mental processing', *Arch. Neurol.*, 47: 151–6.

Kanno I., Uemura K. and Higano S. (1988). 'Oxygen extraction fraction at maximally vasodilated tissue in the ischemic brain estimated from the regional COh2 responsiveness measured by positron emission tomography', *J. CBF Metabol.*, 8: 227–35.

Kawamura J., Meyer J. S., Terayama Y. *et al.* (1991). 'Leukoaraiosis correlates with cerebral hypoperfusion in vascular dementia', *Stroke*, 22: 609–14.

Keller M. B., Lavori P. W., Klerman G. L. *et al.* (1986). 'Low levels and lack of predictors of somatotherapy and psychotherapy received by depressed patients', *Arch. Gen. Psychiatry*, 43: 458–66.
Kellner C. H., Beale M. D., Pritchett J. T. *et al.* (1994). 'Electroconvulsive therapy and Parkinson's disease: the case for further study', *Psychopharmacol. Bull.*, 30: 495–500.
Kertesz A., Black S. E., Tokar G. *et al.* (1988). 'Periventricular and subcortical hyperintensities on magnetic resonance imaging', *Arch. Neurol.*, 45: 404–8.
Kinkel W. R., Jacobs L., Polanchini I. *et al.* (1985). 'Subcortical arteriosclerotic encephalopathy (Binswanger's disease)', *Arch. Neurol.*: 951–9.
Kirkpatrick J. B. and Hayman L. A. (1987). 'White-matter lesions in MR imaging of clinically healthy brains of elderly subjects: Possible pathologic basis', *Radiology*, 162: 509–11.
Kobari M., Meyer J. S. and Ichijo M. (1990). 'Leuko-araiosis, cerebral atrophy, and cerebral perfusion in normal aging', *Arch. Neurol.*, 47: 161–8.
Kobayashi S., Okada K. and Yamashita K. (1991). 'Incidence of silent lacunar lesion in normal adults and its relation to cerebral blood flow and risk factors', *Stroke*, 22: 1379–83.
Kohlmeyer K. (1988). 'Periventricular attenuation of the density of cerebral hemisphere white matter in computerized tomography of neuropsychiatric patients in the second half of life: Diagnostic significance and pathogenesis', *Fortschr. Neurol. Psychiatr.*, 56: 279–85.
Krishnan K. R. (1993). 'Neuroanatomic substrates of depression in the elderly', *J. Geriatr. Psychiatry Neurol.*, 6: 39–58.
Krishnan K. R. and McDonald W. M. (1995). 'Arteriosclerotic depression', *Med. Hypotheses*, 44: 111–15.
Krishnan K. R., Goli V., Ellinwood E. H. *et al.* (1988). 'Leukoencephalopathy in patients diagnosed as major depressive', *Biol. Psychiatry*, 23: 519–22.
Krishnan K. R., McDonald W. M., Escalona P. R. *et al.* (1992). 'Magnetic resonance imaging of the caudate nuclei in depression: Preliminary observations', *Arch. Gen. Psychiatry*, 49: 553–7.
Krishnan K. R., McDonald W. M., Doraiswamy P. M. *et al.* (1993). 'Neuroanatomical substrates of depression in the elderly', *Eur. Arch. Psychiatry Clin. Neurosci.*, 243: 41–6.
Krishnan K. R., Hays J. C. and Blazer D. G. (1997). 'MRI-defined vascular depression', *Am J. Psychiatry*, 154: 497–501.
Kumar A., Newberg A., Alavi A. *et al.* (1993). 'Regional cerebral glucose metabolism in late-life depression and Alzheimer disease: a preliminary positron emission tomography study', *Proc. Natl. Acad. Sci. USA*, 90: 7019–23.

Lechner H., Schmidt R., Bertha G. *et al.* (1988). 'Nuclear magnetic resonance image white matter lesions and risk factors for stroke in normal individuals', *Stroke,* 19: 263–5.

Lesser I. M., Miller B. L., Boone K. B. *et al.* (1991). 'Brain injury and cognitive function in late-onset psychotic depression', *J. Neuropsychiatry Clin. Neurosci.*, 3: 33–40.

Lesser I. M., Mena I., Boone K. B. *et al.* (1994). 'Reduction of cerebral blood flow in older depressed patients', *Arch. Gen. Psychiatry.* 51: 677–86.

Lesser I. M., Boone K. B., Mehringer C. M. *et al.* (1996). 'Cognition and white matter hyperintensities in older depressed patients', *Am. J. Psychiatry*, 153: 1280–7.

Levine R. L., Sunderland J. J., Rowe B. R. *et al.* (1986). 'The study of cerebral ischemic reversibility: Part II. Preliminary preoperative results of fluoromethane positron emission tomographic determination of perfusion reserve in patients with carotid TIA and stroke', *Am. J. Physiol. Imaging*, 1: 104–14.

Leys D., Soetaert G., Petit H. *et al.* (1990). ' Periventricular and white matter magnetic resonance imaging hyperintensities do not differ between Alzheimer's disease and normal aging', *Arch. Neurol.*, 47: 524–7.

Lindgren A., Roijer A., Rudling O. *et al.* (1994). 'Cerebral lesions on magnetic resonance imaging, heart disease, and vascular risk factors in subjects without stroke: A population-based study', *Stroke*, 25: 929–34.

Little J. T., Reynolds C. F. III, Dew M. A. *et al.* (1998). 'How common is resistance to treatment in recurrent, nonpsychotic geriatric depression?', *Am. J. Psychiatry*, 155: 1035–8.

Longstreth W. T. Jr., Manolio T. A., Arnold A. *et al.* (1996). 'Clinical correlates of white matter findings on cranial magnetic resonance imaging of 3301 elderly people: The Cardiovascular Health Study', (*see* comments), *Stroke*, 27: 1274–82.

Lopez O. L., Becker J. T., Rezek D. *et al.* (1992). 'Neuropsychiatric correlates of cerebral white-matter radiolucencies in probable Alzheimer's disease', *Arch. Neurol.*, 49: 828–34.

Lopez O. L., Becker J. T., Reynolds C. F. III *et al.* (1997). 'Psychiatric correlates of MR deep white matter lesions in probable Alzheimer's disease', *J. Neuropsychiatry Clin. Neurosci.*, 9: 246–50.

Manolio T. A., Kronmal R. A., Burke G. L. *et al.* (1994). 'Magnetic resonance abnormalities and cardiovascular disease in older adults: The Cardiovascular Health Study', *Stroke*, 25: 318–27.

Marshall V. G., Bradley W. L. S., Marshall C. E. *et al.* (1988). 'Deep white matter infarction: Correlation of MR images and histopathologic findings', *Radiology*, 167: 517–22.

Martinot J. L., Hardy P., Feline A. *et al.* (1990). 'Left prefrontal glucose hypometabolism in the depressed state: a confirmation', *Am. J. Psychiatry*, 147: 1313–17

Masdeu J. C., Wolfson L., Lantos G. *et al.* (1989). 'Brain white-matter changes in the elderly prone to falling', *Arch. Neurol.*, 46: 1292–6.

Matsubayashi K., Shimada K., Kawamoto A. *et al.* (1992). 'Incidental brain lesions on magnetic resonance imaging and neurobehavioral functions in the apparently healthy elderly', *Stroke*, 23: 175–80.

Matsushita K., Kuriyama Y., Nagatsuka K. *et al.* (1994). 'Periventricular white matter lucency and cerebral blood flow autoregulation in hypertensive patients', *Hypertension*, 23: 565–8.

Mayberg H. S., Starkstein S. E., Sadzot B. *et al.* (1990). 'Selective hypometabolism in the inferior frontal lobe in depressed patients with Parkinson's disease', *Ann. Neurol.*, 28: 57–64.

Mayberg H. S., Starkstein S. E., Peyser C. E. *et al.* (1992). 'Paralimbic frontal lobe hypometabolism in depression associated with Huntington's disease', *Neurology*, 42: 1791–7.

Meguro K., Hatazawa J., Yamaguchi T. *et al.* (1990). 'Cerebral circulation and oxygen metabolism associated with subclinical periventricular hyperintensity as shown by magnetic resonance imaging', *Ann. Neurol.*, 28: 378–83.

Mesulam M. M., Mufson E., Levey A. *et al.* (1983). 'Cholinergic innervation of cortex by the basal forebrain: Cytochemistry and cortical connections of the septal area, diagonal band nuclei, nucleus basalis (substantia innominata) and hypothalamus in the rhesus monkey', *J. Comp. Neurol.*, 214: 170–97.

Mirsen T. R., Lee D. H., Wong C. J. *et al.* (1991). 'Clinical correlates of white-matter changes on magnetic resonance imaging scans of the brain', *Arch. Neurol.*, 48: 1015–21.

Miyao S., Takano A., Teramoto J. *et al.* (1992). 'Leukoaraiosis in relation to prognosis for patients with lacunar infarction', *Stroke*, 23: 1434–8.

Miyazawa N., Satoh T., Hashizume K. *et al.* (1997). ' Xenon contrast CT-CBF measurements in high-intensity foci on T2-weighted MR images in centrum semiovale of asymptomatic individuals', *Stroke*, 28: 984–7.

Moeller J. R. and Strother S. C. (1991). 'A regional covariance approach to the analysis of functional patterns in positron emission tomographic data', *J. Cereb. Blood Flow Metab.*, 11: A121–A135

Moeller J., Strother S., Sidtis J. *et al.* (1987), 'Scaled subprofile model: A statistical approach to the analysis of functional patterns in positron emission tomographic data', *J. Cereb. Blood Flow Metab.*, 7: 649–58.

Moody D. M., Brown W. R., Challa V. R. *et al.* (1995). 'Periventricular venous collagenosis: association with leukoaraiosis', *Radiology*, 194: 469–76.

Munoz D. G., Hastak S. M., Harper B. *et al.* (1993). 'Pathologic correlates of increased signals of the centrum ovale on magnetic resonance imaging', *Arch, Neurol.*, 50: 492–7.

Murphy E., Smith R., Lindesay J. *et al.* (1988). 'Increased mortality rates in late-life depression', *Br. J. Psychiatry*, 152: 347–53.

Nobler M. S. and Sackeim H. A. (1998). 'Machanisms of action of electroconvulsive therapy: Functional brain imaging studies', *Psychiatric Annals.*, 28: 23–9.

Nobler M. S., Sackeim H. A., Prohovnik I. *et al.* (1994). 'Regional cerebral blood flow in mood disorders: III. Effects of treatment and clinical response in depression and mania', *Arch. Gen. Psychiatry*, 51: 884–97.

O'Brien J., Desmond P., Ames D. *et al.* (1996). 'A magnetic resonance imaging study of white matter lesions in depression and Alzheimer's disease', *Br. J. Psychiatry*, 168: 477–85.

O'Brien J., Ames D., Chiu E. *et al.* (1998). 'Severe deep white matter lesions and outcome in elderly patients with major depressive disorder: follow-up study', *BMJ*, 317: 982–4.

Okada K., Kobayashi S., Yamagata S. *et al.* (1997). 'Post-stroke apathy and regional cerebral blood flow', *Stroke*, 28: 2437–41.

Oppenheimer S. M., Bryan R. N., Conturo T. E. *et al.* (1995). 'Proton magnetic resonance spectroscopy and gadolinium-DTPA perfusion imaging of asymptomatic MRI white matter lesions', *Magn. Reson. Med.*, 33: 61–8.

Pantoni L. and Garcia J. H. (1995). 'The significance of cerebral white matter abnormalities 100 years after Binswanger's report: A review', *Stroke*, 26: 1293–1301.

Pappata S., Mazoyer B., Dinh S. T. *et al.* (1990). 'Effects of capsular or thalamic stroke on metabolism in the cortex and cerebellum: A positron tomography study', *Stroke*, 21: 519–24.

Passero S., Nardini M. and Battistini N. (1995). 'Regional cerebral blood flow changes following chronic administration of antidepressant drugs', *Prog. Neuro-Psychopharmacol. Biol. Psychiatry*, 19: 627–36.

Perani D., Di PiV, Lucignani G. *et al.* (1988). 'Remote effects of subcortical cerebrovascular lesions: a SPECT cerebral perfusion study', *J. Cereb. Blood Flow Metab.*, 8: 560–7.

Post F. (1962). *The Significance of Affective Symptoms in Old Age*. London: Oxford University Press, Maudsley Monograph No. 10.

Preskorn S. H., Raichle M. E., and Hartman B. K. (1982). 'Antidepressants alter cerebrovascular permeability and metabolic rate in primates', *Science*, 217: 250–2.

Prudic J., Haskett R. F., Mulsant B. *et al.* (1996). 'Resistance to antidepressant medications and short-term clinical response to ECT', *Am. J. Psychiatry*, 153: 985–92.

Rabins P. V., Pearlson G. D., Aylward E. *et al.* (1991). 'Cortical magnetic resonance imaging changes in elderly inpatients with major depression' (*see* comments), *Am. J. Psychiatry*, 148: 617–20.

Rao S. M., Mittenberg W., Bernardin L. *et al.* (1989). 'Neuropsychological test findings in subjects with leukoaraiosis', *Arch. Neurol.*, 46: 40–4.

Reischies F. M., Hedde J. P. and Drochner R. (1989). 'Clinical correlates of cerebral blood flow in depression', *Psychiatry Res.*, 29: 323–6.

Rezek D., Morris J. and Fulling K. H. (1986). 'Periventricular white matter lucencies in senile dementia of the Alzheimer type and in normal aging', *Neurology*, 36: 1–6.

Ring H. A., Bench C. J., Trimble M. R. *et al.* (1994). 'Depression in Parkinson's disease: A positron emission study', *Br. J. Psychiatry*, 165: 333–9.

Roman G. C. (1987). 'Senile dementia of the Binswanger type: A vascular form of dementia in the elderly', *JAMA*, 258: 1782–8.

Rosenberg R., Vostrup S., Andersen A. *et al.* (1988). 'Effect of ECT on cerebral blood flow in melancholia assessed with SPECT', *Convulsive Therapy*, 4: 62–73.

Rubin E., Sackeim H. A., Nobler M. S. *et al.* (1994). 'Brain imaging studies of antidepressant treatments', *Psychiatric Annals.*, 653–8.

Rubin E., Sackeim H. A., Prohovnik I. *et al.* (1995). 'Regional cerebral blood flow in mood disorders: IV. Comparison of mania and depression', *Psychiatry Research: Neuroimaging*. 61: 1–10.

Sackeim H. A. (1999). 'The anticonvulsant hypothesis of the mechanisms of action of ECT: Current status', *J. ECT* (in press).

Sackeim H. A. and Prohovnik I. (1993). 'Brain imaging studies in depressive disorders', in Mann J. J., Kupfer D. (eds), *Biology of Depressive Disorders*, Plenum: New York, 205–58.

Sackeim H. A. and Steif B. L. (1988). 'The neuropsychology of depression and mania', in Georgotas A., Cancro R. (eds), *Depression and Mania*, Elsevier: New York, 265–89.

Sackeim H. A., Prudic J., Devanand D. P. *et al.* (1990a). 'The impact of medication resistance and continuation pharmacotherapy on relapse following response to electroconvulsive therapy in major depression', *J. Clin. Psychopharmacol.*, 10: 96–104.

Sackeim H. A., Prohovnik I., Moeller J. R. *et al.* (1990b). 'Regional cerebral blood flow in mood disorders: I. Comparison of major depressives and normal controls at rest', *Arch. Gen. Psychiatry*, 47: 60–70.

Sackeim H. A., Prohovnik I., Moeller J. R. *et al.* (1993). 'Regional cerebral blood flow in mood disroders: II. Comparison of major depression and Alzheimer's disease', *J. Nucl. Med.*, 34: 1090–1101.

Salloway S., Malloy P., Kohn R. *et al.* (1996). 'MRI and neuropsychological differences in early- and late-life-onset geriatric depression', *Neurology*, 46: 1567–74.

Sappey-Marinier D., Calabrese G., Hetherington H. P. *et al.* (1992). 'Proton magnetic resonance spectroscopy of human brain: applications to normal white matter, chronic infarction, and MRI white matter signal hyperintensities', *Magn. Reson. Med.*, 26: 313–27.

Schmidt R., Fazekas F., Kleinert G. *et al.* (1992). 'Magnetic resonance imaging signal hyperintensities in the deep and subcortical white matter: A comparative study between stroke patients and normal volunteers', *Arch. Neurol.*, 49: 825–7.

Schmidt R., Fazekas F., Offenbacher H. *et al.* (1993). 'Neuro-psychologic correlates of MRI white matter hyperintensities: a study of 150 normal volunteers', *Neurology*, 43: 2490–4.

Seiderer M., Krappel W., Moser E. *et al.* (1989). 'Detection and quantification of chronic cerebrovascular disease: comparison of MR imaging, SPECT, and CT', *Radiology*, 170: 545–8.

Sette G., Baron J. C., Mazoyer B. *et al.* (1989). 'Local brain haemodynamics and oxygen metabolism in cerebrovascular disease: Positron emission tomography', *Brain*, 112: 931–51.

Silfverskiöld P., Gustafson L., Risberg J. *et al.* (1986). 'Acute and late effects of electroconvulsive therapy: Clinical outcome, regional cerebral blood flow, and electroencephalogram', *Ann. NY. Acad. Sci.*, 462: 236–48.

Simpson S. W., Jackson A., Baldwin R. C. *et al.* (1997). 'Subcortical hyperintensities in late-life depression: acute response to treatment and neuropsychological impairment', *Int. Psychogeriatr.*, 9: 257–75.

Soares J. C. and Mann J. J. (1997). 'The anatomy of mood disorders: review of structural neuroimaging studies', *Biol. Psychiatry*, 41: 86–106.

Solomon A., Yeates A. E., Burger P. C. *et al.* (1987). 'Subcortical arteriosclerotic encephalopathy: Brainstem findings with MR imaging', *Radiology*, 165: 625–9.

Starkstein S. E., Robinson R. G., Berthier M. L. *et al.* (1988). 'Differential mood changes following basal ganglia vs thalamic lesions', *Arch. Neurol.*, 45: 725–30.

Steffens D. C. and Krishnan K. R. (1998). 'Structural neuroimaging and mood disorders: recent findings, implications for classification, and future directions', *Biol. Psychiatry*, 43: 705–12.

Steingart A., Hachinski V., Lau C. *et al.* (1987). 'Cognitive and neurologic findings in subjects with diffuse white matter lucencies on computed tomographic scans (leuko-araiosis)', *Arch. Neurol.*, 44: 32–5.

Strakowski S. M., Wilson D. R., Tohen M. *et al.* (1993). 'Structural brain abnormalities in first-episode mania', *Biol. Psychiatry*, 33: 602–29.

Swayze V. W. II, Andreasen N. C., Alliger R. J. *et al.* (1990). 'Structural brain abnormalities in bipolar affective disorder: Ventricular enlargement and focal signal hyperintensities', *Arch. Gen. Psychiatry*, 47: 1054–9.

Tabaton M., Caponnetto C., Mancardi G. *et al.* (1991). 'Amyloid beta protein deposition in brains from elderly subjects with leukoaraiosis', *J. Neurol. Sci.*, 106: 123–7.

Tachibana H., Meyer J. S., Kitagawa Y. *et al.* (1984). 'Effects of aging on cerebral blood flow in dementia', *J. Am. Geriatr. Soc.*, 32: 114–20.

Tamura A., Graham D. I., McCulloch J. *et al.* (1981). 'Focal cerebral ischaemia in the rat: 2. Regional cerebral blood flow determined by iodoantipyrine autoradiography following middle cerebral artery occlusion', *J. Cereb. Blood Flow Metab.*, 1: 61–9.

Tarvonen-Schroder S., Kurki T., Raiha I. *et al.* (1995). 'Leukoaraiosis and cause of death: a five-year follow-up', *J. Neurol. Neurosurg. Psychiatry*, 58: 586–9.

Tatemichi T. K., Prohovnik I, Mohr J. P. *et al.* (1988). 'Reduced hypercapnic vasoreactivity in moyamoya disease', *Neurology*, 38: 1575–81.

Tohgi H., Chiba K. and Kimura M. (1991). 'Twenty-four hour variation of blood pressure in vascular dementia of the Binswanger type', *Stroke*, 22: 603–8.

Trojanowski J. and Jacobson S. (1976). 'Areal and laminar distribution of some pulvinar cortical efferents in rhesus monkey', *J. Comp. Neurol.*, 169: 371–92.

Upadhyaya A. K., Abou-Saleh M. T., Wilson K. *et al.* (1990). 'A study of depression in old age using single-photon emission computerised tomography', *Br. J. Psychiatry*, 157: 76–81.

van Swieten J. C., Geyskes G. G., Derix M. M. *et al.* (1991a). 'Hypertension in the elderly is associated with white matter lesions and cognitive decline', *Ann. Neurol.*, 30: 825–30.

van Swieten J. C., van den Hout J. H., van Ketel B. A. *et al.* (1991b). 'Periventricular lesions in the white matter on magnetic resonance imaging in the elderly: A morphometric correlation with arteriolosclerosis and dilated perivascular spaces', *Brain*, 114: 761–74.

van Swieten J. C., Kappelle L. J., Algra A. *et al.* (1992). 'Hypodensity of the cerebral white matter in patients with transient ischemic attack or minor stroke: Influence on the rate of subsequent stroke', *Ann. Neurol.*, 32: 177–83.

Volkow N. D., Bellar S., Mullani N. *et al.* (1988). 'Effects of electroconvulsive therapy on brain glucose metabolism: A preliminary study', *Convulsive Ther.*, 4: 199–205.

Vorstrup S. (1988). 'Tomographic cerebral blood flow measurements in patients with ischemic cerebrovascular disease and evaluation of the vasodilatory capacity by the acetazolamide test', *Acta. Neurol. Scand.* 114: (Suppl.): 1–48.

Waldemar G., Christiansen P., Larsson H. B. *et al.* (1994). 'White matter magnetic resonance hyperintensities in dementia of the Alzheimer type: morphological and regional cerebral blood flow correlates', *J. Neurol. Neurosurg. Psychiatry*, 57: 1458–65.

Wehr T. A. and Goodwin F. K. (1987). 'Can antidepressants cause mania and worsen the course of affective illness?', *Am. J. Psychiatry*, 144: 1403–12.

Yamamoto M., Meyer J., Sakai F. *et al.* (1980). 'Aging and cerebral vasodilator response to hypercarbia: responses in normal aging and in persons with risk factors for stroke', *Arch. Neurol.*, 37: 489–96.

Yao H., Sadoshima S., Ibayashi S. *et al.* (1992). 'Leukoaraiosis and dementia in hypertensive patients', *Stroke*, 23: 1673–77.

Ylikoski R., Ylikoski A., Erkinjuntti T. *et al.* (1993). 'White matter changes in healthy elderly persons correlate with attention and speed of mental processing', *Arch. Neurol.*, 50: 818–24.

Zakzanis K. K., Leach L. and Kaplan E. (1998). 'On the nature and pattern of neurocognitive function in major depressive disorder', *Neuropsychiatry, Neuropsychal. Behav. Neurol.*, 11: 111–19.

Zubenko G. S., Sullivan P., Nelson J. P. *et al.* (1990). 'Brain imaging abnormalities in mental disorders of late life', *Arch. Neurol.*, 47: 1107–11.

Chapter 5

The Current Status of Eating Disorders

KIRSTINE POSTMA AND CHRIS P. L. FREEMAN

INTRODUCTION

The last twenty-five years have witnessed much productive research in the field of eating disorders. In 1975, bulimia nervosa was virtually unknown and binge eating, particularly at night, was viewed as an occasional accompaniment of severe obesity and of chronic, treatment-resistant anorexia nervosa. The clinical description of bulimia nervosa crystallized during the late 1970s and early 1980s. More recently, the concept of binge-eating disorder has gained ground. Interestingly, these theoretical advances have been associated with radical changes in clinical presentations.

A large number of well-conducted studies have examined the outcome of bulimia nervosa with different types of drug and psychological treatments; these form the basis for the construction of reasonably firm guidelines for evidence-based practice. There has however been less research on the biological basis of bulimia nervosa, and on the extent to which this disorder may be a socially- and culturally-determined behaviour to which all or nearly all women are vulnerable if they restrain their eating to a sufficient degree.

In contrast, there is much information available on the aetiology of anorexia nervosa; but, despite awareness of the disorder for over a century, there is little evidence to guide its management. A quarter of a century ago, the prevailing view was that anorexia nervosa was an environmentally-determined disorder, and that particular patterns of family interaction played a major role in its causation. Genetic and other biological studies now suggest that particularly in the case of restricting anorexia nervosa, temperament may play an important aetiological role; the well-described family pathology may thus be the result of a severe and chronic disorder rather than its cause. A number of large studies on the treatment of anorexia nervosa are currently under way. Controversies still dog the initial approach to treatment. Is in-patient treatment best? Is coercive treatment necessary, and might such treatment produce short-term gains but long-term harm? Is re-feeding necessary before psychotherapy can begin? How can the long-term adverse consequences of a potentially fatal disorder be prevented? Perhaps the single major challenge in the eating disorder field for the next decade is to improve the effectiveness of treatment for severe anorexia nervosa.

Classification and Diagnosis

Eating disorders have been classically considered to be disturbances of appetite and of ingestive aspects of eating. Classifications of eating disorders have tended to be dichotomous in their approach, and have clustered conditions around increased or decreased eating. Clinical observation as well as advances in behavioural sciences have, however, expanded the understanding of eating, and this behaviour is now viewed as a repertoire of constructs that include appetite, estimation of food required, and satiety. Other factors that influence eating behaviour include motivation, cognitive attitudes towards food, and the linking of food with body image. The situation is complicated by the possible physical disposal of eaten food through vomiting or purging. When all these aspects of eating are considered, it becomes evident that an eating disorder will comprise any disturbance in one or more of these aspects. Thus, the complexity of eating disorders almost certainly extends beyond dichotomous conceptualizations into anorexic and bulimic syndromes; this complexity is perhaps reflected by the large number of atypical and unspecified eating disorder categories in contemporary classificatory systems. For want of adequate guidance from these classificatory systems and research, however, this chapter is constrained to view eating disorders in a largely dichotomous framework. Anorexia nervosa, bulimia nervosa, and binge-eating disorder (a potential new diagnostic category, defined for research purposes) will separately be considered.

Anorexia Nervosa

DSM-IV (American Psychiatric Association, 1994) and ICD-10 (World Health Organization, 1992) present contrasting approaches to the diagnosis of eating disorders. DSM-IV does not permit the simultaneous diagnosis of anorexia nervosa and bulimia nervosa; when criteria for both the conditions are met, anorexia nervosa is deemed to be the primary diagnosis, whether or not patients binge or purge. ICD-10 does not place any restriction in this regard. DSM-IV describes restricting and binge eating or purging subtypes of anorexia nervosa; there are no subsyndromes listed in ICD-10.

DSM-IV requires a body weight that is less than 85 per cent of that expected for age and height; this is a change from DSM-III-R, which required at least 25 per cent weight loss. In consequence, the diagnosis of anorexia nervosa has now become more common. ICD-10 is more detailed and requires the patient to either be 15 per cent under weight or have a body-mass index of 17.5 per cent or less. ICD-10 also gives more details for the symptoms to be expected in pre-pubertal anorexia nervosa.

About 50 per cent of patients who initially meet criteria for anorexia nervosa later graduate to bulimia nervosa. Some patients do move from normal weight bulimia to anorexia nervosa, but this is less common (Freeman, 1999).

Bulimia Nervosa

DSM-IV describes a binge as the consumption of an amount of food that is definitely larger than the amount that most people would eat during a similar period of time under similar circumstances. In DSM-IV, two subtypes of bulimia nervosa are described: purging and non-purging. The former category is used when there is a history of self-induced vomiting or the misuse of laxatives, diuretics, or enemas. The latter category is used when there is other inappropriate compensatory behaviour for overeating, such as fasting or excessive exercise.

ICD-10 notes that bulimia nervosa is often preceded by anorexia nervosa, which may have been fully expressed or cryptic. While DSM-IV merely describes bulimic behaviour, ICD-10 provides reasons for such a behaviour; these include a craving for food and a desire to counteract the fattening effects of eating.

There are moves to tighten the DSM-IV criteria for bulimia

nervosa and to include only the group currently described as bulimia with purging. The non-purging type would then be included under binge-eating disorder.

Binge-Eating Disorder

In a multi-site study involving 1,984 subjects, Spitzer *et al.* (1992) noted that binge-eating disorder was present in 30.1 per cent of subjects attending weight-control programs, and that its prevalence in the community was 2.0 per cent. The disorder was commoner in females than in males, and was linked to severity of obesity and marked weight fluctuations. The DSM-IV Workgroup, therefore, recommended that binge-eating disorder be included in DSM-IV. The outcome of this recommendation was the accommodation of binge-eating disorder in an appendix in DSM-IV; research criteria for its diagnosis are provided.

The chief difference between binge-eating disorder and other eating disorders is that in the former condition there is a lack of inappropriate compensatory behaviours such as purging, fasting, and excessive exercise. Hay and Fairburn (1998) examined the validity of the DSM-IV scheme for classifying recurrent binge eating. Young women (n=250) were interviewed at baseline and again, one year later. The diagnosis of bulimia nervosa was found to have good descriptive and predictive validity. While binge-eating disorder could not be distinguished from the non-purging subtype of bulimia nervosa at the first interview, clear distinctions could be made at reassessment between groups of patients. Hay and Fairburn concluded that bulimic eating disorders exist on a continuum of clinical severity, and range from bulimia nervosa, purging type (most severe) through bulimia nervosa, non-purging type (intermediate in severity) to binge-eating disorder (least severe). These findings support a diagnostic distinction between bulimia nervosa, non-purging type, and binge-eating disorder. Data on binge-eating disorder are gradually accumulating, particularly on the aspects of aetiology, epidemiology, and treatment.

Other Forms of Eating Disorders

Atypical eating disorders are classified in DSM-IV under 'Eating disorders not otherwise specified'. ICD-10 includes six atypical forms: Atypical anorexia nervosa, Atypical bulimia nervosa,

Overeating associated with other psychological disturbances, Vomiting associated with other psychological disturbances, Other eating disorders, and Eating disorder, unspecified. The use of so many additional categories testifies to the diversity of the disturbances associated with eating, as also to the extent of further research required.

Nosology : Future Prospects

The diagnostic criteria for eating disorders are under review. It will be interesting to see the future trends in the DSM and the ICD.

Under threat are the labels of anorexia and bulimia, which mean decreased and increased appetite, respectively; in anorexia and bulimia nervosa, cognitive rather than appetitive changes are central to the disorder (Schweiger and Fichter, 1997). Also under threat is the very differentiation between anorexia and bulimia nervosa; this is because many symptoms are common to these two disorders, and because the course of the two disorders may overlap. The Spectrum Hypothesis of eating disorders considers that these disorders are different sides of the same coin; accordingly, it proposes a unitary diagnosis that is subtyped by the presence or absence of specific symptoms (Andersen, 1983).

Walsh and Kahn (1997) discuss the need for clearer definitions of terms used in the current diagnostic criteria; these terms include 'body image', 'binge', and 'recurrent' and 'inappropriate' compensatory behaviour. Walsh and Kahn argue that patients and clinicians may interpret these terms differently, leading to errors in diagnosis.

Eating disorders involve certain repetitive thoughts about food; this provokes the hypothesis that eating disorders belong to the obsessive-compulsive disorder (OCD) spectrum (Kaye *et al.*, 1992). Body image disturbance in relation to eating further diversifies the possible nosological position of eating disorders. The patient's degree of control over eating behaviour also adds to the complexity; this control is increased in anorexia and intermittently breached in bulimia. Future research will no doubt identify the dimensions which will validly subtype eating disorder. Such research might need to be based on an understanding of normal eating behaviours; curiously, aspects of normalcy are yet to be integrated into psychopathological concepts in the field.

Should amenorrhoea be a criterion for the diagnosis of anorexia nervosa? This is a moot point. It is not uncommon for a young woman to present with all features of anorexia, including a very low body weight, but with intact menstrual function. What is the nosological status of such a patient? As DSM-IV indirectly acknowledges, the criterion of amenorrhoea is also inapplicable to men, and to girls who have not yet attained menarche; this suggests that there may be a scope for separate diagnostic criteria for eating disorders in males and in children.

EPIDEMIOLOGY

The epidemiology of bulimia has been much more extensively studied than that of anorexia. A possible reason is that the diagnostic criteria for bulimia nervosa are easier to apply than those for anorexia; therefore, it is more rewarding to design and conduct studies on bulimia than anorexia. Another reason is that bulimia is commoner than anorexia, and is, therefore, again more rewarding to study.

Few studies have examined the incidence of the two eating disorders. This is because estimation of incidence is difficult in both, as eating disorders tend to begin innocently with dieting or just a wish to lose weight. The incidence of eating disorders is hence usually measured retrospectively.

In their critical review of epidemiology research, Fairburn and Beglin (1990) clearly identified differences in the quality of published studies. They pointed out that observed prevalences vary widely, depending on the survey methods used. They concluded that self-report questionnaires are least likely to provide true estimates of the prevalence of bulimia nervosa. Face-to-face interviews yield prevalence rates that are closest to the true figures.

Anorexia Nervosa

In Western cultures, the prevalence of anorexia nervosa is about 0.5–1 per cent; in a review, Hsu (1996) suggested an average rate of 0.5 per cent, Hoek (1991) obtained an incidence of 6.3 per 100,000 in a large, representative sample of the Dutch population during 1985–89. Lucas *et al.* (1991) determined incidence and prevalence rates as well as long-term trends in the incidence of anorexia nervosa from 13,559 medical records of the Rochester community in Minnesota. During 1935–39, the incidence among female residents was 16.6 per 100,000. During 1950–54, the incidence decreased to 7.0 per 100,000, while during 1980–84 it increased to 26.3 per 100,000. These variations were primarily due to changes in the incidence of the disorder among girls aged 10–19 years. The incidence among men, and women aged 20 years and older remained constant, although a linear increase was found for women aged 15–24 years. The overall incidence rates after correction for age were 14.6 and 1.8 per 100,000 person-years for females and males, respectively. Prevalence rates per 100,000 population were 269.9 for females and 22.5 for males.

Eagles *et al.* (1995) found a substantial increase in the referrals of females with anorexia nervosa in Northeast Scotland between 1965 and 1991. The authors opined that the change reflected a genuine increase in incidence. They based their conclusion on the association between anorexia and affective disorders, which showed increased incidence as well. The data, however, suggest that less severely ill patients are now being referred. Hoek *et al.* (1995) concluded that no time trend existed for anorexia nervosa between 1985 and 1989 in the Netherlands. More detailed research is necessary to clarify the reasons for increased incidence or prevalence, if validly observed.

Epidemiological studies on anorexia nervosa have been summarized in Table 5.1.

Table 5.1: Epidemiological Studies on Anorexia Nervosa

Study	Sample	Period	Findings*
Hoek (1991)	Dutch general population	1985–99	I: 6.3
Lucas *et al.* (1991)	females	1935–39	I: 16.6
	females	1950–54	I: 7.0
	females	1980–84	I: 26.3
	males	1935–84	I: 1.8
	females	1935–84	I: 14.6
	males	1935–84	P: 22.5
	females	1935–84	P: 269.9
Eagles *et al.* (1995)	females	1965–91	Mean annual increase of 5.3 per cent

* abbreviations: I: incidence (per 100,000)
P: prevalence (per 100,000)

Bulimia Nervosa

The private and secretive behaviour of bulimics makes it difficult to detect the true number of patients in the community. Low awareness of the condition may result in general practitioners and physicians missing cases. Such problems have dogged earlier epidemiological research. During the last decade, however, extensive studies have been conducted using strict diagnostic criteria, and these have yielded more reliable figures.

Hoek (1991) reported that one-year prevalence of bulimia nervosa in primary care was 1.5 per cent in the Netherlands. In the same population, he reported a yearly incidence of 11.4 per 100,000 during 1985–89. Interestingly, the general practitioners had detected only 11 per cent of the prevalent cases, and only half of detected cases had been referred to mental health facilities. Fairburn and Beglin (1990) described an average rate of 1 per cent in their epidemiology review, while Hsu (1996) suggested that the figure is closer to 2 per cent.

Kendler *et al.* (1991) observed that the prevalence of bulimia nervosa had increased from 0.8 per cent in 25-years-old females born before 1950 to 1.1 per cent in those born between 1950 and 1959 to 3.7 per cent in those born after 1959. Hoek *et al.* (1995) found that the increasing incidence of bulimia nervosa was specific to the more urbanized areas. Heatherton *et al.* (1995), however, found that the prevalence of bulimia nervosa in American college students reduced between 1982 and 1992. Subjects in 1992 reported healthier eating habits, but were more likely to be overweight.

Fombonne (1996) reviewed epidemiological studies conducted since 1980 and concluded that the prevalence of eating disorders had not changed. He suggested that changes in diagnostic and referral practice may account for the increased numbers of patients seen for treatment. Hsu (1996) observed that eating disorders appear to have become more common during the last ten years, but only in Western cultures. He opined that the rate of increase was not high, and that it may now have reached a plateau. While the recent increase in the diagnosis of bulimia nervosa may be related to increased population size as well as to greater awareness amongst patients and clinicians alike, a true time trend cannot be ruled out; this is, therefore, a question for future research.

Epidemiological studies on bulimia nervosa have been summarized in Table 5.2.

Table 5.2: Epidemiological Studies on Bulimia Nervosa

Study	Sample	Period	Findings*
Hoek (1991)	Dutch general population	1985–99	I: 11.4 P: 1.5
Kendler (1991)	25-years-old females	1974	P: 0.8
	25-years-old females	1975–84	P: 1.1
	25-years-old females	1985	P: 3.7

* abbreviations: I: incidence (per 100,000)
P: prevalence (%)

Binge-Eating Disorder

The diagnosis of binge-eating disorder appears to be becoming commoner, and the disorder prevails in obese persons (Goldfein *et al.*, 1993; Ferguson and Spitzer, 1995); this may merely reflect an increased awareness of the condition amongst clinicians and public alike. Since the available diagnostic criteria are neither definitive nor widely accepted, no reliable data are as yet available about the epidemiology of this disorder. Appropriate studies remain to be conducted.

Special Groups

Males represent about 10 per cent of all cases of eating disorders (Fairburn and Beglin, 1990; Hsu, 1996; Andersen and Holman, 1997). Several studies show a disturbed psychosexual and gender identity development in males with anorexia or bulimia nervosa (Fichter and Daser, 1987; Andersen and Holman, 1997); these may be possible risk factors for eating disorders in males. The small number of cases makes it difficult to describe a distinction between males and females in aetiology and symptomatology.

Turnbull *et al.* (1987) described five cases of men with bulimia nervosa, all of whom had clinically significant and distressing pathology. The illnesses of these patients would have been missed had the most widely used rating scales (Eating Disorder Inventory (EDI) and Eating Attitude Test (EAT)) been used for screening. Therefore, care is necessary when assessing and diagnosing males through the commonly used assessment instruments that have been developed largely for females.

Studies on the epidemiology of eating disorders in *children* are rare and contradictory. Some describe an increase in rates of anorexia, while others show a decrease from an already low figure. Data on the prevalence of bulimia are even scantier. Several studies show a different gender division in children, with estimates for males reaching as much as 30 per cent of all cases of anorexia nervosa (Bryant-Waugh and Lask, 1995). The problems of accurate diagnosis are similar to those that occur with male groups. Amenorrhoea as a symptom can only be applied to post-menarcheal females. Estimating low body weight may be problematic as it can be difficult to decide what a child's normal weight should be. The diagnosis may be further confounded by an impaired growth resulting from the eating disorder. Bryant-Waugh and Lask (1995) suggested specific diagnostic criteria for childhood onset of anorexia nervosa: (a) determined food avoidance, (b) a failure to maintain the steady weight gain expected for age, or actual weight loss, and (c) overconcern with weight and shape.

The epidemiology of eating disorders has been extensively studied in *non-whites*. However, only a few studies have measured prevalences in non-whites in their country of origin. Most studies describe comparisons between white and non-white populations in the same, Western, society. This has resulted in data which are mainly applicable to non-white immigrants to Western societies, who have, to a greater or lesser extent, adapted to cultural standards in their new country. Regrettably, most comparisons between countries have utilized self-report questionnaires; the resultant data are possibly biased (Fairburn and Beglin, 1990). Based on data from the USA, Pike and Walsh (1996) reported that the incidence of anorexia nervosa and bulimia nervosa in non-Caucasian females comprised 2–5 per cent and 1–4 per cent (respectively) of all cases with these diagnoses. Binge-eating disorder was, however, similar in prevalence in both Caucasian and non-Caucasian groups. Reiss (1996) compared African-Caribbean and white British female family planning clinic attendees using the Bulimic Investigatory Test, Edinburgh (BITE) and the General Health Questionnaire. The African-Caribbean group showed a significantly higher level of abnormal eating behaviour, which could not be explained by a significantly higher body-mass index. This may indicate a high prevalence of eating problems in African-Caribbeans. Whether these subjects actually suffer from eating disorders to a similarly high extent requires more detailed assessments.

Mumford *et al.* (1991, 1992) studied the incidence of eating disorders in Asian schoolgirls in Lahore, Pakistan, as well as in Asian schoolgirls in Bradford, UK. In Lahore, girls with high scores on the EAT were interviewed to determine whether they suffered from any DSM-III-R eating disorder. Among 368 girls in English medium schools, one girl met full criteria for bulimia nervosa and five subjects had partial syndrome bulimia nervosa. None was diagnosed with anorexia nervosa. The prevalence of bulimia nervosa among Asian girls in Bradford was 3.4 per cent which was much higher than that in Lahore. However, the Asian community in Bradford came from an underdeveloped region of Pakistan, while Lahore is a large city. In order to rule out socioeconomic factors in aetiopathogenesis, Choudry and Mumford (1992) studied schoolgirls in Mirpur, Pakistan, which is the region from which the families in Bradford hailed. A new Urdu translation of the EAT was used, and girls scoring above 20 were interviewed. Among 271 schoolgirls, one case of bulimia nervosa was identified. The greater vulnerability of the Bradford Asians thus appeared to result from exposure to a Western culture. Cultural stresses within their traditional families could have further contributed to a vulnerability to (or protection against!) eating disorders.

Chaturvedi (1998; personal communication) carried out a large survey among 797 students from different colleges in Bangalore, India. He found no cases of eating disorders using the BITE, and only two subthreshold cases of eating disorders in those who were assessed using DSM-III-R diagnostic criteria.

Lee *et al.* (1989) and Lee (1991) described several cases of anorexia nervosa in Chinese females in Hong Kong. The rapid Westernization of this state may have resulted in an increased adoption of Western ideals of beauty, leading to an increase in dieting behaviour; nevertheless, Lee *et al.* (1989) argued that the rates of eating disorders in Hong Kong are unlikely to reach Western proportions because the Chinese socio-cultural environment tends to protect persons from such disorders. Close family control as well as a slightly obese figure being considered as the ideal body shape both contribute to a lesser likelihood of desire to diet and to be thin.

Lee (1991) found that patients commonly attributed poor food intake to abdominal bloating. Striving for thinness was hardly part of the aetiology found. However, the author expected that with Westernization, clinical patterns might gradually change. Lee *et al.* (1996) stated that 'the typically 'Western' pattern of body dissatisfaction has overshadowed the traditional Chinese notions of female beauty based on the face and other nontruncal features.' Lee and Lee (1996) found that 'disordered eating behaviour was related to body dissatisfaction and, to a lesser extent, to family cohesion and conflict.' They concluded that Western patterns of body dissatisfaction and disordered eating attitudes are increasing among Chinese adolescent females. They expected more weight-control behaviour and eating disorders to arise in Hong Kong in the future. A similar, progressive increase in the prevalence of eating disorders may occur in other Asian countries as well, when Western cultural values mix with the traditional Eastern values.

Co-morbidity

Eating disorders are frequently comorbid with other psychiatric disorders, and this comorbidity has been well studied. The most common comorbid conditions are affective disorders (particularly depression) and OCD. Other anxiety disorders, personality disorders, and substance abuse disorders have also been described as comorbid accompaniments. Opinions have been expressed that eating disorders may be better classified under the psychiatric syndromes with which they are commonly comorbid. However, the characteristics of eating disorders are unique and profound, and eating disorders are clearly comorbid with several different psychiatric conditions rather than just one. Therefore, eating disorders almost certainly deserve an independent nosological status.

Comorbidity studies should be viewed from an age perspective. This is because as age advances, the opportunity for the occurrence of comorbidity increases. In particular, certain psychiatric disorders develop only during later life; thus, comorbidity in older samples may arise out of chance co-occurrence of disorders rather than out of a direct association.

Affective Disorders

Most patients with anorexia nervosa develop symptoms of physical and emotional disturbance at some point during the course of their illness. These symptoms include lack of energy, tiredness, irritability, poor concentration, and social withdrawal. It is often difficult to determine whether such symptoms are due to depression or starvation.

A lifetime history of unipolar mood disorder characterizes a substantial number of patients with eating disorders; major depression is more common in patients with mixed disorder (anorexia/bulimia nervosa) than in those with either eating disorder alone (Halmi *et al.*, 1991; Fornari *et al.*, 1992; Herzog *et al.*, 1992). Major depression occurs more frequently in family members of bulimic patients than can be expected on the basis of chance (Strober and Humphrey, 1987); however, there is no corresponding excess of eating disorders in family members of patients with major depression (Freeman, 1999). This conflicts with the hypotheses that propose a common pathogenesis between major depression and eating disorders. Bipolar disorder is seldom comorbid with eating disorders.

Anxiety Disorders

Halmi *et al.* (1991) reported a 65 per cent lifetime prevalence of anxiety disorders in patients with anorexia nervosa. The most common anxiety disorders were social phobia and OCD. OCD was more common in patients who did not binge. The anxieties generally concerned food and food-related subjects or, in social phobia, food-related situations such as eating in public. Fornari *et al.* (1992) suggested that bulimic anorectics were significantly more likely than restricting anorectics to receive a lifetime diagnosis of OCD. Thiel *et al.* (1995) found that 37 per cent of 93 women with either anorexia or bulimia nervosa met DSM-III-R criteria for OCD. These patients had a significantly higher score on the EDI than eating disorder patients without OCD. As discussed elsewhere in this chapter, Srinivasagam *et al.* (1995) found consistent obsessive behaviour in patients who had recovered from anorexia nervosa. Srinivasagam *et al.*, therefore, suggested that obsessive traits may be related to the onset of the eating disorder rather than arising as a consequence of the disorder or as an unrelated condition.

Personality Disorders

Herzog *et al.* (1992) studied psychiatric comorbidity in 229 female patients seeking treatment for eating disorders. All subjects were interviewed using the Structured Interview for DSM-III-R Personality Disorders. Twenty-seven per cent of the sample aged over 18 years received a diagnosis of at least one personality disorder. Thirty-nine per cent of patients with mixed anorexia/bulimia had at least one personality disorder as compared with 22 per cent of patients with anorexia alone, and 21 per cent of patients with bulimia alone; the difference was statistically significant. Among anorectics, the commonest diagnoses were avoidant (7 per cent) and compulsive (7 per cent) personality disorders. Among bulimics, the commonest diagnoses were borderline (6 per cent) and histrionic (6 per cent) personality disorders. Among patients with mixed anorexia and bulimia, borderline personality disorder was diagnosed to a significantly greater extent (12 per cent) than in the anorectic (0 per cent) and bulimic (6 per cent) patients.

Skodol *et al.* (1993) obtained similar findings: anorexia nervosa was most commonly associated with avoidant personality disorder, and bulimia nervosa with borderline personality disorder. Eating disorder patients who manifested personality disorder comorbidity showed greater chronicity of illness, lower levels of functioning, and possibly poorer treatment outcome at follow-up than patients with eating disorders alone (see also Walsh and Kahn, 1997).

Substance Abuse

Herzog *et al.* (1992) found current substance abuse to be low in patients with eating disorders. While no substance abuse was observed in anorectics, the prevalence was only 5 per cent in bulimics and 8 per cent in subjects with mixed anorexia and bulimia. Lifetime prevalences of substance abuse comorbidity were, however, higher: 12 per cent in anorexia, 31 per cent in bulimia, and 37 per cent in the mixed group. The low rate of substance abuse in anorexia was due to a lower incidence of alcohol consumption.

Wiederman and Pryor (1996) studied 134 women with anorexia and 320 women with bulimia. Even after controlling for age and severity of the eating disorder, bulimics were more likely than anorectics to have used alcohol, amphetamines, barbiturates, marijuana, tranquillizers, and cocaine. For both eating disorders, the severity of caloric restriction was predictive of amphetamine use. Severity of bingeing was predictive of tranquillizer use, and severity of purging was predictive of alcohol, cocaine, and cigarette use. As bulimics have been found to be more impulsive, the authors suggested that the personality styles of these patients may be related to the relatively greater incidence of substance abuse.

In a study on the prevalence of eating disorders in alcohol-dependent men and women, bulimia nervosa, but not anorexia nervosa, was diagnosed more often than expected. Bulimia was significantly more prevalent in females (3.5 per cent) than in males (0.7 per cent) (Schuckit *et al.*, 1996).

Co-morbidity in Males

In anorexia nervosa, low body weight results in lower energy and lower sex drive in both women and men. In men, alterations in sexual orientation may also be observed. In a group of 135 males with eating disorders, Carlet *et al.* (1997) observed diagnosis-related differences in sexual orientation. Among the bulimic patients, 42 per cent were judged to be either homosexual or bisexual; among the anorectics, 58 per cent were deemed to be virtually asexual on account of a very low sexual drive. In this study, comorbid psychiatric disorders were also common: 54 per cent of the patients were diagnosed with major depression disorder, 37 per cent with substance abuse, and 26 per cent with a personality disorder.

In a related context, Fichter and Daser (1987) suggested that atypical gender role behaviour may play a role in the aetiology of eating disorders in males.

AETIOPATHOGENESIS

The aetiopathogenesis of eating disorders can be viewed from many different angles (Table 5.3). Leon *et al.* (1997) classified aetiological factors according to psychological, cultural and familial, developmental, and biological influences. Schweiger and Fichter (1997) provided an even more detailed description; important additions were the influence of dysfunctional cognitions and the effects of cognitive restraint, both of which are found frequently in patients with eating disorders. The authors also mentioned the possible contribution of traumatic experiences and psychiatric comorbidity to the onset and genesis of eating disorders. In interpreting the significant association of various phenomena with eating disorders, it must be kept in mind that such associations may be causal to, resultant from, or coincidental with the eating disorders.

Table 5.3: Aetiopathogenetic Mechanisms Implicated in Eating Disorders

Socioeconomic factors
Familial, cultural, and social factors
Stress and life events
Personality factors
Psychiatric co-morbidity
Body image distortion and body disparagement
Dieting·
Genetic factors
Brain structure and function
Serotonergic dysregulation
Neuroendocrine factors
Opioids
Leptin

Socioeconomic Status

It has long been believed that eating disorders arise chiefly in higher socioeconomic strata. Reviewing the literature on the social class distribution of eating disorders, Gard and Freeman (1996), however, concluded that 'theories of aetiology reliant upon this stereotype must be questioned.' While the relationship between anorexia nervosa and high socioeconomic status has not been proven, there is evidence for a skewed relationship between bulimia nervosa and socioeconomic status, suggesting that bulimia is more common in lower socioeconomic strata (Gard and Freeman, 1996).

The Role of the Family, Culture, and Society

Cultural ideas about beauty, expressed by the media and reinforced by family and friends, undoubtedly motivate young persons to strive for the ideal shape through dieting behaviour. At the same time, poor family relationships may increase a young person's need for control, which could be expressed through abnormal expressions of bodily self-restriction. However, neither of these factors has been consistently found significant across studies.

The prevalence of anorexia nervosa has remained unchanged, while that of bulimia nervosa appears to have risen; therefore, social and cultural factors may be playing a more important role in the aetiology of the latter. Public ideals about body shape may prompt dieting behaviour; since the urge to binge increases with restriction of food intake, bulimic patterns may emerge (Lowe, 1993).

Tiggeman and Pickering (1996) administered questionnaires to 94 adolescent women who reported on the quantity of time that they spent watching television, the type of programs that they watched, and the level of body dissatisfaction that they experienced. Drive for thinness was also assessed. It was found that the time spent watching television did not correlate with body dissatisfaction or drive for thinness. However, the type of programs watched did: watching soap operas and movies correlated positively with body dissatisfaction, while watching sports was correlated negatively. Watching music videos was most strongly related to drive for thinness. Leon *et al.* (1997) pointed out that the media influences body (dis)satisfaction and dieting behaviour only if family and friends reinforce the picture portrayed.

The Influence of Stress and Life Events

The possible contribution of traumatic experiences to the onset of eating disorders has been investigated and discussed by several researchers. The increased likelihood of past physical or sexual abuse among patients with eating disorders is not significantly greater than among those with other psychiatric illnesses (Welch and Fairburn, 1994; Schweiger and Fichter, 1997). More extensive studies have recently been published.

Welch *et al.* (1997) compared the occurrence of specific life events during the year before the onset of bulimia nervosa in 102 bulimic women and 204 control women without an eating disorder. Life events which significantly differentiated bulimic women from controls were a major house move, a significant episode of physical illness, pregnancy, a member joining or leaving the family, physical abuse, and sexual abuse. Life events which did not differ between the two groups were bereavement, a major episode of illness in a close relative or friend, the formation of a new relationship with a partner, or the termination of an existing relationship.

Welch *et al.* suggested that specific life events may play a role in precipitating the onset of bulimia. This hypothesis is probably premature on at least two counts. First, the opinions of Welch *et al.* notwithstanding, there did not appear to be any meaningful pattern distinguishing the life events that were significantly associated with bulimia from the life events that were not. Second, no evidence in psychiatry so far exists to indicate that specific psychosocial stresses induce specific biological changes, thereby predisposing to specific psychiatric disorders.

A more reasonable interpretation of the findings is that bulimia, like many other psychiatric states, may be precipitated by the experience of stress which cumulates non-specifically. This interpretation will remain valid until other retrospective studies (if not prospective research) uncover data that, in support of the Welch *et al.* conjecture, demonstrate that specific stresses are *consistently* associated with specific disorders.

In another study, Schmidt *et al.* (1997) presented data on 72 patients with anorexia nervosa, 29 with bulimia nervosa, and two groups of retrospective community controls. All but two patients were women. Life events and difficulties were studied for the year before the onset of the eating disorder in the patient groups, and in the previous year in the control groups.

The patient groups were observed to have experienced somewhat more stress than controls. The stressors were most commonly interpersonal in nature. Bulimic patients experienced significantly more interpersonal stressors than anorexic patients. Anorexic patients experienced significantly more problems related to sexuality than bulimic patients or controls; these problems resulted in feelings of shame and disgust. If anorexia nervosa is viewed as a form of self-harm, it may represent a reaction to such feelings of bodily shame or disgust.

While it is tempting to speculate that interpersonal and sexual stresses precipitate bulimia and anorexia respectively, simpler explanations must first be considered. Some caveats have already been discussed in the context of Welch *et al.* study. Another possibility which bears consideration is that there may be a common predisposition to the eating disorder and to the experience of a specific stress.

There are two strands of evidence which indirectly support such a common predisposition hypothesis. First, Troop and Treasure

(1997) found that during their childhood, women with eating disorders (n=43) had experienced greater helplessness and lesser mastery than normal controls (n=20). These traits of reduced ability to cope with stress during childhood resemble the poor adjustment during childhood of persons who later manifest neurodevelopmental schizophrenia. Second, Kendler and Karkowski-Schuman (1997) found that genetic risk factors for major depression may increase the probability of experiencing specific interpersonal and occupational or financial stressful life events.

These studies call for a revision of the stance that stress and life events precipitate psychiatric disorders. Apparently, there is a case for the hypothesis that the experience of life events is not as independent as earlier believed. Certain of these thoughts are currently under examination by behavioural geneticists who consider that many behaviours may be genetically predetermined. Clearly, research in this field is poised at an interesting point.

Personality Factors

Among the various psychological factors that may contribute to the aetiology of eating disorders, the most apparent are personality and temperament, more specifically obsessive and neurotic traits. There appears to be a relationship between certain core symptoms of anorexia nervosa (high striving for control over the body) and obsessional personality traits. Srinivasagam *et al.* (1995) investigated the persistence of perfectionistic and obsessive behaviour in 20 patients who had recovered from anorexia nervosa. Subjects were at normal weight and had been menstruating regularly for more than a year. These patients were compared with 16 healthy women using several self-report scales (EDI, Frost Multi-dimensional Perfectionism Scale, and the Yale-Brown Obsessive Compulsive Scale). The recovered anorectics scored significantly higher on all scales, indicating persistence of certain characteristics of anorexia nervosa after recovery. The authors suggested that the higher scores on these scales may describe personality traits that contribute to the pathogenesis of anorexia nervosa. More research, with larger samples of recovered patients, is needed to draw firm conclusions. It would also be interesting to follow-up children with obsessive traits to assess their likelihood of developing eating disorders.

Psychiatric Co–morbidity

Eating disorders and affective disorders are frequently comorbid (Halmi, 1997; Wonderlich and Mitchell, 1997). Therefore, a comparison of eating disorders (particularly bulimia nervosa and binge-eating disorder) and affective disorders may yield valuable insights. It is interesting that physical and psychological treatments that are effective in patients with affective disorders are also effective in patients with bulimia nervosa and binge-eating disorder; this is discussed in more detail later in this chapter. Distorted cognitions have been shown to play an important role in the onset of depression, and cognitive behaviour therapy (CBT) is useful in depressed patients. Since eating disorders (especially bulimia nervosa and binge-eating disorder) often present with many features of depression, cognitive distortions may similarly be involved in their onset. Distorted thoughts about true weight and shape as compared to a perceived ideal body image may initiate dieting behaviour. The discovery of vomiting and the use of laxatives or excessive exercise to compensate for overeating can lead to the disturbed idea that one can eat anything, and as much as one wishes, without putting on extra weight. At first this appears appealing and convenient, but as the amount eaten and the compensatory behaviour increases in frequency and magnitude, the general health of the individual deteriorates, and the diagnosis of an eating disorder becomes inevitable.

Body Image Distortion and Body Disparagement

One of the core features of eating disorders is a lack of satisfaction with the body image. This image is a construct that develops along with physical and cognitive development. The comparison between social ideals of beauty and body image results in a certain degree of body satisfaction or dissatisfaction. This satisfaction or dissatisfaction varies across individuals depending upon actual physical appearance, body image, psychological sensitivity to public opinion, and opinions expressed in social and family circles. In general, women are more inclined to be dissatisfied with the size and shape of their body; those who develop an eating disorder are even less happy and more eager to lose weight.

Bulimic patients who do not wish to reduce their food intake, or who are inclined to binge, are not necessarily unhappy with their body size; however, they fear an increase in body weight as a result of their high food intake. In contrast, anorectics clearly have a distorted picture of an ideal body size and shape; they tend to strive for a body which is thin beyond safety limits for reasonable health. Once ill, anorectics cannot distinguish such a body size from the healthy minimum. Possibly reinforcing the dysfunctional cogntions of anorectic patients is the fact that the body-mass index of fashion models is generally below 20, while the preferred average for minimum mortality is 22.

It is difficult to measure how persons actually perceive and estimate their own body. Smeets (1995) extensively researched this issue and concluded that there is clear evidence that anorectics show a disturbance of body image rather than of body size perception. Smeets (1997) therefore recommended cognitive neurological research on the top-down influence of thoughts and feelings on perception and estimation of visual cues. An interesting case report in this connection is that of a woman who had been totally blind since the age of two. She developed anorexia nervosa when she was 21 (Yager and Hatton, 1986). Thus, visual cues are not essential to feel fat and to wish to be thin.

The Role of Dieting

Several of the aetiopathogenetic mechanisms discussed so far elicit dieting behaviour rather than the eating disorder *per se*. Can dieting cause an eating disorder? Lowe (1993) suggested that dieting increases the urge to binge, thus paving the way for the development of bulimic patterns of eating. Hsu (1997) reviewed the evidence on the subject in a recent editorial. He examined five longitudinal investigations that had studied the evolution of eating disorders; all pointed to the role of dieting behaviour in the pathogenesis of eating disorders.

Not all dieters proceed to develop an eating disorder, and not all persons with an eating disorder have a previous history of pathological dieting; obviously, therefore, other risk factors must also be involved. Hsu identified a family history of eating disorders, mood disorder, and possibly alcohol or substance abuse as other important risk factors. He concluded that dieting may hence be more likely to precipitate an eating disorder if such other risk factors are present.

Genetic Factors

The genetics of eating disorders have been poorly investigated; a possible reason is the difficulty in defining valid phenotypes given the currently available tools and concepts about eating disorders. Reviews of family studies show that there is an increased incidence of anorexia and bulimia nervosa in the family members of probands. After controlling for environmental influences, twin studies (in clinic populations) reveal a definite genetic influence: there is a higher concordance in monozygotic than in dizygotic twins (Spelt and Meyer, 1995; Walters and Kendler, 1995). By way of example, in twins with anorexia nervosa, Holland *et al.* (1984) reported a concordance of 56 per cent for monozygotic twins and 7 per cent for dizygotic twins. In general, however, the data appear more robust for bulimia than for anorexia.

The only population-based twin study revealed a relationship between bulimia nervosa, depression, panic, and phobias (Kendler *et al.*, 1991 and 1995). Surprisingly, though it is known that eating behaviours like total calorie intake and beverage intake appear to have some genetic programming, there have been no major genetic studies of other dysfunctional eating traits.

Brain Structure and Function

A longitudinal magnetic resonance imaging (MRI) study of brain changes in adolescents with anorexia nervosa found that white matter changes were reversible after weight gain, but grey matter volume deficits were not (Katzman *et al.*, 1997).

Unilateral temporal hypoperfusion was discovered in children with anorexia nervosa; in 8 cases, the hypoperfusion was observed in the left temporal lobe, and in 5 cases the hypoperfusion was observed in the right temporal lobe. Three of these patients recovered, but the abnormality persisted in follow-up scans (Gordon *et al.*, 1997).

Patients with anorexia nervosa show general and local hypometabolism, which persists beyond the acute stages of the illness, and which may be a result of starvation (Delvenne *et al.*, 1997a). An increase in caudate nucleus glucose metabolism was noticed in anorexia relative to bulimia (Krieg *et al.*, 1991). Left anterolateral prefrontal cortex hypometabolism varied with the depressive symptoms in bulimia nervosa, but temporal lobe hypermetabolism and asymmetries appeared independent of mood state (Andreason *et al.*, 1992). Parietal cortex metabolism was significantly lower in at least one study of bulimic patients (Delvenne *et al.*, 1997b). In these studies, state-dependent changes, however, could be ruled out.

Regard and Landis (1997) observed that right anterior lesions in cortical, basal ganglia, and limbic regions were associated with preoccupation with food and fine eating. Chipkevitch (1994) found that brain tumours, especially those of the hypothalamus, mimicked typical or atypical anorexia nervosa; in this report, 33 per cent of 19 tumours were germ cell neoplasms.

Serotonin Dysregulation

Evidence for a serotonergic basis for eating disorders comes from both preclinical and clinical studies. The comorbidity of eating disorders, depression, and OCD may reflect underlying serotonergic dysregulation. Pharmacological challenge studies in bulimic patients show a decreased serum prolactin response to both fenfluramine (Jimerson *et al.*, 1997) and mCPP. (Levitan *et al.*, 1997), suggesting decreased serotonergic responsivity. Tryptophan depletion in bulimic patients leads to increased food intake and irritability (Weltzin *et al.*, 1995). Decreased levels of CSF 5-HIAA correlate with severity of bingeing in bulimia (Jimerson *et al.*, 1992). These data further support the notion that decreased serotonergic function is associated with bulimia. Serotonin-amplified platelet aggregation is increased in normal-weight bulimics as compared with healthy controls and restricting anorectics; successful treatment does not alter this response (McBride *et al.*, 1991). This implies an increased 5-HT2 sensitivity in bulimic patients, such as might result from a hyposerotonergic state.

Serotonergic dysfunction has also been reported in anorexia nervosa, but the causal effect of malnutrition herein cannot be ruled out. Weight-restored anorectics and controls show similar responses to d-fenfluramine challenge, suggesting that nutritional factors perhaps underlie the 5-HT abnormalities observed in anorexia (O'Dwyer *et al.*, 1996).

Neuroendocrine Factors

Hypothalamic-pituitary adrenal (HPA) axis abnormalities have been described in eating disorders. Corticotrophin-Releasing Hormone (CRH) blocks Growth Hormone Releasing Hormone (GHRH)-induced Growth Hormone (GH) release in healthy subjects but not in patients with anorexia nervosa and atypical eating disorders (Eating Disorder Not Otherwise Specified) Rolla *et al.*, 1994). Hexarelin stimulation blocks GHRH-induced GH surge in normals and in subjects with weight-loss related amenorrhoea, but not in anorectic children (Popovic *et al.*, 1997). Thus, this HPA abnormality may be anorexia-specific and not just related to weight loss.

In one study, GHRH increased food intake in anorexia nervosa (Vaccarino *et al.*, 1994). Hypercortisolism in anorexia may be associated with increased central CRH levels and normal circulating levels of adrenocorticotrophic hormone (Kaye, 1996).

Sundblad *et al.* (1994) reported high levels of serum testosterone in patients with bulimia, and hypothesized a relationship between testosterone and increased impulsive behaviours such as bingeing; however, it remains to be demonstrated that bulimic subjects with multiple dyscontrol behaviours have elevated testosterone levels. There is an increased incidence of ovarian dysfunction in normal-weight women with bulimia nervosa (Schweiger *et al.*, 1992). A high prevalence of polysystic ovaries has been observed in bulimic women whose weight was restored (McCluskey *et al.*, 1991).

Osmoregulatory dysfunction in bulimia nervosa has also been studied. This dysfunction may result in a compensatory increase in arginine vasopressin levels. Arginine vasopressin has been linked with the obsessional preoccupation with aversive consequences of eating and weight gain (Demitrack *et al.*, 1992). Melatonin levels in patients with anorexia and bulimia nervosa are lower than in controls (Kennedy, 1994). However, in another study melatonin levels were found to be normal in patients with both eating disorders, after depression was controlled for (Mortola *et al.*, 1993).

The Role of Endogenous Opioids

The addiction model of anorexia nervosa proposes that anorectics become addicted to the starvation state; in these patients, food intake produces dysphoria and withdrawal symptoms. Many anorectics report not just a sense of control, but a feeling of being very 'high' when they successfully restrict for long periods.

The addiction model further proposes that high level of endogenous opiods are released during dieting; this reinforces dieting behaviour (Marrazzi *et al.*, 1997). A higher opiod tonus has been described in bulimics as well: Vescovi *et al.* (1996) reported an increased 24-hour beta endorphin secretion in normal-weight bulimic women as compared with controls.

The Role of Leptin

Leptin is a 167 amino acid peptide coded by 'ob' (obesity genes). Autosomal recessive ob/ob mutation in mice gives rise to infertile, hyperphagic, obese strains. While leptin infusion leads to weight loss in mice, the presence of obesity makes leptin ineffective (Considine, 1997).

Low leptin levels have been associated with amenorrhoea (Kopp *et al.*, 1997). Serum leptin levels show a linear association with body-mass index (Ferron *et al.*, 1997). Leptin levels in plasma and CSF are low during the acute phase of anorexia nervosa, and normalize with weight gain (Hebebrand *et al.*, 1997a; Mantzoros *et al.*, 1997); the underlying mechanism may be a change in the body-mass index. Thus, leptin may not be aetiopathogenetically related to anorexia. The relationship of leptin to bulimia is even more tenuous as serum leptin levels do not differ between binge-eating and non-binge-eating obese women (Karhunen *et al.*, 1997).

TREATMENT

Treatment studies of eating disorders have largely focused on drug therapy versus psychotherapy. The results have been varied. Some drugs were effective for certain symptoms only, while others were effective for only one of the eating disorders, usually bulimia nervosa. With psychotherapy, only the later, structured therapies were effective in eating disorders; again, bulimic patients appeared to respond better. The better response of bulimia to treatment may be because it is easier to handle positive symptoms (such as bingeing and vomiting) than negative ones (such as food restriction). This section presents an overview of interesting findings in the treatment of anorexia nervosa, bulimia nervosa and, to the extent possible, binge-eating disorder. For a more comprehensive overview, the reader is referred to the American Psychiatric Association (1993) guidelines.

Anorexia Nervosa

Patients who suffer from anorexia nervosa often strongly feel that they do not want or need treatment. This makes treatment programmes difficult to implement. General principles for the treatment of anorectics may therefore be enunciated as follows (Freeman, 1999):

1. The initial interview, assessment, and subsequent engagement and treatment are of vital importance, and need time and considerable skill.
2. Psychological treatment is the treatment of choice. Experience in treating anorectic patients is probably more important than the type of psychotherapy used.
3. In-patient treatment may be required for some patients, and a small number will require compulsory treatment to prevent them from dying.
4. Psychological treatment is impractical and of little benefit in severely starving patients. Such patients first require a degree of weight restoration.
5. The treatment needs to involve significant others (family of origin and/or partner), though this does not need to be in the form of systematized family therapy.
6. Treatment needs to be flexible, and should be adapted to suit the patient's needs. Treatment approaches in the past have been too rigid.
7. Treatment cannot be brief. Treatment services therefore need to be organized so as to provide continuity of care throughout the various phases of treatment.

There are few data to support any specific treatment for anorexia nervosa. The pharmacotherapy and psychotherapy research is limited to a few studies conducted on small samples. It is therefore a common practice to combine both forms of therapy to treat anorectics; however, no empirical data support this strategy.

Brambilla and colleagues studied the efficacy of combined cognitive behaviour therapy (CBT), nutritional counselling and antidepressant drug therapy in 22 female patients with anorexia nervosa, restricted type (Brambilla *et al.*, 1995a) and 13 female patients with anorexia nervosa, binge-eating/purging type (Brambilla *et al.*, 1995b). In the first group, during the four months of therapy patients who had received nortriptyline (n=7) as well as those who had received fluoxetine (n=15) improved significantly and comparably on body-mass index and on ratings of depression and anxiety. While the EDI scores also improved, ratings on the BITE did not change. Similar results were obtained in the binge eating/purging patients who had received amineptine (n=7) or fluoxetine (n=6). Findings in both groups need to be validated in larger samples and across longer courses of therapy. Long-term follow-up also requires investigation.

While Gwirtsman *et al.* (1990) found that fluoxetine reduced depressive symptoms and induced weight gain in six patients with anorexia nervosa, Strober *et al.* (1997) found no additional benefit with fluoxetine in the follow-up treatment of anorexia patients who had participated in an intensive, multi-disciplinary treatment program.

The Maudsley group of studies is the best known amongst trials of psychotherapy for anorexia nervosa; the results available to-date have been presented by Dare and Eisler (1995). Study I compared individual and family therapy in 80 patients of all ages. The group with early onset (less than 19 years) and short history (less than 3 years) of anorexia had much better 1-year follow-up results with family therapy as compared with individual therapy. Patients with short history but late onset of illness, however, showed better follow-up weight maintenance after individual supportive therapy rather than family therapy. These findings were confirmed at 5-year follow-ups.

Study II examined the treatment of 100 severely ill adult patients with anorexia nervosa and low-weight bulimia nervosa. At the time the Dare and Eisler (1995) chapter was written, patients who had received family therapy appeared to have a better outcome than those who had received individual therapy: nearly two-thirds of the family therapy group had either a good or an intermediate outcome at 1-year follow-up. Outcome with family therapy was good in bulimic patients as well, but the small sample precludes confident conclusions.

Study III compared family therapy and family counselling in adolescent patients. There were no significant differences between treatments at the end of therapy; the trends that were observed favoured the simpler, counselling treatment. Interestingly, families with high criticality of the ill child appeared to benefit more from family counselling than from family therapy; this was thought to be because during counselling there is more time and opportunity to address such issues. Follow-up data on this study are as yet unavailable.

Study IV is currently under way; it addresses family therapy as compared to individual focal therapy and standard out-patient treatment.

Bulimia Nervosa

Research has highlighted the usefulness of antidepressant drugs in the treatment of bulimia nervosa. These drugs improve mood and reduce unhealthy eating behaviour, but may not completely stop bulimic symptoms. In the short term, antidepressants appear to be almost as effective as cognitive behaviour therapy. Long-term effects require more research, and the issue of how long treatment should last also remains to be resolved.

Pope *et al.* (1983) found a good response to imipramine, as compared to placebo, in 11 chronically bulimic women. The subjects had been recruited from different sources, and were not necessarily depressed at intake. A significant reduction in binge eating was maintained even after 8 months of treatment. In a 12-week trial, McCann and Agras (1990) randomized 23 female, non-purging bulimics to desipramine (n = 10) or placebo (n = 13) treatment categories. There was a 63 per cent reduction in binge eating in the former group, and only 16 per cent reduction in the latter.

Walsh *et al.* (1991) studied the effect of desipramine in 80 bulimic patients. During the first 8 weeks, desipramine reduced binge eating to a significantly greater extent than did placebo (47 per cent vs 7 per cent). Less than half of these patients, however, met the response criteria for entry into the maintenance phase. During 4 months of maintenance treatment, 29 per cent of the patients entering the maintenance phase relapsed. There were too few patients during the final phase to permit conclusion on the long-term effects of desipramine in the treatment of binge eating.

Fairburn *et al.* (1993) compared CBT with behaviour therapy (BT) and interpersonal therapy (IPT) in the treatment of bulimia nervosa. BT resulted in a strong reduction of behavioural symptoms; at follow-up, however, the results were not well sustained. CBT and IPT treatments made equivalent, substantial, and lasting changes across all symptom areas. Improvement through IPT took slightly longer to develop than improvement through CBT. In a 6-year follow-up of these patients, as well as patients from another trial, patients who had received CBT or IPT were found to fare far better than those who had received BT (Fairburn *et al.*, 1995).

In bulimic patients, the combination of drug therapy and psychotherapy appears to work better than either treatment alone. Agras *et al.* (1994) randomly assigned 61 patients diagnosed with DSM-III-R bulimia nervosa into one of five treatment groups: desipramine alone for 16 weeks, desipramine alone for 24 weeks, CBT alone for 18 sessions, desipramine combined with CBT for 16 weeks, or desipramine combined with CBT for 24 weeks. Patients were followed-up for one year. In the 16-week desipramine group, only 18 per cent of patients were free of binge-eating behaviour at 1-year follow-up; in contrast, this figure was 78 per cent in the 24-week combined treatment group. For the symptom of bingeing alone, 24-week desimpramine was almost as effective as CBT alone and the combined treatment. However, overall symptomatology was best reduced by the 24-week combined treatment; depression, purging, emotionally-driven eating as well as dietary restraint were all reduced.

Walsh *et al.* (1997) randomized 120 women with bulimia nervosa to receive CBT with placebo (n=25), CBT with medication (n=23), supportive therapy with placebo (n=22), supportive therapy with medication (n=22), or medication alone (n=28). The supportive therapy was psychodynamically oriented. The medication used was desipramine; fluoxetine was prescribed if desipramine proved ineffective or occasioned adverse effects. There were several findings of interest. CBT reduced behavioural symptoms (binge eating and vomiting) and improved attitudes towards eating better than did supportive therapy. CBT plus medication (but not supportive therapy plus medication) was superior to medication alone. Medication with either psychological treatment led to greater reduction in binge eating and depression as compared to placebo with psychological treatment. Garner *et al.* (1993) had earlier obtained similar results when comparing CBT and supportive-expressive therapy: the former was moderately more effective in the short term. However, the sample in this study consisted of a group of 60 referred patients who may not have been representative of the bulimia nervosa population.

Recent studies have suggested that medication may contribute little incremental improvement over CBT alone (Marcus and Levine, 1998; Wilson, 1999); if so, medication may be more helpful for comorbid anxiety and depression than for bulimic symptoms *per se* (Wilson, 1999).

Family therapy for bulimics has not yet been extensively studied. The Maudsley studies (Dare and Eisler, 1995) comparing individual and family therapy showed contradicting results at 5-year follow-up: the first study showed a better outcome for patients who had received individual therapy, while the second showed a better outcome for those who had received family therapy.

Several unconventional treatments of bulimia have been studied. Treasure *et al.* (1994) found that a *self-treatment manual* may be useful as a first intervention for bulimia nervosa. In their study, full remission was obtained in 24 per cent of patients receiving CBT, in 22 per cent of those using the manual, and in just 11 per cent of a waiting list control group. Lam *et al.* (1994) studied the effectiveness of *light therapy* in the treatment of bulimia nervosa. Relative to dim light, bright light produced a significantly greater improvement in both mood and eating behaviour. It is conceivable that a greater effect may be found in patients who show a seasonal pattern in the severity of their illness. Beumont *et al.* (1997) described good results with *nutritional counselling* for bulimics. The counselling was provided by a dietician, but was not clearly described in the report. Fluoxetine was a useful adjunct, but its use was associated with higher relapse when treatment was stopped.

While Carter and Fairburn (1998) described how *cognitive-behavioural self-help* can be useful in the treatment of bulimia nervosa, Wilson (1999) argued that the manuals alone are insufficient. He suggested that results with CBT could be improved using '*guided mirror exposure*' to facilitate emotional processing of body shape and weight concerns. Davis *et al.* (1999) obtained good results with *brief group psycho-education* followed by individual CBT.

Binge-Eating Disorder

Binge-eating disorder is not yet accepted as a clinical diagnosis; therefore, studies investigating its treatment are rare. However, as most studies investigating treatment for bulimia nervosa focus on the symptom of bingeing, some extrapolations can be made; this stance has been adopted by other authors as well (for example, Hudson *et al.*, 1996; Agras, 1997; Wilfley and Cohen, 1997). Available data suggest that antidepressant drugs may be useful for binge-eating disorder, and drug therapy combined with psychotherapy may be the most effective.

Prognosis and Predictors of Outcome

Prognosis, and clinical characteristics that predict the outcome of anorexia and bulimia nervosa were partly discussed in the section on treatment; this section will, therefore, focus only on studies that have not already been considered.

Anorexia Nervosa

For many reasons, including the rarity of the disorder, little is known about the natural history of untreated anorexia nervosa. Ratnasuriya *et al.* (1991) described a 20-year follow-up of 41 anorectics admitted to the Maudsley Hospital between 1959 and 1966. Twelve subjects (29 per cent) had a favourable outcome with normal body weight and menstruation, 13 (32 per cent) had an intermediate outcome with near normal body weight and/or menstrual abnormalities, and 15 (37 per cent) had a poor outcome with low body weight and absent or scanty menstruation. Data from one patient were unavailable. Of the 15 with poor outcome, 8 were chronically ill while 7 had died (6 from causes related to anorexia). In this sample, the results of 5-year follow-up tallied with that of the 20-year follow-up. Poor outcome was associated with later age of onset, history of neurotic and personality disturbances, disturbed relations in the family, and a longer duration of the illness.

Steinhausen and Seidel (1993) studied 60 subjects with eating disorders 41–80 weeks after in-patient treatment; these patients comprised 48 subjects with anorexia nervosa, 1 subject with partial anorexia, 5 subjects with bulimia nervosa, and 6 subjects with combined anorexia and bulimia. At follow-up, 4 subjects (6.7 per cent) were found to have died, 2 as a direct result of the disorder and 2 of suicide or it's consequences, with the disorder still florid. Five (8.3 per cent) subjects still suffered from anorexia nervosa,

2 (3.3 per cent) from anorexia and bulimia nervosa, 7 (11.7 per cent) from partial syndromes of anorexia, and 2 (3.3 per cent) from partial syndromes of bulimia. Thirty-four subjects (56.7 per cent) had recovered. The remaining 6 subjects (10 per cent) refused to co-operate or could not be traced. Only limited conclusions can be drawn from this report because of the widely varying duration of treatment (4–60 weeks) and time of follow-up (41–80 weeks); furthermore, the in-patient treatment was not described in detail, and initial and follow-up diagnoses were not directly compared.

In general, findings indicate that mortality is higher in subjects with anorexia nervosa than in subjects with other psychiatric disorder or in members of the general population (Sullivan, 1995). Prognosis improves when patients have an initial body-mass index that is higher than 13 (Baran *et al.*, 1995; Hebebrand *et al.*, 1997b); a lower value indicates a 'substantial risk for chronic anorexia nervosa and death related to emaciation' (Hebebrand *et al.*, 1997b). Brief hospitalization for patients who are severely underweight may not be cost-effective as the majority will need to be re-hospitalized later (Baran *et al.*, 1995). Laboratory findings may aid prognosis: Herzog *et al.* (1997) found that low weight at initial examination (less than 60 per cent of expected weight) and low serum albumin level (less than 3.6 g/L) best predicted a lethal course. High serum creatinine and uric acid levels predicted chronicity of illness.

In the most recent study, Strober *et al.* (1999) found that the absence of weight phobia and body image disturbance predicts a less malignant course of illness and a better outcome. The authors considered such patients to suffer from an atypical form of anorexia, and argued that their outcome data validate the need to distinguish typical and atypical diagnostic subtypes of the disorder.

Reviewing the literature, Schoemaker (1997) was unable to draw reliable conclusions on outcome following early intervention; one reason was that most studies considered duration of illness rather than early intervention *per se*.

Bulimia Nervosa

In patients with bulimia nervosa, Rossiter *et al.* (1993) found that Cluster B personality disorders (antisocial, borderline, histrionic, and narcissistic) predicted a significantly poorer outcome after 16 weeks of treatment with desipramine, CBT, or a combination of the two. Fairburn *et al.* (1995) found that premorbid and paternal obesity predicated a poor 6-year outcome of bulimia nervosa.

Keel and Mitchell (1997) reviewed 88 studies that reported follow-up data on patients with bulimia nervosa. Important findings were:

1. The crude mortality rate due to all causes of death was 0.3 per cent. This may, however, be an underestimate because of methodological issues related to the reviewed studies.
2. Six months after the initial presentation, follow-up studies reported that 28–33 per cent of women were in remission, compared to 21–75 per cent reported by treatment outcome studies. This advantage for treatment continued for the first 5 years following the initial presentation. Subsequently, remission rates flattened out to about 50 per cent in both follow-up and treated groups.
3. Five to ten years after the initial presentation, nearly 20 per cent of women continued to meet the full criteria for the disorder, indicating chronicity of the disease course.
4. About 30 per cent of women who improved experienced relapse into bulimic symptoms; the risk of relapse appeared to decline 4 years after the initial presentation.
5. Few prognostic factors were consistently identified across studies. Inconsistent prognostic indicators include comorbid axis I disorders, such as depression and substance abuse, past history of anorexia nervosa, age of onset and presentation, severity, and duration of symptoms. Personality traits such as impulsivity were, however, found likely to lead to poorer outcome.

Prevention

Any form of preventive work is always based upon and developed according to the needs of the population of interest. Both quantitative (for example, incidence and prevalence of a disorder in a population) and qualitative (for example, how the disorder affects daily life) data are required to determine the focus of intervention. All that is presently known for certain is that eating disorders are rare, that they chiefly affect young females, and that they disrupt a wide range of functions in direct proportion to the severity of symptoms. Possible aetiopathogenetic factors have been described, but only a few have been clearly shown to influence the development of eating disorders; no all-important single factor has been found, and it is unlikely that there is any. Intervention programs can, therefore, focus only on the assumed factors involved. In such circumstances, no prevention program can be complete, and effectiveness should be evaluated with these issues in mind.

Killen *et al.* (1993) carried out a randomized controlled trial with an intervention that was designed to modify eating attitudes and unhealthy weight regulation practices of young adolescent girls. A total of 963 girls aged 11–13 years were assigned to intervention-based classes or no-treatment control classes. The intervention program focused on education about the harmful effects of unhealthy weight regulation, promotion of healthy weight regulation measures, and development of coping skills to resist undesirable social pressure. The only positive finding was that there was a small increase in knowledge at 7-month follow-up. The authors concluded that this disappointing result stemmed from their expectation that the incidence of disturbed eating attitudes and weight concerns would increase in the course of time; they discovered, instead, that such aberrant attitudes and concerns did not increase in either experimental or control groups.

Carter *et al.* (1997) evaluated a school-based eating disorder prevention program that was designed to reduce dietary restraint. The sample consisted of 46 girls, aged 13–14 years. The intervention comprised eight 45-minute, once-weekly, educational sessions; topics discussed included social pressure to achieve a certain body shape and weight, the development of eating disorders and their characteristics, getting help for eating disorders, and healthy eating habits. The intervention resulted in an increase in knowledge as well as a decrease in target behaviour and attitudes. However, these effects fades at 6-month follow-up, and an increase in dietary restraint was observed at that time.

Other studies have also obtained similar findings. It appears that primary intervention programs for eating disorders are not suitable for the general population. Even if the highest-risk age group is approached, intervention does not result in much difference in the later incidence of the disorders; as a result, Rosenvinge and Borresen (1999) argue for the use of a health promotion paradigm for primary and secondary prevention of eating disorders. It is important to identify more specific risk groups, and to focus primary prevention programs on these groups. Such prevention programs may then be more useful and cost effective. Aetiological research is of course required to help design and improve on the contents of such intervention programs.

SERVICES

Patterns of health care, and the perceived need and demand for health services vary much from country to country. This section will therefore highlight the main elements that any comprehensive service should consider in planning service delivery for eating disorders.

The largest change in service during the last 15 years has been a move towards shorter and less coercive treatment regimes for anorexia nervosa. This has occurred partly because of an ideological backlash against the very strict operant conditioning treatments that were popular during the sixties and seventies and partly because of the advent of managed care in the USA, funding only relatively short admissions a few weeks in duration. There are now many centres at which it is not possible to have lengthy, 6–12 month admissions during which most of the re-feeding and weight gain occurs. This has led to an increasing use of intensive out-patient treatment programs or day care partial hospitalization. There is no firm evidence base to support these changes, although there is an increasing disillusionment with the effectiveness of intensive in-patient treatment programmes.

One of the most useful services that a specialist eating disorder facility can offer is the provision of a comprehensive physical and nutritional assessment. The vast majority of individuals with eating disorders of mild or moderate severity can be treated in individual practice, such as by a single, medically-qualified therapist. While a non-medical therapist may be just as well or even better qualified to deliver psychological treatment, there is a concern that the physical problems of many patients will be neglected. Assessments of osteoporosis, reproductive function, electrolyte status, and cardiac status is important; it is also important to provide an objective feedback of these results to the patient. A recent survey carried out in the United Kingdom (Health Advisory Service, 1996) showed that eating disorder patients and their families overwhelmingly preferred to be treated in a specialist centre rather than as part of a general psychiatry or psychology service. Patients preferred individual to group treatment, and were prepared to travel for such treatments for up to an hour each way, per appointment. Group treatment was acceptable if it were to be an adjunct to individual therapy, but not if it was the main treatment on offer.

Most specialist centres now offer a many-tiered approach to the treatment of bulimia, beginning with-help or guided self-help, and culminating with individual cognitive therapy that is supplemented by drug treatment, if appropriate. A few, severely ill or intractable patients may require day care or even in-patient treatment. No information is as yet available on how patients are affected by having to pass through various filters, progressing to the next stage of treatment only when failure has occurred at a lower level. Nevertheless, the finding that between 30 and 50 per cent of cases of bulimia nervosa can be successfully treated with a guided self-help program involving a specially prepared manual and only 2–5 hours of therapist contact is an important one, and it seems reasonable that it should be the first stage of treatment for most individuals.

References

Agras W. S. (1997). 'Pharmacotherapy of bulimia nervosa and binge-eating disorder: longer-term outcomes', *Psychopharmacol. Bull.*, 33: 433–6.

Agras W. S., Rossiter E. M., Arnow B. *et al.* (1994). 'One-year follow-up of psychosocial and pharmacologic treatments for bulimia nervosa', *J. Clin. Psychiatry*, 55: 179–83.

American Psychiatric Association (1993). 'Practice guideline for eating disorders', *Am. J. Psychiatry*, 150: 207–28.

——— (1994). *Diagnostic and Statistical manual of mental Disorders*, 4th ed., Washington, D. C.: American Psychiatric Association.

Andersen A. E. (1983). 'Anorexia nervosa and bulimia: a spectrum of eating disorders', *J. Adol. Health care*, 4: 15–21.

Andersen A. E. and Holman J. E. (1997). 'Males with eating disorders: challenges for treatment and research', *Psychopharmacol Bull.*, 33: 391–7.

Andreason P. J., Altemus M., Zametkin A. J. *et al.* (1992). 'Regional cerebral glucose metabolism in bulimia nervosa', *Am. J. Psychiatry*, 149: 1506–13.

Baran S. A., Weltzin T. E., and Kaye WH (1995). 'Low discharge weight and outcome in anorexia nervosa', *Am. J. Psychiatry*, 152: 1070–2.

Beumont P. J. V, Russel J.D., Touyz S.W. *et al.* (1997). 'Intensive nutritional counselling in bulimia nervosa: a role for supplementation with fluoxetine?', *Aust. N. Z. J. Psychiatry*, 31: 514–24.

Brambilla F., Draisci A., Peirone A. *et al.* (1995a). 'Combined cognitive-behavioural, psychopharmacological and nutritional therapy in eating disorders. 1: Anorexia nervosa-restricted type', *Neuropsychobiology*, 32: 59–63.

——— (1995b). 'Combined cognitive-behavioural, psychopharmacological and nutritional therapy in eating disorders. 2: Anorexia nervosa-binge-eating/purging type', *Neuropsychobiology*, 32: 64–7.

Bryant-Waugh R. and Lask B. (1995). 'Eating disorders in children', *J. Child Psychol. Psychiatry*, 36: 191–202.

Carlet D. J., Camargo C. A., and Herzog D. B. (1997). 'Eating disorders in males: a report on 135 patients', *Am. J. Psychiatry*, 154: 1127–32.

Carter J. C., Steward D. A., Dunn V. J. *et al.* (1997). 'Primary prevention of eating disorders: might it do more harm than good?', *Int. J. Eat. Disord.*, 22: 167–72.

Carter J. C. and Fairburn C. G. (1998). 'Cognitive-behavioural self-help reduces binge eating in women', *J. Consult. Clin. Psychol.*, 66: 616–23.

Chipkevitch E. (1994). 'Brain tumours and anorexia nervosa syndrome', *Brain Development*, 16: 175–9.

Choudry I. Y. and Mumford D. B. (1992). 'A pilot study of eating disorders in Mirpur (Pakistan) using an Urdu version of the Eating Attitude Test', *Int. J. Eat. Disord.*, 11: 243–51.

Considine R. V. (1997). 'Leptin and obesity in humans', *Eating and Weight Disorders*, 2: 61–6.

Dare C. and Eisler I. (1995). 'Family Therapy', in G. Szmukler, C. Dare, and J. Treasure (eds), *Handbook of Eating Disorders: Theory, Treatment and Research*, Chicester: John Wiley and Sons, 333–49.

Davis R., McVey G., Heinmaa M. *et al.* (1999). 'Sequencing of cognitive-behavioural treatments for bulimia nervosa', *Int. J. Eat. Disord.*, 25: 361–74.

Delvenne V., Goldman S., Biver F. *et al.* (1997a). 'Brain hypometabolism of glucose in low-weight depressed patients and in anorectic patients: a consequence of starvation? *J. Affect. Dis.*, 44: 69–77.

Delvenne V., Goldman S, Simon Y. *et al.* (1997b). 'Brain hypometabolism of glucose in bulimia nervosa', *Int. J. Eat. Disord.*, 21: 313–20.

Demitrack M. A., Kalogeras K. T., Altermus M. *et al.* (1992). 'Plasma and cerebrospinal fluid measures of arginine vasopressin secretion in patients with bulimia nervosa and in healthy subjects', *J. Clin. Endocrin. Metabol.*, 74: 1277–83.

Eagles J. M., Johnston M. I., Hunter D. *et al.* (1995). 'Increasing incidence of anorexia nervosa in the female population of Northeast Scotland', *Am. J. Psychiatry*, 152: 1266–71.

Fairburn C. G. and Beglin S. J. (1990). 'Studies of the epidemiology of bulimia nervosa', *Am. J. Psychiatry*, 147: 401–8.

Fairburn C. G., Jones R., Peveler R. C. *et al.* (1993). 'Psychotherapy and bulimia nervosa', *Arch. Gen. Psychiatry*, 50: 419–28.

Fairburn C. G., Norman P. A., Welch S. L. *et al.* (1995). 'A prospective study of outcome in bulimia nervosa and the long-term effects of three psychological treatments', *Arch. Gen. Psychiatry*, 52: 304–12.

Ferguson K. J. and Spitzer R. L. (1995). 'Binge-eating disorder in a community-based sample of successful and unsuccessful dieters', *Int. J. Eat. Disord.*, 18: 167–72.

Ferron F., considine R. V., Peino R. *et al.* (1997). 'Serum leptin concentrations in patients with anorexia nervosa, bulimia nervosa and non-specific eating disorders correlate with the body-mass index, but are independent of the respective disease', *Clin. Endocrin.*, 46: 289–93.

Fichter M. M. and Daser C. (1987). 'Symptomatology, psychosexual development and gender identity in 42 anorexic males', *Psychol. Med.*, 17: 409–18.

Fombonne E. (1996). 'Is bulimia nervosa increasing in frequency?', *Int. J. Eat. Disord.*, 19: 287–96.

Fornari V., Kaplan M., Sandberg D. E. *et al.* (1992). 'Depressive and anxiety disorders in anorexia nervosa and bulimia nervosa', *Int. J. Eat. Disord.*, 12: 21–9.

Freeman C. P. L. (1999). 'Eating disorders', in E. C. Johnstone, C. P. L. Freeman, A. K. Zealley (eds), *Companion to Psychiatric Studies*, Edinburgh: Churchill Livingstone (in press).

Gard M. C. and Freeman C. P. L. (1996). 'The dismantling of a myth: a review of eating disorders and socioeconomic status', *Int. J. Eat. Disord.*, 20: 1–12.

Garner D. M., Rockert W., Davis R. *et al.* (1993). 'Comparison of cognitive-behavioural and supportive expressive therapy for bulimia nervosa', *Am. J. Psychiatry*, 150: 37–46.

Goldfein J. A., Walsh B. T., LaChaussie J. L. *et al.* (1993). 'Eating behaviour in binge-eating disorder', *Int. J. Eat. Disord.*, 14: 427–31.

Gordon I., Lask B., Bryant-Waugh R. *et al.* (1997). 'Childhood-onset anorexia nervosa; towards identifying a biological substrate', *Int. J. Eat. Disord.*, 22: 159–65.

Gwirtsman H. E., Guze B. H., Yager J. *et al.* (1990). 'Fluoxetine treatment of anorexia nervosa: an open clinical trail', *J. Clin. Psychiatry*, 51: 378–82.

Halmi K. A. (1997). 'Comorbidity of the eating disorders', in D. Jimerson and W. H. Kaye (eds), *Baillière's Clinical Psychiatry, International Practice and Research, Edition Eating Disorders*, London: Baillière Tindall, 3: 291–302.

Halmi K. A., Eckert E., Marchi P. *et al.* (1991). 'Comorbidity of psychiatric diagnoses in anorexia nervosa', *Arch. Gen. Psychiatry*, 48: 712–18.

Hay P. J. and Fairburn C. G. (1998). 'The validity of the DSM-IV scheme for classifying bulimic eating disorders', *Int. J. Eat. Disord.*, 23: 7–15.

Health Advisory Service Report (1996). *Services for Eating Disorders*, Special publication, Brighton: Health Advisory Service.

Heatherton T. F., Nichols P., Mahamedi A. L. M. *et al.* (1995). 'Body weight, dieting and eating disorder symptoms among college students, 1982 to 1992', *Am. J. Psychiatry*, 152: 1623–9.

Hebebrand J., Blum W. F., Barth N. *et al.* (1997a). 'Leptin levels in patients with anorexia nervosa are reduced in the acute stage and elevated upon short-term weight restoration', *Molecular Psychiatry*, 2: 330–4.

Hebebrand J., Himmelmann G. W., Herzog W. *et al.* (1997b). 'Prediction of low body weight at long-term follow-up in acute anorexia nervosa by low body weight at referral', *Am. J. Psychiatry*, 154: 566–9.

Herzog D., Keller M., Sacks N. *et al.* (1992). 'Psychiatric comorbidity in treatment-seeking anorexics and bulimics', *J. Am. Acad. Child Adol. Psychiatry*, 31: 810–18.

Herzog W., Deter H. C., Fiehn W. *et al.* (1997). 'Medical findings and predictors of long-term physical outcome in anorexia nervosa: a prospective, 12-year follow-up study', *Psychol. Med.*, 27: 269–79.

Hoek H. W. (1991). 'The incidence and prevalence of anorexia nervosa and bulimia nervosa in primary care', *Psychol. Med.*, 21: 455–60.

Hoek H. W., Bartelds A. I. M., Bosveld J. J. F. *et al.* (1995). 'Impact of urbanization on detection rates of eating disorders', *Am. J. Psychiatry*, 152: 1272–8.

Holland A. J., Hall A. and Murray R. (1984). 'Anorexia nervosa, a study of 32 twin pairs and one set of triplets', *Br. J. Psychiatry*, 145: 414–19.

Hsu L. K. (1996). 'Epidemiology of the eating disorders', *Psychiatr. Clin. North Am.*, 19: 681–700.

Hsu L. K. G. (1997). 'Can dieting cause an eating disorder?', *Psychol. Med.*, 27: 509–13.

Hudson J. I., Carter W. P. and Pope H. G. (1996). 'Antidepressant treatment of binge-eating disorder: Research findings and clinical guidelines', *J. Clin. Psychiatry*, 57 (suppl. 8): 73–9.

Jimerson D. C., Lesem M. D., Hegg A. P. *et al.* (1992). 'Low serotonin and dopamine metabolite concentration in cerebrospinal fluid from bulimic patients with frequent binge episodes', *Arch. Gen. Psychiatry*, 49: 132–8.

Jimerson D. C., Wolfe B. E., Metzer E. D. *et al.* (1997). 'Decreased serotonin function in bulimia nervosa', *Arch. Gen. Psychiatry*, 54: 529–34.

Karhunen L., Haffner S., Lappalainen R. *et al.* (1997) 'Serum leptin and short-term regulation of eating in obese women', *Clin. Science*, 92: 537–8.

Katzman D. K., Zipursky R. B., Lambe E. K. *et al.* (1997). 'A longitudinal magnetic resonance imaging study of brain changes in adolescents with anorexia nervosa', *Arch. Ped. Adol. Med.*, 151: 793–7.

Kaye W. H. (1996). 'Neuropeptide abnormalities in anorexia nervosa', *Psychiatry Res.*, 62: 65–74.

Kaye W. H. Weltzin T. E., Hsu L. K. G. *et al.* (1992). 'Patients with anorexia nervosa have elevated scores on the Yale-Brown Obsessive-Compulsive Scale', *Int. J. Eat. Disord.*, 12: 57–62.

Keel P. K. and Mitchell J. E. (1997). 'Outcome in bulimia nervosa', *Am. J. Psychiatry*. 154: 313–21.

Kendler K. S. and Karkowski-Schuman L. (1997). 'Stressful life events and genetic liability to major depression: genetic control of exposure to the environment?', *Psychol. Med.*, 27: 539–47.

Kendler K. S., MacLean C., Neale M *et al.* (1991). 'The genetic epidemiology of bulimia nervosa', *Am. J. Psychiatry*, 148: 1627–37.

Kendler K. S., Walters E. E., Neale M. C. *et al.* (1995). 'The structure of genetic and environmental factors for six major psychiatric disorders in women: phobia, generalized anxiety, panic disorder, bulimia, major depression and alcoholism', *Arch. Gen. Psychiatry*, 52: 374–83.

Kennedy S. H. (1994). 'Melatonin disturbances in anorexia nervosa and bulimia nervosa', *Int. J. Eat. Disord.*, 16: 257–65.

Killen J. D., Taylor C. B., Hammer L. D. *et al.* (1993). 'An attempt to modify unhealthy eating attitudes and weight regulation practices of young adolescent girls', *Int. J. Eat. Disord.* 13: 369–84.

Kopp W., Blum W. F., von Prittwitz S. *et al.* (1997). 'Low leptin levels predict amenorrhoea in underweight and eating disordered females', *Molecular Psychiatry*, 2: 335–40.

Krieg J. C., Holthoff V., Schreiber W. *et al.* (1991). 'Glucose metabolism in the caudate nuclei of patients with eating disorders, measured by PET', *Eur. Arch. Psychiatry Clin. Neurosci.*, 240: 331–3.

Lam R.W., Goldner E. M., Solym L. *et al.* (1994). 'A controlled study of light therapy for bulimia nervosa', *Am. J. Psychiatry*, 151: 744–50.

Lee S. (1991). 'Anorexia nervosa in Hong Kong: A Chinese perspective', *Psychol. Med.*, 21: 703–11.

Lee A. M. and Lee S. (1996). 'Disordered eating and its psychosocial

correlates among Chinese adolescent females in Hong Kong', *Int. J. Eat. Disord.*, 20: 177–83.
Lee S., Chiu H. F. K., and Chen C-N. (1989). 'Anorexia nervosa in Hong Kong: Why not more Chinese?', *Br. J. Psychiatry*, 154: 683–8.
Lee S., Leung T., Lee A. M. *et al.* (1996). 'Body dissatisfaction among Chinese undergraduates and its implications for eating disorders in Hong Kong', *Int. J. Eat. Disord.*, 20: 77–84.
Leon G. R., Keel P. K., Kelly A.B. *et al.* (1997). 'The future risk factor research in understanding the etiology of eating disorders', *Psychopharmacol. Bull.*, 33: 405–11.
Levitan R. D., Kaplan A. S., Joffe R. T. *et al.* (1997). 'Hormonal and subjective responses to intravenous metachlorophenylpiperazine in bulimia nervosa', *Arch. Gen. Psychiatry*, 54: 521–7.
Lowe M. (1993). 'The effects of dieting on eating behaviour: a three factor model', *Psychol. Bull.*, 114: 100–21.
Lucas A. R., Beard C. M., O'Fallon W. M. *et al.* (1991). '50-year trends in the incidence of anorexia nervosa in Rochester, Minn.: A population-based study', *Am. J. Psychiatry*, 148: 917–22.
Mantzoros C., Flier J. S., Lesem M. D. *et al.* (1997). 'Cerebrospinal fluid leptin in anorexia nervosa: correlation with nutritional status and potential role in resistance to weight gain', *J. Clin. Endocrin. Metabol.*, 82: 1845–51.
Marcus M. D. and Levine M.D. (1998). 'Eating disorder treatment: an update', *Current Opinion in Psychiatry*, 11: 159–63.
Marrazzi M.A., Luby E. D., Kinzie J *et al.* (1997). 'Endogenous codeine and morphine in anorexia and bulimia nervosa', *Life Sci.*, 60: 1741–7.
McBride P. A., Anderson G. M., Khait V. D. *et al.* (1991). 'Serotonergic responsivity in eating disorders', *Psychopharmacol. Bull.*, 27: 365–72.
McCann U. D. and Agras W. S. (1990). 'Successful treatment of nonpurging bulimia nervosa with desipramine: a double-blind, placebo-controlled study', *Am. J. Psychiatry*,, 147: 1509–13.
McCluskey S., Evans C., Lacey J. H. *et al.* (1991). 'Polycystic ovary syndrome and bulimia', *Fertility and Sterility*, 55: 287–91.
Mortola J. F., Laughlin G. A., and Yen S. S. (1993). 'Melatonin rhythms in women with anorexia nervosa and bulimia nervosa', *J. Clin. Endocrin. Metabol.*, 77: 1540–4.
Mumford D. B., Whitegouse A. M., and Platts M. (1991). 'Sociocultural correlates of eating disorders among Asian schoolgirls in Bradford', *Br. J. Psychiatry*, 158: 222–8.
Mumford D. B., Whitehouse A. M, and Choudry I. Y. (1992). 'Survey of eating disorders in English-medium schools in Lahore, Pakistan', *Int. J. Eat. Disord.*, 11: 173–84.
O'Dwyer A. M., Lucey J. V. and Russel G. F. (1996). 'Serotonin activity

in anorexia nervosa after long-germ weight restoration: response to d-fenfluramine challenge', *Psychol. Med.*, 26: 353–9.

Pike K. M. and Walsh B. T. (1996). 'Ethnicity and eating disorders: implications for incidence and treatment', *Psychopharmacol. Bull.*, 32: 265–74.

Pope H. G., Hudson J. I., Jonas J. M. *et al.* (1983). 'Bulimia treated with imipramine: a placebo-controlled,, double-blind study', *Am. J. Psychiatry*, 140: 555–8.

Popovic V., Micic D., Djurovic M. *et al.* (1997). 'Absence of desensitization by hexarelin to subsequent GH releasing hormone-mediated GH secretion in patients with anorexia nervosa', *Clin. Endocrin.*, 46: 539–43.

Ratnasuriya R. H., Eisler I., Szmukler G. I. *et al.* (1991). 'Anorexia nervosa: outcome and prognostic factors after 20 years', *Br. J. Psychiatry*, 158: 495–502.

Regard M. and Landis T. (1997). '"Gourmand Syndrome" eating passion associated with right anterior lesions', *Neurology*, 48: 1185–90.

Reiss D. (1996). 'Abnormal eating attitudes and behaviours in two ethnic groups from a female British urban population', *Psychol. Med.*, 26: 289–99.

Rolla M., Andreoni A., Bellitte D. *et al.* (1994). 'Corticotrophin releasing hormone does not inhibit growth hormone-releasing hormone-induced release of growth hormone in control subjects but is effective in patients with eating disorders', *J. Endocrin.*, 140: 327–32.

Rosenvinge J. H. and Borresen R. (1999). 'Preventing eating disorders time to change programmes or paradigms?', *Eur. Eat. Disord. Rev.*, 7: 5–16.

Rossiter E. M., Agras W.S. , Telch C. F. *et al.* (1993). 'Cluster B personality disorder characteristics predict outcome in the treatment of bulimia nervosa', *Int. J. Eat. Disord.*, 13: 349–57.

Schmidt U., Tiller J., Blanchard M. *et al.* (1997). 'Is there a specific trauma precipitating anorexia nervosa?', *Psychol. Med.*, 27: 523–30.

Schoemaker C. (1997). 'Does early intervention improve the prognosis in anorexia nervosa? A systematic review of the treatment-outcome literature', *Int. J. Eat. Disord.*, 21: 1–15.

Schuckit M. A., Tipp J. E., Anthenelli R. M. *et al.* (1996). 'Anorexia nervosa and bulimia nervosa in alcohol-dependent men and women and their relatives', *Am. J. Psychiatry*, 153: 74–82.

Schweiger U., Pirke K. M., Laessle R. G. *et al.* (1992). 'Gonadotropin secretion in bulimia nervosa', *J. Clin. Endocrin. Metabol.*, 74: 1122–7.

Schweiger U. and Fichter M. (1997). 'Eating disorders: clinical presentation, classification and aetiological models', in D. Jimerson and

W. H. Kaye (eds), *Bailièrre's Clinical Psychiatry, International Practice and Research, edition Eating Disorders*, London: Bailliere Tindall, 3: 199–216.

Skodol A. E., Oldham J. M., Hyler S. E. *et al.* (1993). 'Comorbidity of DSM-III-R eating disorders and personality disorders', *Int. J. Eat. Disord.*, 14: 403–16.

Smeets M. A. M. (1995). *Body size estimation research in anorexia nervosa-breaking the deadlock*, Dissertation, Utrecht, The Netherlands: ISOR Publishers.

——— (1997). 'The rise and fall of body size estimation research in anorexia nervosa: review and reconceptualization', *Eur. Eating Disord. Rev.*, 5: 75–97.

Spelt J. and Meyer J. M. (1995). 'Genetics in eating disorders', in J. R. Turner, L. R. Cardon, and J. K. Hewiit (eds), *Behaviour Genetic Approaches in Behavioural Medicine*, New York: Plenum Press, 167–85.

Spitzer R.L. Devlin M., Walsh B. T. *et al.* (1992). 'Binge-eating disorder: a multi-site field trial of the diagnostic criteria', *Int. J. Eat. Disord.*, 11: 191–203.

Srinivasagam N. M., Kaye W. H., Plotnicov K. H. *et al.* (1995). 'Persistent perfectionism, symmetry, and exactness after long-term recovery from anorexia nervosa', *Am. J. Psychiatry*, 152: 1630–4.

Steinhausen H. C. and Seidel R. (1993). 'Outcome in adolescent eating disorders', *Int. J. Eat. Disord.*, 14: 487–96.

Strober M. and Humphrey L. L. (1987). 'Familial contributions to the aetiology and course of anorexia nervosa and bulimia', *J. Consult. Clin. Psychol.*, 55: 654–9.

Strober M., Freeman R., DeAntonio M. *et al.* (1997). 'Does adjunctive fluoxetine influence the post-hospital course of restrictor-type anorexia nervosa? A 24-month prospective, longitudinal follow-up and comparison with historical controls', *Psychopharmacol. Bull.*, 33: 425–31.

Strober M., Freeman R., and Morrell W. (1999). 'Atypical anorexia nervosa: separation from typical cases in course and outcome in a long-term prospective study', *Int. J. Eat. Disord.*, 25: 135–42.

Sullivan P.F. (1995). 'Mortality in anorexia nervosa', *Am. J. Psychiatry*, 152: 1073–4.

Sundblad C., Bergman L., and Eriksson E. (1994). 'High levels of free testosterone in women with bulimia nervosa', *Acta. Psychiatr. Scand.*, 90: 397–8.

Thiel A., Broocks A., Ohlmeier M. *et al.* (1995). 'Obsessive-compulsive disorder among patients with anorexia nervosa and bulimia nervosa', *Am. J. Psychiatry*, 152: 72–5.

Tiggeman M. and Pickering A. S. (1996). 'Role of television in adolescent women's body dissatisfaction and drive for thinness', *Int. J. Eat. Disord.*, 20: 199–203.

Treasure J., Schmidt U., Troop N., *et al.* (1994). 'First step in managing bulimia nervosa: a controlled trial of a therapeutic manual', *BMJ*, 308: 686–9.

Troop N. A. and Treasure J. L. (1997). 'Setting the scene for eating disorders. II: Childhood helplessness and mastery', *Psychol. Med.*, 27: 531–8.

Turnbull D. J., Freeman C. P. L., Barry F. *et al.* (1987). 'Physical and psychological characteristics of five male bulimics', *Br. J. Psychiatry*, 150: 25–9.

Vaccarino F. J., Kennedy S. H., Ralevski E. *et al.* (1994). 'The effects of growth-hormone releasing factor on food consumption in anorexia nervosa patients and normals', *Biol. Psychiatry*, 35: 446–51.

Vescovi P. P., Rastelli G., Volpi R. *et al.* (1996). 'Circardian variations in plasma ACTH, cortisol and beta-endorphin levels in normal-weight bulimic women', *Neuropsychobiology*, 33: 71–5.

Walsh B. T. and Kahn C. B. (1997). 'Diagnostic criteria for eating disorders: current concerns and future directions', *Psychopharmacol. Bull.*, 33: 369–72.

Walsh B. T., Hadigan C. M., Devlin M. J. *et al.* (1991). 'Long-term outcome of antidepressant treatment for bulimia nervosa', *Am. J. Psychiatry*, 148: 1206–12.

Walsh B. T., Wilson G. T., Loeb K. L. *et al.* (1997). 'Medication and psychotherapy in the treatment of bulimia nervosa', *Am. J. Psychiatry*, 154: 523–31.

Walters E .E. and Kendler K. S. (1995) 'Anorexia nervosa and anorexia-like syndromes in a population-based female twin sample', *Am. J. Psychiatry*, 152: 64–71.

Welch S. L. and Fairburn C. G. (1994). 'Sexual abuse and bulimia nervosa; three integrated case control comparisons', *Am. J. Psychiatry*, 151: 402–7.

Welch S. L., Doll H. A., and Fairburn C. G. (1997). 'Life events and the onset of bulimia nervosa; a controlled study', *Psychol. Med.*, 27: 515–22.

Weltzin T. E., Fernstrom M. H., Neuberger S. K. C. *et al.* (1995). 'Acute tryptophan depletion and increased food intake and irritability in bulimia nervosa', *Am. J. Psychiatry*, 152: 1668–71.

Wiederman M. W. and Pryor T. (1996). 'Substance use among women with eating disorders', *Int. J. Eat. Disord.*, 20: 163–8.

Wilfley D. E. and Cohen L. R. (1997). 'Psychological treatment of bulimia nervosa and binge-eating disorder', *Psychopharmacol. Bull.*, 33: 437–54.

Wilson T. G. (1999). 'Treatment of bulimia nervosa: the next decade', *Eur. Eat. Disord. Rev.*, 7: 77–83.

Wonderlich S. A. and Mitchell J. E. (1997). 'Eating disorders and comorbidity: empirical, conceptual and clinical implications', *Psychopharmacol. Bull.*, 33: 381–90.

World Health Organization (1992). *International Classification of Diseases*, 10th rev., Geneva: World Health Organization.

Yager J. and Hatton C. A. (1986). 'Anorexia nervosa in a women totally blind since the age of two', *Br. J. Psychiatry*, 149: 506–9.

Chapter 6

Perspectives on Somatization

R. RAGURAM

During the past decade, much research has been conducted on somatization in view of the recognition of its prevalence and its importance in both primary care and psychiatric settings. This review will focus on areas of contemporary interest in the field, and on issues concerning cultural aspects of the phenomenon.

DEFINITIONS AND CONCEPTS

The concept of somatization is in disarray. When Stekel introduced the term in the early part of this century, it was considered to be a defense mechanism akin to conversion. Recently, however, somatization was atheoretically described as the tendency to experience and communicate somatic distress in response to psychosocial stress, and the disposition to seek medical help in consequence (Lipowski, 1988). Since the inclination to preferentially communicate somatic rather than psychological distress is common, the crucial issue is to decide when such behaviour becomes pathological. Lipowski resolved the issue by emphasizing certain cognitive and behavioural components. He considered somatization to be abnormal if :

1. the individual attributes it to a physical illness; and
2. the individual consequently engages in persistent medical help-seeking.

In addition, Lipowski stressed that patients who somatize usually feel uncomfortable about and resist attempts to consider the possibility of psychological causation. In a similar vein but seeking semantic precision, Escobar *et al.* (1987) operationally defined somatization as medically unexplained physical symptoms.

Though largely adopted by many investigators, there are several inadequacies in both these definitions. The attributory styles of individuals can be substantially governed by cultural beliefs concerning health and sickness; in many cultures, somatic distress is often viewed within a framework of spiritual or humoural influences, and not exactly as an indication of physical illness. Few rural patients in developing societies engage in persistent medical help-seeking; this is primarily because such facilities are often inadequate or unaffordable for their use. The locus of resistance to examine psychological causation may reside not within the individual but in the interpersonal and social arena. As a result of inexperience, or because of a negative attitude towards possible psychological antecendents, clinicians may also resist considering psychological mechanisms. Lee (1997) therefore argued that somatization is best considered as a 'co-creative process that involves physicians as much as patients positioned in particular sectors of a socio-economically constrained health care system'.

Bridges and Goldberg (1991) defined somatizers as patients who met four essential criteria:

1. Consulting behaviour: The patient sought medical help for somatic manifestations of a psychiatric illness, and did not present with psychological symptoms.
2. Attribution : The patient considered these somatic complaints to be due to physical rather than psychiatric disease.
3. Diagnosis: No psychiatric disorder was detectable using standard research criteria.
4. Likely response to intervention: In the opinion of the research psychiatrist, treatment of the psychiatric disorder would alleviate the somatic symptoms.

These operational criteria appear attractive because they are based primarily on behavioural aspects of the condition. However, the previously discussed problem of an attributory style remains, and a fresh problem arises: the subjective bias of the investigator who has to opine that the somatic symptoms would improve with treatment of the psychiatric disorder. A further problem is that these criteria identify only the subset of somatizers who have an identifiable psychiatric disorder in addition to their somatic complaints.

In this context, it is important to remember that the presence of somatization does not imply that the individual manifesting it must necessarily suffer from a psychiatric ailment. Among the psychiatric disorders where it is prominently present, somatization disorder constitutes a specific subset with a cluster of characteristic symptoms.

Nosology

Initially subsumed under hysteria, somatization disorder was later called Briquet's syndrome. The term, somatization disorder, itself first appeared in DSM-III (American Psychiatric Association, 1980), based on the work of the St. Louis group, which had demonstrated high reliability, stability, and validity for the condition (Perley and Guze, 1962; Guze, 1975). Somatization disorder did not find a specific place in the International Classification of Diseases in its ninth edition (ICD-9; World Health Organization, 1978); however, Briquet's disorder was cited as an inclusion term under 'Other Neurotic Disorders' in ICD-9. DSM-III guidelines for the diagnosis of somatization disorder required the clinician to ask the patient about the presence of various physical complaints from a lengthy list of thirty-seven potential symptoms. This list was marginally modified in DSM-IIIR (American Psychiatric Association, 1987), and the total number of symptoms was scaled down to thirty-five. A firm diagnosis required the presence of thirteen symptoms.

The diagnostic approach in DSM-IV (American Psychiatric Association, 1994) was substantially altered, based on the recommendations of Cloninger and Yutsky (1993) that the symptoms be classified into clinically meaningful clusters. The physical complaints were accordingly categorized into four groups: reports of pain, gastrointestinal discomfort, sexual symptoms, and pseudoneurological symptoms. In addition, the diagnostic threshold for the disorder was brought down drastically to a requirement for the presence of just eight symptoms. The additional criterion in DSM-IIIR that there should be 'positive evidence, or a strong presumption, that the symptoms are linked to psychological disorder or conflicts' was abandoned since it proved difficult to operationalize in many clinical situations.

The category of somatization disorder was first introduced in the ICD in its tenth edition (World Health Organization, 1992). Tyrer (1989) expressed reservations about the inclusion of somatization disorder in the ICD. He wrote, 'the introduction of the term somatization disorder has been an American initiative, and the ICD-10 has been somewhat reluctantly carried in its wake'. Though the ICD-10 delineation of the construct of somatization is similar to that of DSM-IV, the description is much broader, and a firm diagnosis requires the presence of just six symptoms.

Both ICD-10 and DSM-IV suggest the diagnosis of undifferentiated somatoform disorder for patients who do not fulfil the criterion requirements for somatization disorder, and yet continue to have disabling physical complaints. Curiously, in many community surveys undifferentiated somatoform disorder has been found to be much more prevalent than somatization disorder itself (Escobar *et al.*, 1987).

Since the description of somatization disorder has varied in the DSM, and since the disorder has only recently been included in the ICD, it is important to examine the degree of congruence between different definitions. Yutzy *et al.* (1995) found high concordance between DSM-III, DSM-IIIR and DSM-IV; ICD-10 showed poor concordance with the DSM definitions. The authors suggested that the low concordance between the ICD and DSM systems could have been due to variable interpretations of the three questions on health-care utilization in the ICD-10 definition.

Somatization disorder as defined by DSM-IV and ICD-10 is uncommon in clinical practice. Prior to the publication of these two classificatory systems, Escobar *et al.* (1989) had introduced the concept of Somatic Symptom Index (SSI). This construct of an 'abridged' somatization disorder required six lifetime medically unexplained symptoms in women, and four lifetime medically unexplained symptoms in men. The SSI was shown to be associated with functional impairment and excess health-care use (Katon *et al.*, 1984; Escobar *et al.*, 1989; Swartz *et al.*, 1991; Smith *et al.* 1995). A limitation to the operationalization of the SSI is that the clinician has to enquire about the lifetime prevalence of somatoform symptoms from a long list of thirty-seven symptoms; this could prove difficult in a busy primary care setting. Another limitation is the possible unreliability of the documentation of a lifetime symptom.

In an interesting recent study (Kroenke *et al.*, 1997), another less restrictive version of somatoform disorder was outlined. Termed as multisomatoform disorder, it was defined as three or more current somatoform symptoms reported from a 15-symptom checklist, and the presence of somatoform symptoms for at least two years. In their study of 1000 primary care patients, Kroenke *et al.* found the prevalence of multisomatoform disorder to be 8.2 per cent. Patients diagnosed with this disorder experienced much disability. Kroenke *et al.* suggested that this disorder could be a valid diagnosis, potentially more useful than the DSM-IV diagnosis of undifferentiated somatoform disorder. While studies are needed to confirm the validity of this construct, it raises the issue of what constitutes an appropriate symptom threshold to define a disorder. One suggestion is that thresholds should be anchored at points at which therapy has been proven effective (Fletcher *et al.*, 1988). It remains to be seen whether variations in the threshold that is necessary to define somatization influence therapeutic response and long-term outcome.

Another important nosological issue is the relationship between somatization disorder and personality disorders. Early investigations focused on the association between somatization disorder and histrionic or antisocial personality disorders (Lilienfeld, 1992). The existence of such an association was in consonance with the speculations of the St. Louis school, and was based mainly on research conducted in psychiatric settings. A weak association of somatization disorder with antisocial personality was found in the Epidemiological Catchment Area (ECA) study (Simon and von Korff, 1990). When Smith (1991) examined somatization disorder in a primary care setting, he found that the most common comorbid personality disorders were avoidant, paranoid, self-defeating, and obsessive personality disorders. In another study, Stern *et al.* (1993) reported a higher prevalence of personality disorders among patients with somatization disorder than among controls; the three commonest diagnoses were passive-aggressive, obsessive-compulsive, and paranoid personality disorders. Since somatization disorder often begins early in life and persists through adulthood, and since it frequently co-exists with personality disorders, might it be a disorder of development? Over half of the respondents in a survey of senior British psychiatrists reported the belief that patients with somatization disorder suffer primarily from personality problems (Stern *et al.*, 1993).

DEVELOPMENTAL PERSPECTIVES

Recently, there has been an attempt to view somatoform disorders within a developmental framework. Craig *et al.* (1993) speculated that inadequate parenting early in life and disproportionate experience of illness during childhood are separate risk factors that combine in adulthood to result in somatization. In a carefully designed study, these workers found that somatizers were more likely to report physical illness and poor parental care during childhood. While the lack of parental care increases the risk for the development of an emotional disorder, the disproportionate experience of childhood illness increases the likelihood that the individual will interpret innocuous bodily sensations as bodily dysfunctions.

Other studies have also examined possible childhood antecedents of adult somatization behaviour. For example, Hartvig and Sterner (1985) reported that during childhood, adults with somatization had experienced more illness and more physical debility in family members; and, Morrison (1989) found that women with somatization were more likely to report childhood sexual abuse.

Much research indicates that somatizers hail from dysfunctional homes; nevertheless, little is known about the specific dimensions of family functioning that may increase the risk for somatization. In a study of student volunteers, Terre and Ghiselli (1997) reported that at different developmental stages different aspects of family life were associated with the report of somatic complaints; for instance, at the undergraduate level, family conflict and family achievement orientation predicted somatic emphasis. Since this study was conducted on a non-clinical sample, inferences about the significance of these factors in clinical populations must be drawn with caution.

Despite the tentative nature of the findings, developmental and life-span approaches to somatization offer a promising paradigm to explore the processes which contribute to the origin of the phenomenon. Regrettably, the available studies are cross-sectional or retrospective. Though difficult to conduct, longitudinal research is essential to unravel both causative and protective factors that are involved in the origins of somatization.

The International Study of Somatoform Disorders

Two long-held myths about somatization have recently been exploded: that somatization occurs predominantly in non-Western cultures or developing societies, and that somatization is an expression of emotional distress in persons whose verbal skills are less developed. It is now reasonably clear that somatization is also commonly encountered in primary care settings in the developed world (Bridges and Goldberg, 1991; Bridges *et al.*, 1991). Furthermore, the recent World Health Organization study on presentation of mental illness in general health care settings has convincingly demonstrated that 'in both developed and developing countries, most of the patients with definite psychological disorder presented with a complaint similar to those usually associated with somatic illness, such as back pain, shortness of breath, and dizziness' (Ustun and Sartorius, 1995). Therefore, if somatization is universal in its occurrence, the issue that needs to be addressed is whether the pattern of somatic symptoms and the meanings attached to these symptoms vary across cultures. In order to clarify these issues, the World Health Organization launched the International Study of Somatoform Disorders. The objectives of the investigation were (Janca *et al.*, 1995a):

1. To test the cross-cultural applicability of the ICD-10 and DSM-IV somatoform disorder criteria.
2. To develop a set of instruments for the assessment of somatoform disorders and to test the applicability, reliability, and validity of these instruments in different cultures.
3. To assess the rates and characteristics of somatoform disorders in different parts of the world.
4. To develop a set of educational tools for teaching physicians about the characteristics and management of somatoform disorders in different cultures.
5. To develop and evaluate a programme of intervention for somatoform disorders in various settings.

As a starting point of the study, a mail questionnaire survey involving 42 experts from 23 countries was conducted to elicit opinions about the applicability of the ICD-10 somatoform dis-order criteria in different cultural settings. While the ICD-10 concept of somatoform disorder was generally found acceptable, the criteria for somatization disorder were felt to be restrictive; most experts emphasized the need to retain the more inclusive category of undifferentiated somatoform disorder (Janca *et al.*, 1995b). This stance is easily understood when one considers the presentation of somatization in different settings. Psychiatrists usually see severe forms of somatization syndromes, characterized by a long-standing history of various somatic symptoms. Severe and chronic somatization disorders are, however, relatively rare in the general population (Escobar *et al.*, 1987). In contrast, acute forms of somatization often arise in various primary care settings, and are associated with a disproportionate number of consultations and investigations (Barsky *et al.*, 1986). A pertinent view that has herein been expressed is that somatization disorder may represent the extreme end of the somatization spectrum (Katon *et al.*, 1991); the utility of this construct outside psychiatric settings may hence be limited.

The participating experts in the WHO survey were provided with a list of sixty-nine diagnostically important somatic symptoms from DSM-III, DSM-IIIR, DSM-IV, and ICD-10. The experts were asked to rate the symptoms on four measures: the frequency of the symptom, the extent to which the symptom was suggestive of somatization, the likelihood that the patient would refuse to accept the absence of a medical explanation for the symptom, and the appropriateness of the symptom for a particular culture. Based on these assessments, the investigators also evaluated the usefulness of a particular symptom for the broader diagnoses of somatoform disorders in ICD-10. The most useful symptoms were deemed to be those which the experts considered to be frequent, strongly suggestive of somatization, and very likely to provoke a refusal of a psychological explanation. The five physical complaints which emerged as most useful as rated on these parameters were back pain, chest pain, dyspepsia, experience of muscular aches and pains, and palpitations. Most of these symptoms do not appear in the ICD-10 description of somatization disorder. In contrast, the experience of abnormal skin sensations, which has been assigned prominence in ICD-10, did not appear in the list of symptoms considered diagnostically useful by the experts in the study. Similarly, sexual and pseudoneurological complaints, considered diagnostically important for somatization disorder in DSM-IV, were rarely seen across cultures, and were also deemed to be cross-culturally inappropriate by the experts.

In the first phase of the actual study that followed, three instruments were developed: the Somatoform Disorders Schedule (SDS), the Screener for Somatoform Disorders, and the Somatoform Symptom Checklist. The instruments were found to be acceptable and reliable (Janca *et al.*, 1995c). Preliminary analysis of data from Phase I of the study revealed that aches and pains in different parts of the body were the most frequent somatic symptoms across cultures. Contrary to expectations, the average number of somatic symptoms experienced was not found to be higher among patients from the developing countries; this is evident from Table 6.1 which presents the frequency of medically unexplained somatic symptoms across sites. A significant proportion of patients also reported temporal association of the somatic symptoms with stressful life events. More importantly, subjective content analysis of the patients' reports revealed that attitudes and beliefs concerning health and sickness largely determined the interpretation and attribution of the symptoms (Isaac *et al.*, 1995).

This WHO study of somatoform disorders is an important ongoing project; the results of the next two phases, dealing with intervention and the development of educational materials,

Table 6.1: Frequency of Medically Unexplained Somatic Symptoms across sites in the International Study of Somatoform Disorders (Isaac *et al.*, 1995).

City (country)	Range of frequency of symptoms*#
Bangalore (India)	23–68 per cent
Cagliari/Milan (Italy)	48–85 per cent
Harare (Zimbawe)	33–66 per cent
Sao Paulo (Brazil)	49–80 per cent
Temple (U.S.A.)	18–56 per cent

* The data presented are the frequencies of the least common and the most common symptoms at each site.

\# Somatic symptoms encountered included headache, back pain, pain in the limbs, pain in the joints, chest pain, belly pain, sensations of tingling, numbness, creeping or crawling, body shakes, weakness, dizziness, hot/cold sweats, trouble with walking, palpitations, breathlessness, fast breathing, dryness of mouth, nausea, lump in the throat, intolerance of food, epigastric discomfort, sensation of bloating, and loose bowels.

will provide much úseful information. Attempts to examine psychological phenomena across cultures in a reliable manner are a worthwhile pursuit and the WHO has been vigorously pursuing this strategy for the past several years. However, its earlier investigations such as the International Pilot Study of Schizophrenia, which had been criticized for paying insufficient attention to the range and complexity of meanings attached to psychological distress, and for focusing attention on a narrow range of clinical attributes of illnesses that are deemed to be culturally invariant (Fabrega, 1989). It is disheartening to note that inspite of this criticism the WHO has not incorporated any cultural varibles in its multinational study of somatoform disorders.

Modern psychiatry struggles to remove meanings and contexts from diagnostic processes not because these are unimportant, but because problems arise out of their incorporation into the diagnostic processes. This observation is particularly true with regard to notions involving the aetiology of illnesses. In the attempt to increase the reliability of the psychiatric symptoms used in diagnosis, meanings associated with such symptoms have been expunged from nosological systems. But, what exactly constitutes a symptom? Will not the definition of the symptom itself be determined by the contexts in which the distress occurs, and the meanings assigned to it? Especially in the area of somatization, attribution and interpretation of bodily symptoms in different cultures is likely to be significantly influenced by patients' cultural beliefs concerning health and sickness. It is therefore surprising that no effort has been made in the International Study of Somatoform Disorders to specifically examine this dimension. In the absence of such an initiative, the attempt to relate the higher prevalence of somatic symptoms in Brazil to 'Latin culture' (Isaac *et al.*, 1995) appears superficial and lacks conviction. There is an imperative need to examine phenomena such as somatization in a way that is contextually sensitive, and yet relevant for comparative examinations.

SOMATIZATION AND THE NEW CROSS-CULTURAL PSYCHIATRY

For long, cultural psychiatry had an arcane image, dominated by a neo-colonial view of the native. The focus was on the display, promotion and consumption of ethnic psychological ware, determined predominantly by mental health professionals from the West. Striking changes have, however, occurred during the past decade (Lewis-Fernandez and Kleinman, 1995). The cultural psychiatrist of today is no more the Faustus of the modern world, journeying through nations and cultures, hungering forever after knowledge. In contrast, he is a scientist who is keen to examine the contextual factors which shape and influence psychiatric illnesses; he wishes to explore the range of meanings associated with these factors in everyday locales and in routine clinical encounters rather than in far-way, exotic places,

This approach has often been referred to as the 'new cross-cultural psychiatry'. The emergence of this approach has also signalled the coming together of psychiatry and anthropology. In many ways, anthropology offered psychiatry an innovative means to examine cultural factors without becoming unduly enmeshed in the form/content dilemma. The relationship between the two disciplines has nevertheless been uneasy (Skultans, 1991); difficulties arise from the differing orientations of the two disciplines. The concerns of the psychiatrist are pragmatic: to identify and delineate symptoms, and to evolve methods of handling them clinically. The concerns of the anthropologist, in contrast, are focused on individual distress alone, but embrace a wider context of beliefs and practices that influence and shape human suffering. The challenge is how the universalistic approach of the medically-oriented psychiatrist and the particularistic perspective of the anthropologist can be employed in a complementary way. Since somatization is universal and at the same time considerably influenced by cultural factors, the coming together of psychiatry and anthropology should not only promote an understanding of cultural factors that affect somatization in specific contexts, but also facilitate culturally informed comparative research. Such an approach is crucial now as we live in a period in which the investigation of context-free biological universals and the quest for a common, uniform diagnostic language prominently engage the attention of mental health professionals. The impediment may not be just one of theoretical integration but one of evolving appropriate methodologies to examine psychological problems within and across cultures.

When we shift from the clinical to the cultural aspects of somatization, the referent changes. The focus is on the contexts in which somatization occurs and the meanings ascribed to somatization. These in turn depend on the beliefs, knowledge, and practices concerning the human body in a particular culture. Cross-cultural explorations cannot be undertaken by merely viewing somatization as a clinical phenomenon, or as an item in a research questionnaire. The personal significance of physical symptoms has to be unravelled against the background of a general schema of meanings concerning the human body in health and in sickness. Representations of the body in turn are related to the structure of the society. As Douglas (1982) observed, 'the social body constrains the way the physical body is perceived. The physical experience of the body is always modified by the social categories through which it is known, and sustains a particular view of the society.'

The perception of bodily distress is modified by influences that are transmitted culturally; hence, the body in pain contains within it an image as well as a message. Parts of the body may be imbued with emotional qualities. For instance, in traditional Chinese medical practice expressions such as the 'angry liver', the 'anxious heart' and the 'melancholic spleen' are common. When Chinese patients report with complaints related to the liver or the spleen, the traditional healers attend to the physical complaints and additionally take cognizance of the associated emotional states that the organs represent. Based on these observations, Ots (1990) argued that bodily symptoms can be considered as correspondents or equivalents of emotions, and not as psychological experiences transformed into somatic symptoms. It has also been suggested that somatic symptoms are best viewed as metaphors of self/society relations, with the body acting as a mediating symbolic device (Kirmayer, 1992), the meaning of which resides within a particular cultural context and in the background of individual life-worlds. Metaphors communicate not just the cultural meanings but also indicate the commonalties in human suffering across cultures.

Many psychiatrists may consider an exploration into these dimensions of somatization a difficult task for which they are ill-equipped. It may not really be so. The most common method of data collection employed in medical encounters is the same as that employed in anthropology: talking to people. The difference lies only in the scope of enquiry. One of the noteworthy attempts to integrate psychiatric and anthropological research methods has been the work of Krause (1989) among Sikh and Punjabi patients in Bedford, UK. Emphasizing that these patients do not view physical symptoms in isolation from the meanings attributed to them, she points out, 'Punjabi patients do not simply somatize; rather, the physical symptoms about which these patients seek medical help are expressions of end outcomes of a range of contexts and processes affecting them in their daily lives.' For instance, the term *garam* refers not just to heat, but also to energy in food, humours in the body, mental states, and a certain kind of body disposition. Although at one level the term refers to a physical sensation, at other levels it draws attention to multiple psychological and social issues and themes. Focusing merely on the somatic complaint would address only one component of this physical-psychological-cultural continuum.

Whatever be the cultural contexts studied, somatization bears a close temporal relationship to stressful life events (Isaac *et al.*, 1995), and the disability associated with it is also considerable (Gurjee *et al.* 1997). In these times of dramatic changes worldwide in economic, political, and social arenas, the resultant turmoil and stress is likely to increase the burden of somatization. For instance, somatization was found to be particularly common among refugees who had experienced significant psychosocial trauma (Castillo *et al.*, 1994). The processes by which culture modulates the effects of traumatic stress to produce somatoform symptoms (as opposed to more overt psychologic disturbance) is poorly understood and researched. Waitzkin and Magana (1996) argued that the mechanism by which psychological trauma is transformed into somatic symptoms often involves an 'incoherence' in narrative structure; in consequence, the traumatic experience cannot be told as a coherent whole that encompasses both stress and symptoms. The transformation of a traumatic narrative into somatic symptoms may constitute the culturally sanctioned 'way of knowing' and of processing the stress in some cultural contexts. The crucial question then is whether bringing these narratives of trauma into consciousness will have a therapeutic effect for patients with somatization. This also raises the issue of what constitutes a culturally sensitive strategy to handle somatization.

THEORIES OF SOMATIZATION: THE ROLE OF STIGMA

Various theories have been advanced to explain the processes involved in somatization across cultures (Kirmayer, 1984). Most of the theories focus on the balance between the expression of somatic and psychological distress, and the factors governing these. A prominent explanatory model invokes the construct of alexithymia. According to this model, some patients lack the linguistic skills that are necessary to articulate emotional distress, and therefore experience their distress in somatic terms. The Toronto Alexithymia Scale (TAS) was developed to provide empirical support for this model. Bagby *et al.* (1994) demonstrated that the TAS has satisfactory validity; however, the study was carried out on samples of college students, and this limits the application of the TAS in clinical situations.

One of the few studies to examine the relationship between alexithymia and somatization in clinical settings was conducted by Bach *et al.* (1994). The authors did not find prominent alexithymic characteristics in patients with somatoform disorder. They also observed that a substantial proportion of somatoform patients actually had scores in the non-alexithymic range. Thus, at present there is no convincing evidence to support a strong relationship between alexithymia and clinical manifestations of somatization.

The salience of psychological introspection in the West has been considered to reflect greater sophistication and differentiation in linguistic dimensions (Leff, 1977). Accordingly, the erstwhile notion that somatization is chiefly prevalent in the developing world led to the explanation that it results from linguistic deficits which do not allow the patient to express his psychological state. This view of somatization indicated the privileged position accorded to the Western cultural tradition—(of which medicine is a product)—over the cultures and health system practices of a vast majority of mankind. Challenging this view, however, is the observation that all over the world, in diverse cultural settings, somatic symptoms constitute a common pattern of clinical presentation to Western-style physicians and traditional healers alike. In addition, contrary to expectations, somatic distress and emotional distress do not always bear an antithetical relationship to each other: many patients who initially present with somatic symptoms can recognize and identify psychological distress when directly asked (Weiss *et al.*, 1995). Similar observations have been made by Cheung *et al.* (1981) among Chinese patients seeking treatment in general practice settings. Patients 'somatization is less a denial of the underlying psychological affliction than a locally appropriate strategy of engaging physicians' concern (Lee, 1997). Somatization is perhaps best construed as a communicative act that is woven into the fabric of culture which needs to be studied with culturally appropriate approaches.

Stigma has emerged as a prominent cultural explanation for somatization. It is conceivable that the patterning of felt distress in somatic rather than psychological idioms might be due to a powerful social stigma attached to the expression of emotional problems in a particular cultural context. For years, social research into stigma was guided by the concept of spoiled identity (Goffman, 1963); this concept describes the adverse effect that stigma (associated with illness) has on the patient's social status. Recent research has considered a more ethnographic view of stigma in contrast with the view of spoiled identity alone. (Kleinman *et al.*, 1995). Stigma is associated with fears of decreased self-esteem and power, jeopardized marital prospects, and shame in social and marital life. The fear of disclosure is also a vital aspect of perceived stigma which arises from perturbations in the local worlds of affected persons.

The role of stigma needs to be examined through approaches that integrate clinical and anthropological paradigms. Weiss and colleagues (1992) operationalized this framework through a semi-structured interview—the Explanatory Model Interview Catalogue (EMIC). EMIC explores aspects of illness experiences, causal explanations, and patterns of help-seeking within an ethnographic framework. Using EMIC, Raguram *et al.* (1996) examined the relationship between somatization and stigma about illness in a sample of depressed patients. Stigma scores were found to be low in patients with a primary somatoform diagnosis as compared with those with a primary depressive diagnosis. Greater severity of depression was associated with higher stigma scores; in contrast, greater severity of somatization was associated with lower stigma scores. While both depressive and somatic symptoms were distressing to the patients, qualitative analysis showed that patients viewed depressive rather than somatic symptoms as socially disadvantageous. Somatic symptoms were considered less stigmatizing since they resembled illness experiences that most persons in society have from time to time. Depressive symptoms were considered to compromise self-esteem, diminish social status, and interfere with marriage.

Besides stigma, other social factors may also influence the pattern of expression of psychological symptoms. Reports from the West indicate that in some clinical settings the social desirability and availability of psychotherapy as a viable treatment option may favour the reporting of psychological rather than physical symptoms (Mechanic, 1980; Olfson and Pincus, 1994). Thus, explanations of somatization need to be attuned to analyses that emphasize and incorporate cultural influences; it is fallacious to merely pay attention to cultural differences and to hypothesize linguistic or other deficits.

Management Issues

Most patients with somatization disorder have had multiple, unsuccessful medical consultations. When these patients are advised to meet a psychiatrist, many feel reluctant and apprehensive about the consultation. Hence, the psychiatrist's first session with the client is a crucial one. Creed and Guthrie (1993) offered many useful suggestions for interviewing a patient with somatization disorder. Prior to the first meeting, the psychiatrist should familiarize himself with all the background information concerning the patient. If possible, the psychiatrist should discuss with the referring clinician the reasons for the referral, and whether the patient has been told that he/she would be meeting a psychiatrist. During the clinical interview, the psychiatrist should strive to establish the therapeutic alliance early. Detailed enquiry about the physical symptoms and an empathic response to the felt distress would contribute to establishing an effective rapport at this stage. It is also important to look for subtle verbal and non-verbal cues that indicate the emotional state of the individual. If the psychiatrist is not sure about the psychological aspects of the illness during the initial interview, it is best to be honest and suggest further sessions for exploration. This interview process is a prelude to formulating specific treatment strategies; if the patient is well-prepared and feels comfortable with the rationale and approach of the clinician, his/her adherence to the treatment programme will be better. The broad issues in the treatment of somatizing patients have been outlined by Bass and Benjamin (1993). These authors also emphasize the importance of engaging the patient early in therapy.

Many specific therapeutic strategies have been suggested for somatization. An often quoted method emphasizes the technique of reattribution (Goldberg *et al.*, 1989). This method essentially encourages the patient to reattribute the somatic symptoms not to causes within the physical body but to psychosocial problems. Goldberg *et al.* developed a videotaped training package to educate general practitioners in the techniques involved. The appeal of reattribution lies in its simplicity and ease of application even in general practice settings. Apart from this initial description in which the authors stress that the model is provisional and at an early stage of development, no further reports are available about its modification, applicability, and effectiveness. It is likely that reattribution would be an appropriate technique only in those patients with somatization who have a comorbid anxiety or depressive disorder; this would limit the utility of the intervention. Also, an issue which Goldberg *et al.* sidestep is how reattribution can be effected without examining the general health beliefs and attributory styles of patients.

Recently, cognitive behaviour therapy (CBT) has been used to treat somatization (Bertagnolli *et al.* 1994). A practical guide to its usage has been provided by Sharpe and colleagues (1992). The major focus of CBT is to monitor and alter dysfunctional cognitions that may be associated with innocuous somatic complaints. Although the approach holds promise, few studies have actually examined distorted cognitions associated with somatization, and whether clinical improvement occurs in tandem with changes in these cognitions. CBT is further limited by the paucity of trained therapists, especially in the Third World countries. Modifications in the methods may also be necessary to suit the needs and requirements of general practitioners who are principally involved in the care of these patients.

An important issue in the treatment of somatization is how these psychological techniques can be usefully employed in cultural settings other than the ones from which they originate. The psychological techniques outlined essentially focus on changing the way a person thinks about his/her bodily sensations. Such an orientation reflects a Western reductionistic epistemology which privileges the mind over the body. As thinking and feeling has been located within the mind in Western biomedicine, there is an understandable difficulty among its practitioners to acknowledge that the physical body could also be a locus of experience. Therefore, when a person assigns importance to distress in the body and is reluctant to acknowledge the assumed distress in the mind, he/she is viewed to be 'pathological'.

Ontological distinctions between the disorders of the mind and those of the body are not prevalent in non-Western schools of medicine. While the impact of these theoretical orientations might be weakening with the advent of market economy and rapid urbanization, many people in the non-Western societies still make use of traditional or local healers because of poor access to modern medical facilities. We have little information on how such patients are managed in these traditional sectors of care. Inexplicably, the WHO International Study of Somatoform Disorders has not evinced much enthusiasm to examine the traditional methods of care, even though one of its stated aims is to evolve intervention programmes for somatization in different settings. Logically, before treatment alternatives from developed countries are unquestioningly applied, it is necessary to explore how somatization is handled in specific social settings, particularly those which labour under meagre economic and manpower resources.

Relevant to this discussion is the moving ethnography that Scheper-Hughes (1992) has written on the travails of everyday life in Brazil. In Brazil, people see themselves as doubly cursed by drought and famine. Most of their daily activities are devoted to relieving hunger, a task in which they often do not succeed. A common folk diagnosis for their resultant distress is *delirio de fome*, that is, madness from hunger. This local frame of reference has undergone change consequent upon the Western medicalization of the Brazilian society. The focus has now shifted: starvation cannot be cured, but madness may be relived with medication. *Delirio de fome* has gradually given way to another folk concept, *nervos*, which is characterized by multiple somatic complaints, including aches and pains. This way, 'the madness, the *delirio de fome*, once understood as the terrifying endpoint in the experience of collective starvation, is transformed into a personal and psychological problem, one that requires medication' (Scheper-Hughes 1992, p 169). The new, enforced medical awareness persuades people to buy medicines that do not address the primary problem of hunger. The result is that people are left with even less money for food than ever before, ensuring the continuation of collective misery. Viewed against this background, the ongoing trials of drug treatment of somatization and the pharmaceutical organizational support to the WHO International Study of Somatoform Disorders, indicate an unsettling trend in the management of somatization. Prescribing pills for personal pains may not suffice to address the complexities of somatization.

In Conclusion

Significant advances have taken place in the field of somatization during the past decade. Major initiatives have examined the nosological aspects, epidemiological correlates, and developmental antecedents of the problem. The findings of the ongoing multinational study on somatoform disorders are eagerly awaited. Explorations into the cultural dimensions of the disorder inform us that somatization is not a disorder of the inarticulate mind but is one of an emergent bodily consciousness, grounded in a particular sociocultural reality. Consequently, management strategies evolved to address somatization need to be consciously local so as to be sufficiently relevant and innovative to handle its complex origins.

References

American Psychiatric Association (1980). *Diagnostic and Statistical Manual*, 3rd edition, Washington, D. C.: American Psychiatric Press.

——— (1987). *Diagnostic and Statistical Manual*, 3rd edition (revised), Washington, D. C.: American Psychiatric Press.

——— (1994). *Diagnostic and Statistical Manual*, 4th edition, Washington, D. C: American Psychiatric Press.

Bach M., Bach D., Bohmer F. *et al.* (1994). 'Alexithymia and somatization: relationship to DSM-IIIR Diagnosis', *J. Psychosom. Res.*, 38: 529–38.

Bagby R. M., Parker G. J. and Taylor J. D. A. (1994). 'The 20-item TAS-1: item selection and cross-validation of the factor structure', *J. Psychosom. Res.*, 38: 33–40.

Barsky A. J., Wyshak G. and Klerman G. I. (1986). 'Medical and psychiatric determinants of outpatient medical utilization', *Med. Care*, 24: 548–63.

Bass C. and Benjamin S. (1993). 'The management of chronic somatization', *Br. J. Psychiatry*, 162: 472–80.

Bertagnolli A., Harris S. and Arean P. A. (1994). 'Treating somatization disorders with cognitive behaviour therapy', *Beh. Therapy*. 17: 55–9.

Bridges K. W. and Goldberg D. P. (1991). 'Somatic presentation of DSM-III psychiatric disorders in primary care', *J. Psychosom. Res.*, 29: 563–9.

Bridges K., Goldberg D., Evans B. *et al.* (1991). 'Determination of somatization in primary care', *Psychol. Med.*, 21: 473–83.

Castillo R., Waitzkin H. and Escobar J. I. (1994). 'Somatic symptoms and mental health disorders in immigrant and refugee populations', in Miranda J, Hohmann, Atkinson C *et al.* (eds), *Mental Health Disorders in Primary Care*, San Francisco: Josey-Bass, 163–85.

Cheung F., Lau B. W. and Waldman E. (1981). 'Somatization among Chinese depressives in general practice', *Int. J. Psychiatry Med.*, 10: 361–74.

Cloninger C. R. and Yutzy S. (1993). 'Somatoform and dissociative disorders: a summary of changes for the DSM-IV', in Dunner D. L. (ed.) *Current Psychiatric Therapy*, Philadelphia: WB Saunders.

Craig T. K. J., Boardman A. P., Mills K. *et al.* (1993). 'The South London Somatization Study: I. Longitudinal course and the influence of early life experience', *Br. J. Psychiatry*: 163: 579–88.

Creed F. and Guthrie E. (1993). 'Techniques for interviewing the somatizing patient', *Br. J. Psychiatry*, 162: 467–71.

Douglas M. (1982). *Natural Symbols-Explorations in Cosmology*, New York: Pantheon Books.

Escobar J. L., Burnan A, Karno M. *et al.* (1987). 'Somatization in the community', *Arch. Gen. Psychiatry*, 44: 713–18.

Escobar J. L., Rubio-Stipec M., Canino G. *et al.* (1989). 'Somatic Symptom Index (SSI): a new and abridged somatization construct', *J. Nerv. Mental Dis.*, 177: 140–6.

Fabrega H. Jr (1989). 'Cultural relativism and psychiatric illness', *J. Ment. Nerv. Dis.*, 162: 415–25.

Fletcher R. H., Fletcher SW and Wagner EH (1988). *Clinical Epidemiology: The Essentials*, Baltimore, MD: Williams and Wilkins.

Goffman E. (1963). *Stigma: Notes on the Management of Spoiled Identity*, Englewood cliffs, NJ: Prentice Hall.

Goldberg D., Gask L. and O'Down T. (1989). 'The treatment of somatization: teaching techniques of reattribution', *J. Psychos. Res.*, 33: 689–95.

Gurjee O., Simon G. E., Ustun T. B. *et al.* (1997). 'Somatization in cross-cultural perspective: a WHO study in primary care', *Am. J. Psychiatry*, 154: 984–95.

Guze S. B. (1975). 'The validity and significance of hysteria (Briquet's syndrome)', *Am. J. Psychiatry*, 132: 138–41.

Hartvig P. and Sterner G. (1985). 'Childhood psychological environmental exposure in women with diagnosed somatoform disorders', *Scand. J. Soc. Med.*, 13: 153–7.

Isaac M., Janca A., Burke K. C. *et al.* (1995). 'Medically unexplained somatic symptoms in different cultures: a preliminary report from Phase I of the World Health Organization International Study of Somatoform Disorders', *Psychother. Psychosomatics*, 64: 88–93.

Janca A., Isaac M. and Costa e Silva J. A. (1995a). 'World Health Organization International Study of Somatoform Disorders-background and rationale', *Eur. J. Psychiatry*, 9: 100–10.

Janca A. , Isaac M., Bennett L. A. *et al.* (1995b). 'Somatoform disorders in different cultures—a mail questionnaire survey', *Soc. Psychiatry Psychiatr. Epidemiol.*, 30: 44–8.

Janca A., Burke K. C., Isaac M. *et al.* (1995c). 'The World Health Organization Study of Somatoform Disorders Schedule: a preliminary report on design and reliability', *Eur. J. Psychiatry*, 10: 373–8.

Katon W., Ries R. K. and Kleinman A. (1984). 'The prevalence of somatization in primary care', *Compr. Psychiatry*, 25: 208–15.

Katon W., Lin E., Von Korff M. *et al.* (1991). 'Somatization: a spectrum of severity', *Am. J. Psychiatry*, 148: 34–40.

Kirmayer L. J. (1984). 'Culture, affect and somatization', *Transcult. Res. Review*, 21: 154–262.

Kirmayer L. (1992). 'The body's insistence on meaning: metaphor as a presentation and representation in illness experience', *Med. Anthropol. Quarterly*, 6: 323–46.

Kleinman A. (1980). *Patients and Healers in the Context of Psychiatry*, Berkeley: University of California Press.

Kleinman A., Wang W. Z., Li S. C. *et al.* (1995). 'The social course of epilepsy: chronic illness as social experience in interior China', *Soc. Sci. Med.*, 40: 1319–30.

Krause I. B. (1989). 'Sinking heart: a Punjabi communication of distress', *Soc. Science Med.*, 29: 563–75.

Kroenke K., Spitzer R. L., de Gruy F. V. *et al.* (1997). 'Multisomatoform disorder: an alternative to undifferentiated somatoform disorder for the somatizing patient in primary care', *Arch. Gen. Psychiatry*, 54: 352–8.

Lee S. (1997). 'A Chinese perspective of somatoform disorders', *J. Psychos. Res.*, 43: 115–19.

Leff J. (1977). 'The cross-cultural study of emotions', *Cult. Med. Psychiatry*, 1: 317–50.

Lewis-Fernandez R., Kleinman A. (1995). 'Cultural psychiatry-theoretical, clinical and research issues', *Psychiatr. Clin. N. Am.*, 18: 433–48.

Lilienfeld S. O. (1992). 'The association between antisocial personality and somatization disorders: a review and integration of theoretical models', *Clin. Psychol. Rev.*, 12: 641–62.

Lipowski Z. J. (1988). 'Somatization-the concept and its clinical applications', *Am. J. Psychiatry*, 145: 1358–68.

Mechanic D. (1980). 'The experience and report of common physical symptoms', *J. Health Soc. Beh.*, 21: 146–55.

Morrison J. (1989). 'Childhood sexual histories of women with somatization disorder', *Am. J. Psychiatry*, 146: 239–41.

Olfson M. and Pincus H. A. (1994). 'Outpatient psychotherapy in the United States: I. Volume, costs, and user characteristics', *Am. J. Psychiatry*, 151: 1281–8.

Ots T. (1990). 'The angry liver, the anxious heart and the melancholic spleen', *Cult. Med. Psychiatry*, 14: 21–58.

Perley M. G. and Guze SB (1962). 'Hysteria: the stability and usefulness of clinical criteria', *N. Engl. J. Med.*, 266: 421–6.

Raguram R., Weiss M. and Channabasavanna SM (1996). 'Stigma, depression and somatization—a report from South India', *Am. J. Psychiatry*, 153: 1043–9.

Scheper-Hughes N. (1992). *Death Without Weeping: The Violence of Everyday Life in Brazil*, Berkeley: University of California.

Sharpe M., Peveler R. and Mayou R. (1992). 'The psychological management of patients with functional somatic symptoms—a practical guide', *J. Psychosom. Res.*, 36: 515–29.

Simon G. E. and Von Korff M. (1990). 'Somatization and psychiatric disorders in the NIMH Epidemiology Catchment Area study', *Am. J. Psychiatry*, 148: 1494–1500.

Skultans V. (1991). 'Anthropology and Psychiatry—the uneasy alliance', *Transcult. Psychiatr. Res. Rev.*, 28: 5–24.

Smith G. R. (1991). *Somatization Disorder in the Medical Setting*, Washington, D. C.: American psychiatric Association Press.

Smith G. R., Monson R. A. and Ray D. C. (1995). 'A trial of the effect of a standardized psychiatric consultation of health outcomes and cost in somatizing patients', *Arch. Gen. Psychiatry*, 52: 238–43.

Stern J., Murphy M. and Bass C. (1993). 'Attitudes of British psychiatrists to the diagnosis of somatization disorder: a questionnaire survey', *Br. J. Psychiatry*, 162: 463–6.

Swartz M., Landerman R. and George L. (1991). 'Somatization disorder', in Robins L., Regier D. A. (eds), *Psychiatric Disorders in America*, New York: Free Press, 220–57.

Terre L. and Ghiselli W. (1997). 'A developmental perspective on family risk factors in somatization', *J. Psychos. Res.*, 42: 197–208.

Tyrer P. (1989). *Classification of Neurosis*, Chichester: John Wiley and Sons.

Ustun T. B. and Sartorius N. (1995). *Mental Illness in General Health Care: an International Study*, Chichester: John Wiley and Sons.

Waitzkin H. and Magana H. (1996). 'The black box in somatization: unexplained physical symptoms, culture, and narratives of trauma', *Soc. Sci. Med.*, 45: 811–25.

Weiss M., Doongaji D. R., Siddhartha S. *et al.* (1992). 'The Explanatory Model Interview Catalogue (EMIC): contribution to cross-cultural research methods from a study of leprosy and mental health', *Br. J. Psychiatry*, 160: 819–30.

Weiss M., Raguram R. and Channabasavanna S. M. (1995). 'Cultural dimensions of psychiatric diagnosis: a comparison of DSM-IIIR and illness explanatory models in South India', *Br. J. Psychiatry*, 166: 353–9.

World Health Organization (1978). *Mental Disorders: Glossary and Guide to Their Classification in Accordance with the Ninth Revision of the International Classification of Diseases (ICD-9)*, Geneva: World Health Organization.

——— (1992). *The ICD-10 Classification of Mental and Behavioural Disorders*, Geneva: World Health Organization.

Yutzy S. H., Cloninger C. R., Guze S. B. *et al.* (1995). 'DSM-IV field trial: testing a new proposal for somatization disorder', *Am. J. Psychiatry*, 152: 97–101.

Chapter 7

Major Mental Illness in Women: Clinical Issues

PRABHA S. CHANDRA AND
KAVITHA VIJAYALAKSHMI

INTRODUCTION

During recent years, there has been an increase in the interest paid to gender differences in psychiatry, possibly as a result of the political processes that have been initiated by women themselves (Bennet, 1993). While the information available is as yet limited, it is already evident that major gender differences exist in the prevalence, clinical manifestations, response to treatment, and course of all major psychiatric disorders.

In many matters related to women and chronic mental illness, serious lacunae in knowledge exist; for example, when new psychotropic drugs are released, little information is available about gender-specific effects of these drugs, and their impact on menstruation, pregnancy, and lactation (Merkata *et al.*, 1993). Furthermore, psychosocial programmes rarely keep issues specific to women on their agenda; most rehabilitation settings have common programmes for men and women without incorporating aspects specifically relevant to women. Psychopharmacological and psychosocial issues are both of concern because it is becoming increasingly apparent that female psychiatric patients require a different approach to management.

The scope of this chapter, therefore, is to highlight aspects of importance in the field of chronic mental illness in women; disorders considered are depression, bipolar disorder, and schizophrenia. Special attention is paid to endocrine and reproductive events, and to drug and psychosocial issues in management.

The Course of Major Mental Illness in Women

Depression

Women are twice as likely as men to be diagnosed with depressive symptoms. Women with depression appear to have an earlier age of onset than men, and often become symptomatic during adolescence. There is also evidence to suggest that women are more likely to develop recurrent depression, and that the average length of an episode is longer in women. Reproductive events such as the premenstrual syndrome and postpartum depression may often be a starting point for more chronic psychiatric disorders (Weissman and Offson, 1995; Kornstein *et al.*, 1996).

Bipolar Disorder

The most clearly documented difference between men and women with bipolar disorder is that rapid cycling is approximately three times more common in women (Leibenluft, 1996). Women may also have more depressive episodes than men. In a 16-year follow-up study, Angst (1978) reported that 60 per cent of the episodes experienced by women were depressive as compared with 36 per cent in men. Roy-Byrne *et al.* (1985) found that bipolar men had more hospitalizations for mania while bipolar women had more hospitalizations for depression. Other gender differences have also been reported: dysphoric or mixed mania appear to show a female preponderance (McElroy, 1992); however, the data are inconsistent.

Schizophrenia

Pioneers such as Bleuler and Kraeplin believed that the clinical picture of early-onset schizophrenia associated with poor premorbid development, emotional blunting, and poor outcome occurred more frequently in males than in females. Nevertheless, until recently most research ignored issues specific to women. One explanation is that in women there is a potential confound introduced by cyclical variations in hormonal levels (Kulkarni, 1997). Another reason is that there are fewer female as compared with male in-patients with schizophrenia (Hafner *et al.*, 1989; Sartorius *et al.*, 1986).

Most studies focusing on women and schizophrenia report a later age of onset and a longer interval between onset of illness and hospitalization in women. The later age of onset has been linked to neuroleptic-responsiveness (Meltzer *et al.*, 1997). Many studies have reported that women have a less severe course of illness than men, and experience fewer hospitalizations with shorter in-patient stays. Women have fewer negative symptoms, better social adaptation, and better response to lower doses of neuroleptic drugs (Childers *et al.*, 1990).

There is also evidence to suggest that when women do not make a good recovery, the course of their illness is worse than that of men in the same situation. Major social stresses, such as homelessness, poverty, and victimization, create a very poor quality of life for women with chronic psychotic illness. Domestic conflicts and violence from family sources also lead to difficulties in chronically psychotic women (Milburn and D'Ercole, 1991; Walter and Kenward, 1985).

Interestingly, female schizophrenic patients aged 20–40 years appear to require lower doses of neuroleptic drugs than older females or males of the same age group (Kulkarni, 1997); higher oestrogen levels in women of reproductive age may explain this finding. The role of oestrogen is discussed in a later section.

The Menstrual cycle and Major Mental Illness

Depression

A constellation of severe premenstrual symptoms is experienced by 3.1–9.0 per cent of women (Rivera-Tovar and Frank, 1990; Chaturvedi *et al.*, 1993; Bancroft, 1993). The most common symptoms are depressed mood, mood swings, anxiety, irritability, decreased interest in everyday activities, and sleep and appetite changes (Hurt *et al.*, 1992; Bancroft *et al.*, 1994). During the premenstrual phase, many women experience depression amounting to atypical major depressive disorder. Not only is a history of mood disorder common among women with premenstrual dysphoric disorder, but these women are also at a high risk for eventually developing Major Depression. Likewise, most women with Major Depression experience severe premenstrual exacerbation of their symptoms. Halbreich (1997) presents an interesting discussion on the possibility that premenstrual symptoms are an expression of vulnerability traits to depression. The lifetime comorbidity rates of depression in women with premenstrual dysphoric disorder are high, and range from 30–70 per cent (Freeman *et al.*, 1994; Harrison *et al.*, 1989; Steinberg *et al.*, 1994).

Prospective ratings of mood are important in women with mood disorders, particularly depression, in order to establish premenstrual exacerbation. This is particularly important given the fairly high prevalence of suicidal ideation and intent reported in the premenstrual phase (Chaturvedi *et al.*, 1995; Endicott, 1993; Halbreich and Endicott, 1985). While drugs such as fluoxetine, buspirone, and alprazolam are useful in women with premenstrual dysphoric disorder, women with chronic or recurrent depression should be monitored for premenstrual worsening, and appropriate drug or dose modification should be implemented as necessary. Nonpharmacological techniques such as dietary changes and stress management are useful therapeutic adjuncts.

Bipolar Disorder

The relationship between the menstrual cycle and bipolar disorder has been described chiefly in the form of case reports. There have however been a few systematic studies. Diamond *et al.* (1976) found an increase in hospitalization rates during the menstrual phase. A somewhat similar finding was reported by Prema *et al.* (1991) that emergency admissions increase during the premenstrual phase in women with bipolar disorders. Price and DiMarzio (1986) found a high rate of retrospective report of premenstrual mood changes in women with rapid-cycling disorder; 60 per cent of the women in the study had a past history of severe premenstrual syndrome. In contrast with these studies, Wehr *et al.* (1988) found no relationship between the menstrual cycle and bipolar disorder. Brockington *et al.* (1988) described a series of women with puerperal bipolar disorder and premenstrual relapses. The general consensus thus appears to be that women with bipolar disorder are more likely to experience premenstrual dysphoric disorder and relapses during the menstrual or premenstrual phase.

Schizophrenia

Oestrogens are known to modulate the sensitivity of the dopamine receptor and potentiate the action of neuroleptics in laboratory animals. Oestrogens appear to be antidopaminergic in humans as well (Gordon *et al.*, 1980; Behrens *et al.*, 1992). These effects suggest that oestrogen may have a therapeutic role to play in schizophrenia, and indeed clinical evidence seems to support such a conclusion. This evidence is briefly reviewed here and elsewhere (Kulkarni, 1997).

The severity of psychotic symptoms has long been known to fluctuate cyclically in women with schizophrenia; mild exacerbation or even the occurrence of psychotic symptoms may be observed premenstrually, during the late luteal phase, when levels of oestrogen drop substantially (Dalton, 1959; Endo *et al.*, 1978; Berlin *et al.*, 1982). Seeman (1983) hypothesized that oestrogen may protect against early onset of severe psychosis in women, and that this may account for increased vulnerability to psychosis during both monthly- and lifetime- low oestrogen phases. Supporting this hypothesis in part, Goldstein (1988) reported that late menarche was associated with earlier onset of psychosis; this suggests that early menarche with greater lifetime exposure to oestrogen may delay the onset of psychoses. It has also been reported that schizophrenic women have a lower requirement for neuroleptic drugs during their reproductive life-span; presumably, the explanation lies in the higher oestrogen levels that are observed during this period of life (Kulkarni, 1997). Therapeutic applications of oestrogen in postpartum depression, in depression associated with menopause, and in schizophrenia are discussed in later sections.

Riecher-Rossler *et al.* (1992) studied the relationship between schizophrenic symptomatology and oestradiol in 32 women during different phases of the menstrual cycle. There was a significant relationship between oestradiol levels and psychopathology scores: with increasing oestradiol levels symptoms improved while with decreasing levels symptoms worsened. This relationship was evident in other areas as well, including ward behaviour and general well-being. Depression, however, did not show any such variation, Studies on psychiatric admissions in relation to the menstrual cycle have yielded similar results. Riecher-Rossler *et al.* 1992) reported an excess of premenstrual admissions while Prema *et al.* (1991) reported excess admissions in both menstrual and premenstrual phases.

These findings may have treatment-related implications. Yonkers *et al.* (1992) suggested that the requirement for neuroleptic drugs and the adverse effects of these drugs may vary across the menstrual cycle. Women may require higher doses premenstrually and lower doses in the intermenstrual period; and, neuroleptic adverse effects may decrease during those phases of the menstrual cycle when oestrogen levels are high. From the practical point of view, however, it may not always be convenient to vary neuroleptic dosage depending on the phase of the menstrual cycle. However, in those women in whom psychopathology shows cyclical changes, appropriate dose variations should be considered. If the patients' understanding and compliance are good, and if adequate monitoring and follow-up are feasible, neuroleptic dose variation across the menstrual cycle may prove a viable treatment strategy in female schizophrenic patients. Adequate neuroleptic protection can thus be provided during the vulnerable periods of the cycle, and unnecessary neuroleptic exposure can be avoided during the low-risk periods.

Pregnancy and Major Mental Illness

Depression

Clinical lore considers pregnancy to be a time of well-being and decreased psychiatric morbidity; nevertheless, various studies have shown that 10–16 per cent of pregnant women fulfil criteria for depression (Kumar and Robson, 1984; Klein and Essex, 1995). Several risk factors for depression during pregnancy have been identified; these include past history of depression, family history of depression, presence of marital discord, experience of recent adverse life-events, and occurrence of an unwanted pregnancy (O'Hara, 1986; Kitamura *et al.*, 1993).

Bipolar Disorder and Schizophrenia

There are surprisingly few data on the effect of pregnancy on bipolar illness and schizophrenia. Affective episodes have been reported to arise in all trimesters of pregnancy; however, Lier *et al.* (1989) found that pregnancy did not influence hospitalization rates in bipolar women. Mania during pregnancy is of concern because overactivity and excitement may lead to exhaustion and foetal problems; therefore, rapid control of symptoms is necessary. Early hospitalization and careful monitoring of foetal status are recommended.

During pregnancy, improvement may be observed in chronic psychoses such as schizophrenia; high oestrogen levels may be responsible for the favourable changes (Kulkarni, 1997). The effects of oestrogen in schizophrenia have already been discussed.

THE POSTPARTUM PERIOD AND MAJOR MENTAL ILLNESS

Depression

Postpartum depression affects between 10 per cent and 22 per cent of women. During the postpartum period, women with a past history of an episode of depression are at a 13–50 per cent risk for recurrence of the illness (Frank *et al.*, 1987; Kendell *et al.*, 1987). Anxiety and depression during pregnancy are potential predictors of postpartum depression (O'Hara, 1986). While the many hormonal changes occurring during and after pregnancy have long been considered as aetiopathogenetic factors, changes involving the hypothalamic-pituitary-thyroid axis were recently suggested to play a role: Harris *et al.* (1992) showed that women positive for antithyroid antibodies at 16 weeks of pregnancy were at a 50 per cent risk for the development of hypothyroidism during the postpartum period. This is significant because hypothyroidism is well-known to be associated with risk for depression. Later, Harris (1994) reported that women with antithyroid antibodies during pregnancy and the puerperium were at a higher risk of developing depression after delivery.

Pharmacological prophylaxis of postpartum depression may need to be considered in women who have one or more of the following risk factors: past history of postpartum depression, past history of nonpuerperal major depression, development of anxiety or depression during pregnancy, and absence of adequate marital and social support. Pharmacological prophylaxis usually involves the use of tricyclic antidepressant drugs, commencing very early during the postpartum period and continued for at least 6 weeks. Relapse rates are significantly reduced with such prophylaxis (Wisner and Perel, 1988). In a controlled study of women with a past history of postpartum depression, Wisner and Wheeler (1994) found a recurrence of depression in only 6.7 per cent of women who underwent antidepressant prophylaxis as compared with 62.5 per cent in those who did not. Antidepressant prophylaxis is safe but does carry a small risk to the child in the event of breast-feeding.

Pharmacological prophylaxis with non-antidepressant drugs has also been considered. Harris (1994) suggested the possible use of thyroxine in women with risk factors for postpartum depression, and who are also thyroid antibody-positive. Oestrogen, administered either orally or through a skin patch, has been tried in low doses with a gradual tapering over 6 weeks; while favourable results have been obtained in treating severe postpartum depression (Gregorie *et al.*, 1996), adequately designed controlled studies are required before oestrogen can be recommended as a viable prophylactic measure.

Bipolar Disorder

A number of studies show that women with bipolar illness are at high risk for postpartum recurrences (Parry, 1989). Kendell *et al.* (1987) reported that bipolar women had a 21.4 per cent risk for psychiatric admission within the first month after childbirth. Early postpartum euphoria predicted the development of depression weeks later. Women with histories of both puerperal and nonpuerperal mania were at more than 50 per cent risk for the experience of an affective episode following delivery. Reviewing the literature, Leibenluft (1996) stated that there is probably no other time in the life of a male or female bipolar patient when the risk of an episode is higher than the risk that a female bipolar patient faces during the postpartum period.

Schizophrenia

Kendell *et al.* (1987) reported that postpartum exacerbation of schizophrenia occurred in 3.4 per cent of women; however, in a prospective study of psychiatric disorders in the puerperium, McNeil (1987) found that women with an earlier episode of schizophrenia had as high as a one in four chance of developing postpartum psychosis.

Schizophrenia in the postpartum period often has a late onset (more than 3 weeks postpartum) and may be missed if restrictive definitions of the postpartum period are used. Confusion is a common symptom. Most women who develop a postpartum recurrence have had a longer duration of previous psychiatric hospitalization, and more active disturbance during the 6 months preceding the current pregnancy (McNeil, 1987).

MENOPAUSE AND MAJOR MENTAL ILLNESS

Depression

Women who experience premenstrual or postpartum depression are at an increased risk for the development of depression during menopause (Stewart and Boydell, 1993); pre-existing depression is also a risk factor (Pearce *et al.*, 1995). It is not clear whether the increased risk for depression is a consequence of psychological changes during menopause or is related to hormonal changes. While hormone replacement therapy is a much discussed subject across a wide range of medical disciplines, it is probably indicated in depression during natural menopause only if physical symptoms are present; these include vasomotor symptoms, or sexual difficulties due to vaginal dryness or decreased libido. In depression associated with artificial menopause (related to bilateral oophorectomy), hormone replacement may have a more positive role (Pearce *et at.*, 1995). However, hormone replacement therapy, particularly the progesterone component, has also been reported to occasion depression in postmenopausal women (Kornstein, 1997).

Bipolar Disorder

Opinions on the effect of menopause on bipolar disorder are conflicting. Kukopulos *et al.* (1980) found that a third of bipolar women start rapid cycling or continuous cycling during the perimenopause or menopause phase. Wehr *et al.* (1988), however, reported no such effect.

Schizophrenia

Watt *et al.* (1983) and Seeman and Lang (1990) described an increased risk for the development or exacerbation of schizophrenia during the postmenopausal period. While this phase of life is associated with numerous life stresses, it is also a phase when the circulating levels of oestrogen are low. It is conceivable that the increased risk for the occurrence or deterioration of schizophrenia may be due to the loss of the protective influence of oestrogen on psychological functioning. This mechanism may also explain why neuroleptic does requirement in psychotic women has been reported to rise during menopause (Seeman, 1996).

EXOGENOUS SEX HORMONES AND MAJOR MENTAL ILLNESS

Many women use exogenous sex hormones for contraception or as replacement therapy after menopause. Issues that therefore require consideration include the effects of these hormones on the course of major mental illness, and the interactions between these hormones and psychotropic agents. With regard to the former, patients have been described in whom rapid cycling may have been induced by conjugated oestrogens (Dawkins and Porter, 1991); with regard to the latter, several clinically relevant findings have been reported.

Ellinwood *et al.* (1983) found that in female patients who were receiving both benzodiazepines and oral contraceptives, cognitive and psychomotor functions were more impaired during the week that the patients were off the contraceptives. The authors suggested that oral contraceptives decrease the rate of absorption of benzodiazepines, leading to a slower and smaller peak in blood levels, and correspondingly less cognitive and psychomotor dysfunction.

Oral contraceptives decrease the oxidative metabolism of benzodiazepines such as chlordiazepoxide, diazepam, alprazolam, and flurazepam, leading to increased steady state levels (Watsky and Salzman, 1991; Sands *et al.*, 1995). Oral contraceptives may not have much effect on benzodiazepines such as clonazepam, lorazepam, and oxazepam, which are metabolized by nitro-reduction, hydroxylation, or conjugation (Sands *et al.*, 1995).

Oral contraceptives also inhibit the hepatic metabolism of antidepressant drugs such as imipramine, thereby increasing their half-life (Abernethy *et al.*, 1984).

In women who take both oral contraceptives and carbamazepine, an important drug interaction arises: carbamazepine increases hormone metabolism, thereby necessitating higher doses of oral contraceptives to ensure protection against pregnancy; oral contraceptives have a similar effect on carbamazepine, necessitating monitoring of carbamazepine levels (Watsky and Salzman, 1991). Phenytoin may similarly decrease the efficacy of oral contraceptives (Ciraulo and Slattery, 1995).

Lithium and oral contraceptives do not interact (Wilder, 1992). No major interactions have been reported between oral contraceptives and other drugs such as antipsychotics.

Woman may be prescribed sex hormones as a specific treatment for major mental illness. The beneficial effects of oestrogen have been studied in women with schizophrenia, mood disorders, and psychosis related to the menstrual cycle (Felthous *et al.*, 1980; Korhonen *et al.*, 1995; Kulkarni *et al.*, 1996). Both oral oestradiol and percutaneous oestradiol gel have been used with good results; the data are, however, too preliminary for firm recommendations to be made.

Other hormone-related effects have also been described. Reviewing the literature, Leibenluft (1996) described several studies in which treatment with exogenous steroids and clomiphene citrate appeared to have mood-stabilizing effects in women.

Major Mental Illness and Sexuality

Women with major mental illness have the same kind of sexual fantasies, urges and feelings, and face the same problems related to sexuality that healthy women do (Apfel and Handel, 1996). There is, therefore, a felt need for the treating psychiatrist to address these matters. Several additional issues also assume importance in patients with major mental illness. Certain of these concerns are dealt with in the sections that follow.

General Sexual Knowledge and Behaviour

Women with schizophrenia may have many misunderstandings about sexual anatomy and physiology, and may lack the basic vocabulary for discussing sex; discussions about sexuality may consequently prove difficult in such patients (Rozensky and Berman, 1984; Kalichman *et al.*, 1994). In a study of schizophrenic women, 52 per cent of subjects were found to have been sexually active during the previous 6 months; sexual activity was greater in women with greater psychopathology, in younger women, in women with lower levels of functioning, and in women with delusions (Kalichman *et al.*, 1994).

High-Risk Behaviour

The prevalence of Human Immunodeficiency Virus (HIV) infection in persons with severe and persisting mental illness is 10–76 times greater than the rate found in the general population.

Estimates indicate that 4–23 per cent of chronic mentally ill women are infected with HIV as compared with 0.3–0.4 per cent of women in the general population (Carey *et al.*, 1995; Weinhardt *et al.*, 1998a).

Research has begun to examine HIV-related high-risk behaviour in mentally ill women. Studies of community-based samples have found a significant prevalence of high-risk sexual behaviours in women with long-standing schizophrenia; such behaviours include having multiple sexual partners, engaging in sex for money, and participating in homosexual encounters. For example, in a study of 47 chronic mentally ill women in New York, Cournos *et al.* (1994) found that 29 per cent reported having had multiple sexual partners, 21 per cent reported having been involved in coercive sex, and 9 per cent reported having had sex with an intravenous drug-user during the previous year. These women were, in general, unlikely to use condoms. A history of sexually transmitted diseases was present in many women, as also a history of current alcohol and drug use in conjunction with sex. Many women reported sexual contacts with unfamiliar persons, such as persons encountered in bars and psychiatric clinics. Many women were also often involved in sex in exchange of money or drugs. There were no differences in risk behaviour between women diagnosed with paranoid schizophrenia, other schizophrenic categories, schizoaffective disorder, or bipolar disorder.

Studying 61 women with severe mental illness in the USA, Weinhardt *et al.* (1998a) found that 54 per cent had been sexually active during the past 2 months; 38 per cent reported at least one of the following risk factors during that period: having more than one male partner; having anonymous male partner(s); having intercourse without a condom with a known or suspected polygamous partner; having sex with a person after alcohol or drug use; having sex with a parenteral drug user; trading sex for money, drugs or lodging; being forced into sex; and/or, receiving drugs of addiction by a parenteral route. Twenty-three per cent of the sample reported two or more of these risk factors, and 16 per cent reported three or more risk factors. Among those with multiple sexual partners, condom use was rare.

In a study from the developing world, Chopra *et al.* (1998) reported high-risk sexual behaviour among women psychiatric patients in Bangalore, India. Many patients had experienced sexual abuse; many patients also expressed an inability to insist on safe sex in their partners and spouses. These studies clearly indicate that identifying and combating high-risk behaviour in sexually active mentally ill women is an important issue all over the world.

Knowledge about and Attitudes Towards HIV Infection

It is necessary to study female patients' knowledge about and attitudes towards HIV infection as this information would help in the development of appropriate management strategies. In a study on this subject, Weinhardt *et al.* (1998a) found that women with chronic mental illness rated insufficient money, unemployment, relationship problems, transportation needs, psychiatric care, and health care as more serious concerns than the risk for HIV infection.

Though patients with severe mental illness may have a reasonable basic knowledge about HIV transmission and the methods of prevention thereof, several misconceptions may exist: a common misconception is that confidentiality about an HIV-positive test will not be maintained. Misconceptions can interfere with important HIV-preventive behaviours. Even in the absence of misconceptions, individuals with adequate information and the necessary motivation to engage in HIV preventive behaviour may not do so due to deficits in safe sex negotiation skills, or the fear of loss of an emotionally or financially supportive relationship.

Management of High-Risk Behaviour

GENERAL ISSUES

The following general issues need to be kept in mind when managing women with long-standing mental illness:

1. Like healthy women, these women have sexual needs, and require to learn how to express their sexuality in a safe way.
2. High-risk behaviour in mentally ill women usually occurs in the context of limited knowledge, unawareness of personal risks, or the existence of other concerns which override the concern for guarding against HIV infection.
3. Mentally ill women may experience symptoms such as hypersexuality, impulsivity, and poor judgement; these can compromise the likelihood of safe sex.

4. Mentally ill women often lack the assertive skills necessary to have safe sex.
5. Unstable and transient interpersonal relationships can predispose to high-risk behaviour in mentally ill women.
6. Mentally ill women are often forced into sex; this compromises their ability to guard against HIV infection.
7. Mentally ill women and their partners may use alcohol or drugs before sex; this lessens the likelihood that safe sex will be practised.

EDUCATION

In general, when educating patients about sex, it is necessary to discuss aspects of sexuality as well as the risk of HIV infection; care must be taken to teach methods for the practice of safe sex. Sex education of this nature has been imparted to schizophrenic patients with successful short-term results (Berman and Rozensky 1984; Kalichman *et al.*, 1995). However, unless the desired behaviour is reinforceed or contextualized, the acquired knowledge and skills decay over time (Kalichman *et al.*, 1995),

Often, it is necessary to provide appropriate education to health-care staff as well. In an in-patient unit or in a community setting, the staff may ignore some obvious or inappropriate intimacies that arise between the patients (Cournos *et al*, 1990). Cohen and Tanenbaum (1985) developed an interdisciplinary sex education programme for staff in long-term psychiatric hospitals. The programme sought to enhance comfortable discussions about sexuality and patient care, to guide personnel in the assessment of risk behaviour, and facilitate their ability to implement intervention strategies.

When educating patients, information regarding HIV transmission, risk behaviours and risk situations, condom use and the effectiveness thereof, the course of HIV infection, consequences of HIV infection, and issues related to HIV testing need to be communicated. Misconceptions which may prevent risk-reducing behaviours need to be identified and addressed. Risk sensitization can be encouraged through the presentation of a videotaped interview of a local woman infected with HIV. Motivation for the practice of safe sex should be encouraged. Personalized education must be provided rather than a standard package of information with do's and don'ts.

ACQUISITION OF SELF-MANAGEMENT SKILLS

Patients should learn self-management skills, such as how to buy, keep, and use condoms. They should learn to identify the high-risk situations in which they are vulnerable to unprotected sex; for example, patients are less likely to take precautions if they have sex alter using alcohol or illicit drugs, if they have sex during periods of anxiety or depression, or if they venture into situations in which they are likely to be coerced into sex. Fears about or negative attitudes towards the implementation of various safe sex measures should be identified and tackled; for example, some women may be anxious about their partners' response should they insist on the use of a condom. Motivational issues should be addressed.

ACQUISITION OF ASSERTIVE SKILLS

Women with severe mental illness typically have extensive social skills deficits (Dilk and Bond, 1996); sexual assertive skills training may therefore help these women reduce their risk for HIV infection. Such assertive training can help women learn how to persuade unwilling male partners to use a condom. Assertive training can be accomplished through simulated interactions by the group facilitators, participant practice and instructive feedback. The generalization of acquired skills to actual sexual interactions needs to be monitored. The importance of sexual assertiveness is recognised by leading theoretical models of risk-taking such as the information-motivation-behavioural skills model (Fisher and Fisher, 1992). According to this model, a deficit in sexual assertiveness skills hinders risk-reduction efforts in a woman who is motivated to change her behaviour; this is because the woman finds it difficult to negotiate for safer sex behaviour with her partner.

A study incorporating these management methods showed that women with chronic mental illness can acquire and maintain the information and skills needed to reduce their chances of infection with HIV. Treated women enhanced their sexual assertiveness skills and maintained this improvement over a 4-month follow-up period (Weinhardt *et al.*, 1998b).

OTHER SIGNIFICANT ISSUES

Management programmes should attempt to modify the social contexts in which high-risk behaviour occurs. Special contexts are those related to vulnerable interpersonal relationships, substance abuse, and sexual abuse. Women may be reluctant to initiate a conversation about condoms because of the fear that this may result in an aggressive confrontation, injury, or the end of the relationship; realistic risk-reducing practices therefore need to be built within these contexts. Chronic mental illnesses are often comorbid with drug and alcohol abuse disorders (Regier *et al.*, 1990). Alcohol and drug use prior to risky sex may be common among adults with a chronic mental illness (Carey *et al.*, 1997). Therefore, the association between the use of alcohol and illicit drugs on the one hand and unsafe sexual behaviour on the other hand needs to be addressed. Whether this association is direct or results from a third variable such as impulsivity requires exploration. Sexual abuse is more common among women with chronic mental illness than in the general population (Rosenberg *et al.*, 1996); interventions need to be developed to address this problem. Patients should be helped to break abusive relationships. Referral to domestic abuse shelters should be made if such facilities are available.

Finally, therapists should encourage patients to seek testing if there is a history of unprotected anal or vaginal intercourse with a partner whose HIV serostatus is unknown or positive, or if there is a history of substance abuse using shared needles. Depending on the client's level of functioning, therapists should consider assisting with the scheduling of the test and co-ordinating counselling efforts with the testing site. With the prospect of testing, clients may experience an increase in anxiety and other psychiatric symptoms. Intensive therapist support, increased attention to suicidal ideation and, possibly, increased pharmacotherapeutic cover may be necessary for some clients.

Practical issues Related to Pregnancy

In women with chronic mental illness, as in other stigmatized and marginalized groups, the desire to become pregnant may be intensified because child-bearing is one source of self-esteem that can be pursued despite multiple losses in role functioning as a consequence of the illness. However, pregnancy poses several problems to the mentally ill woman. Certain of these problems are considered in the sections that follow.

Diagnosis of Pregnancy

The diagnosis of pregnancy may be difficult as mentally ill women are poor self-observers or may deny pregnancy. Clinicians should therefore keep records of patients' contraceptive practices and menstrual cycles. Clinicians should also maintain a high level of alertness for possible pregnancy, and should ask for pregnancy tests whenever there is a suspicion that a patient may be pregnant.

Prenatal Concerns

Women with chronic mental illness are more likely to have unwanted pregnancies, and are more likely to be older, unemployed, and homeless (Miller *et al.*, 1992). Poor prenatal care is consequently common. Risk for pregnancy-related complications therefore increases, and this risk is compounded by the increased prevalence of substance abuse, poverty, and poor nutrition in such patients (Rudolph *et al.*, 1990).

Psychotic denial of a confirmed pregnancy is rare but potentially dangerous; it is associated with a diagnosis of schizophrenia, a history of loss of custody of children, and a fear of future loss of custody (Miller, 1990). Potential risks involved in the denial of pregnancy are poor prenatal care, foetal abuse, precipitous labour or unassisted delivery, neonaticide, and/or postpartum emotional disturbance (Apfel and Handel, 1996). Psychotic denial should be treated with an intensification of monitoring; in-patient management may be required, particularly during the third trimester of pregnancy, or during crises.

In-patient care with integrated psychiatric and obstetric services has shown to improve perinatal outcome in women with chronic mental illness; sometimes, involuntary in-patient care may be needed. Indications for hospitalization include threats of violence towards the foetus, neglect of prenatal care due to delusions, inability to meet the special nutritional needs of pregnancy, risk of precipitous delivery, and attempts to prematurely self-deliver.

Wherever indicated and possible, temporary guardianship for the baby may need to be planned for. Supportive psychotherapy may be necessary to help the patient deal with the grief over an anticipated loss of custody.

Abortion

Abortions are commoner in women with chronic mental illness than in women in the general population. Spontaneous abortions are commoner because of poor prenatal self-care, and medical terminations of pregnancy are commoner because of poor contraceptive practice and the high risk for an unwanted pregnancy associated with an impaired capacity to care for the child.

Post-abortion psychological reactions are likely to be more severe in women with mental illness. This is true even if the abortion occurs with the consent of the patient. Following an abortion, the patient needs to mourn, and needs help to do so. She also needs help in acknowledging her loss, and in planning for future contraception to prevent an unwanted pregnancy.

Intranatal and Postnatal Concerns

Severely psychotic women may ignore or may not express the experience of labour pains. As a result, early admission may be necessary to monitor the onset and progress of labour. Sometimes, even a well-prepared patient can harbour aggressive feelings towards her baby, or become anxious during actual childbirth. As discussed earlier in this chapter, there is a high incidence of recurrence or exacerbation of mental illness during the postpartum period (McNeil, 1987). Psychiatric deterioration has an impact on the mother-infant relationship. Acute symptoms after childbirth may include denial of childbirth, delusions that the baby is dead or abnormal, and hallucinations commanding the mother to harm the baby (Steward, 1984); these may provoke infanticide. Guilt may occur in women who realize that they are unable to care for their babies. Hence, supportive treatment should be constantly provided until well after delivery.

It can be difficult to treat the patient postpartum as the patient may refuse or postpone the needed hopitalization due to a lack of insight (often aggravated by the withholding of psychotropic medication during pregnancy) and a lack of mother-baby units in psychiatric facilities. The ability of a patient to take her baby home should be based on her mental state and on the presence of at least one other adult in the environment who can take care of both the mother and the child. The patient's mental state can be best assessed by observing mother-child interactions in the maternal units.

Guidance can be obtained from nursery staff and obstetric staff reports. Decisions should be guided by evidence of abilities for childcare in previous pregnancies. Hospitalization in psychiatric hospitals may facilitate bonding, or mourning for custody loss, or may permit more supervision and intervention when there is ambiguity (Stewart and Gangbar, 1989).

Practical Issues Related to Parenting

Proper parenting is vital for the normal intellectual, emotional, and physical development of the child. The parenting abilities of women with chronic mental illness can be enhanced by the availability of support from the primary family, medical facilities (including psychiatrists, gynaecologists, and paediatricians), and tertiary organization. Appropriate guidance should be available to the patient to help her care for her child and attend to its medical needs. The mother-child units should be monitored for early signs of neglect or abuse (Apfel and Handel, 1996).

Illness characteristics impair parenting skills. For instance, schizophrenic patients have a reduced ability to discern non-verbal cues as well as a compromised capacity to recognize affects from facial expressions; these deficits can impair mother-child interactions (Corrigan and Green, 1993). As compared with healthy mothers who are not mentally ill, schizophrenic mothers touch less and play less with children (Gamer *et al.*, 1976), and exhibit withdrawal or inappropriate involvement (Abernethy and Grunebaum, 1972). Treatment with neuroleptic drugs can complicate matters because these drugs may decrease spontaneity (Nicholson and Blanch, 1994).

Some problems in parenting may arise from offspring characteristics. Children of schizophrenic mothers may be 'difficult' and slow to warm up. Contact with and separation from their mothers both have the potential to disturb normal emotional development in these children. If parenting is adequate, it is probably advisable to leave the child with its mother (Walker and Emory, 1983).

Problems in parenting may also arise from practical aspects of living . Homelessness among mentally ill mothers is common. This problem requires the attention of governmental and non-governmental organizations so that group homes or houses for such mothers may be made available (Nicholson *et al.*, 1993; Goering *et al.*, 1992). Unemployment and financial difficulties are also common among mentally ill mothers; they may require assistance with money management (O'Hara, 1986). These matters thus become necessary elements in rehabilitation programmes.

Programmes may be necessary to enhance a patients's parenting skills. These programmes need to be individually tailored with the patient's assets and liabilities in mind. Emphasis should be laid on self-reliance and on enhancement of self-esteem; both can improve confidence in parenting. A model programme developed in the Denver Mothers and Children Project (Waldo *et al.*, 1987) teaches parenting skills to schizophrenic mothers, monitors the developmental progress of the children, and allows for early intervention if needed. The programme provides developmental education to promote awareness of possible developmental delays, and to allay anxieties about the child's development. The programme also teaches good communication skills, techniques for disciplining children, techniques for toilet-training, and techniques for contraception. Themes which can be addressed in the programme are the effects of illness on parenting, and maternal feelings of ambivalence.

Major Mental Illness and Gynaecological Care

General Issues

Women with major mental illness require gynaecological care as do all other women; mental health professionals should regularly assess the need for such care because many patients may never seek assistance even if the need arises. A good reproductive history should be obtained at the initial contact with the patient, and symptoms related to the reproductive system should be asked after during the first, and at all subsequent consultations. Appropriate gynaecological care should be negotiated for depending on the need (D'Ercole *et al.*, 1991). Implementation of the gynaecologist's recommendations should be monitored (Handel, 1985). Preventive measures should be undertaken as required, such as counselling about regular breast examination for suspicious lumps, annual cervical smear examinations after the age of 40, and annual mammograms after the age of 50.

The institution of such measures of care conveys to both patients and staff that a woman's concerns about her body are important. For women with chronic mental illness, for whom much of the treatment is genderless and focused on thought and behaviour, visits to the gynaecologist can become a place to discuss concerns about their bodies.

Family Planning

The family planning needs of women with chronic mental illness should be understood in relation to the outcome of pregnancy in these women. Coverdale and Aruffo (1989) found that 33 per cent of patients who were sexually active did not want to become pregnant, yet did not use birth control methods; 31 per cent of patients had at least one abortion to terminate an unwanted pregnancy, and 60 per cent of the babies born to these patients were being reared by people other than the mothers. These data indicate that women with chronic mental illness may require counselling services for family planning and contraception because they experience difficulties in coping with the stress of parenthood. Most health professionals agree that suitable family planning information should be provided to women with mental illness (Coverdale *et al.*, 1992).

Grunebaum *et al.* (1971) found that most female patients preferred to obtain family planning counselling in mental health settings. Follow-up studies of patients who received such counselling in psychiatric hospitals have shown that most patients continue contraception after discharge, and many patients upgrade to safer, more effective methods of contraception (Abernethy *et al.*, 1975). Yet, despite the need and the desire for services with demonstrated efficacy, the provision of family planning counselling in mental health settings is relatively rare. As a striking example, Rudolph *et al.* (1990) observed that family planning and contraceptive measures were not mentioned in most charts of women with psychotic disorders who were hospitalized during pregnancies.

Offering family planning services together with mental health services has many advantages. The first advantage is one of convenience: women with chronic mental illness may find it hard to tackle the practical problems associated with attending separate psychiatric and family planning clinics; in fact, for many women, the psychiatrist may be the only contact with the health care system. The second advantage relates to consent: during periods of mental stability, women can provide their psychiatrists with an advance informed consent for interventions related to various reproductive events that may occur during a psychotic period. The third advantage is related to skills training: mental health professionals are in an ideal position to offer skills training on how to reduce unwanted sex and how to practice safe sex.

Although this is a delicate issue, eugenics should also be considered: children of mentally ill women have an increased risk of developing mental illness. Family planning counselling should therefore provide information about the heritability of the illness; patients can then make better informed decisions about family planning (Packer, 1992). It must be kept in mind that women with bipolar illness may minimize the burden of their illness and deny the possibility that it could be inherited (Targum *et al.*, 1981).

Guidelines for Family Planning Services

Coverdale *et al.* (1992) have provided practical guidelines for family planning services for women with chronic mental illness. First, a meticulous history should be obtained about sexual behaviour and experiences, pregnancies, and ability to care for children. Next, education about various contraceptive methods should be provided; it must, however, be kept in mind that patients with cognitive deficits or thought disorder will have impaired ability to use such information. Therefore, an attempt should also be made to discuss family planning with the patients' sexual partners. Wherever necessary and feasible, sexual assertiveness training should also be provided to the patients.

Some practical problems may arise; these must be identified and tackled. For example, women with chronic mental illness often do not take their pills as scheduled; oral contraceptives may therefore be an unsuitable method for contraception. Oral contraceptives may also induce mood changes, potentially leading to impaired drug compliance. Schizophrenics have an increased threshold for pain and may not recognize or admit early symptoms of pelvic inflammation; the use of intrauterine devices may therefore be associated with medical risks (Bachrach, 1985). Sometimes, contraceptive implants and intrauterine devices may become a focus of delusions of control (Coverdale *et al.*, 1993). Barrier methods of contraception may be unwise considering the high likelihood of unplanned and pressured sex among women with schizophrenia (Miller and Finnerty, 1996), and the difficulties that schizophrenic women experience in negotiating with their partners for the use of such methods; however, condom use has the advantage of conferring protection against HIV infection. For many women, depot contraception with medroxyprogesterone acetate, a long-acting injectable preparation, is optimal.

Finally, decisions must be made about whether family planning counselling should be provided to the patient alone or whether the patient's spouse, guardian, sexual partner, and/or family (as applicable) should also be involved. While greater participation is obviously preferrable, all decisions must be made on a casewise basis, in consultation with the patient.

In Conclusion

All issues related to women are also applicable to women with mental illness; illness, however, amplifies many issues and creates new ones. Therefore, special attention needs to be paid to the special, gender-based needs of women with major mental illness. Good psychiatric care should therefore integrate aspects related to sexuality, reproduction, and parenting into the management package in order to lessen the adverse consequences for women as well as children. Various phases in a woman's life, such as the premenstrual period, pregnancy, the postpartum period, and menopause, need special consideration with regard to both psychosocial and pharmacological management. In addition, biological and hormonal aspects of a woman's physiology need to be considered in treatment, especially when using psychotropic drugs.

References

Abernethy V. D. and Grunebaum H. (1972). 'Towards a family planning program in psychiatric hospitals', *Am. J. Public Health*, 62: 1638–45.

Abernethy V. D., Grunebaum H., Groover B. *et al.* (1975). 'Contraceptive continuation of hospitalized psychiatric patients', *Fam. Plann. Perspect.*, 7: 231–4.

Abernethy D. R., Greenblatt D. J. and Shader R. I. (1984). 'Imipramine disposition in users of oral contraceptive steroids', *Clin. Pharmacol. Ther.*, 35: 792–7.

Angst J. (1978). 'The course of affective disorders: II. Typology of bipolar manic depressive illness: life chart data from research patients from NIMH', *Arch. Psychiatr. Nervenkr.*, 226: 65–73.

Apfel R. and Handel M. (1996). 'Women with long-term mental illness: a different voice', in Soreff S. M. (ed.), *Handbook for the Treatment of the Severely Mentally Ill*, Seattle: Hograge and Huber, 326–49.

Bachrach L. L. (1985). 'Chronic mentally ill women: Emergence and legitimisation of programme issues', *Hosp. Community Psychiatry*, 36: 1063–9.

Bancroft J. (1993). 'The premenstrual syndrome: a reappraisal of the concept and the evidence', *Psychol. Med.*, 24 (suppl.): 1–46.

Bancroft J., Rennie D. and Warner P. (1994). 'Vulnerability to perimenstrual mood change: the relevance of a past history of depressive disorder', *Psychosom. Med.*, 56: 225–31.

Behrens S. Hafner H., De Vry J. *et al.* (1992). 'Oestradiol attenuates dopamine-mediated behaviour in rats: Implication for sex differences in schizophrenia', *Schizophr. Res.*, 6: 114.

Bennett J. C. (1993). 'Inclusion of women in clinical trials: policies for population subgroups', *N. Engl. J. Med.*, 4: 292–6.

Berlin F. S., Berger G. K. and Money J. (1982). 'Periodic psychosis of puberty: a case report', *Am. J. Psychiatry*, 139: 1119–1207.

Berman C. and Rozensky R. H. (1984). 'Sex education for the chronic psychiatric patient: the effect of sexual issues group on knowledge and attitudes', *Psychosoc. Rehab. J.*, 8: 28–34.

Brockington I. F., Kelly A., Hall P. *et al.* (1988). 'Premenstrual relapse of puerperal psychosis', *J. Affective Disord.*, 14: 287–92.

Carey M. P., Weinhardt L. S. and Carey K. B. (1995). 'Prevalence of infection with HIV among the serious mentally ill: Review of research and implications for practice', *Prof. Psychol. Res. Prac.*, 26: 262–8.

Carey M. P., Carey K. B. and Kalichman S. C. (1997). 'Risk for human immunodeficiency virus (HIV) infection among persons with severe mental illness', *Clin. Psychol. Review*, 17: 271–91.

Chaturvedi S. K., Chandra P. S. and Issac M. K. (1993). 'Premenstrual Experiences: the four profiles and factorial patterns', *J. Psychosom. Obstet. Gynecol.*, 14: 223–35.

Chaturvedi S. K., Chandra P. S., Gururaj G. *et al.* (1995). 'Suicidal ideas during the premenstrual phase', *J. Affective Disord.*, 34: 193–9.

Childers S. E. and Harding C. M. (1990). 'Gender, premorbid social functioning and long-term outcome in DSM-III schizophrenia', *Schizophr. Bull.*, 16: 309–18.

Chopra M. P., Savitha Sri E. V. and Chandra P. S. (1998). 'HIV-related risk among psychiatric inpatients from India', *Psychiatr. Serv.*, 49: 823–5.

Ciraulo D. A. and Slattery M. (1995). 'Anticonvulsants', in Ciraulo D. A., Shader R. I., Greenblatt D. J., Creelman W. (eds), *Drug Interactions in Psychiatry*, 2nd ed., New Delhi; B. I. Waverly Pvt Ltd, 249–310.
Cohen D. and Tanenbaum R. (1985). 'Sexuality education for staff in long-term psychiatric hospitals', *Hosp. Community Psychiatry*, 36: 187–9.
Corrigan P. W. and Green M. F. (1993). 'Schizophrenic patients, sensitivity to social cues: the role of abstraction', *Am. J. Psychiatry*, 150: 589–94.
Cournos F., Empfield M. and Horwarth E. (1990). 'HIV infection in state hospitals: case reports and long-term management strategies', *Hosp. Community Psychiatry*, 43: 942–3.
Cournos F., Guido J. R., Coomaraswamy S., Meyer-Bahlburg H., Sugden R. and Horwath E (1994). 'Sexual activity and risk of HIV infection among patients with schizophrenia', *Am. J. Psychiatry*, 151: 228–32.
Coverdale J. H. and Aruffo J. A. (1989). 'Family planning needs of female chronic psychiatric outpatients', *Am. J. Psychiatry*, 146: 1489–91.
Coverdale J. H., Aruffo J. A. and Grunebaum H (1992). 'Developing family planning services for female chronic mentally ill outpatients', *Hosp. Community Psychiatry*, 43: 475–8.
Coverdale J. H., Bayer T. L., McCullough L. B. *et al.* (1993). 'Respecting the autonomy of chronic mentally ill women in decisions about contraception', *Hosp. Community Psychiatry*, 44: 671–6.
Dalton K. (1959). 'Menstruation and acute psychiatric illness', *BMJ*, 1: 148–9.
Dawkins K. and Potter W. Z. (1991). 'Gender differences in psychokinetics and pharmacodynamics of psychotropic drugs: focus on women', *Psychopharmacol. Bull.*, 27: 417–26.
Diamond S. B., Rubinstein A. A., Dunner D. L. *et al.* (1976). 'Menstrual problems in women with primary affective illness', *Compr. Psychiatry*, 17: 541–8.
Dilk M. N. and Bond G. R. (1996). 'Meta-analytic evaluation of skills training research for individuals with severe mental illness', *J. Consult. Clin. Psychol.*, 64: 1337–46.
D'Ercole A., Skodol A. E., Stuening E. *et al.* (1991). 'Diagnosis of physical illness in psychiatric patients using Axis III and a standardised medical history', *Hosp. Community Psychiatry*, 42: 395–400.
Ellinwood E. H., Easier M. E., Linnoila M. *et at.* (1983). 'Effects of oral contraceptive-and diazepam-induced psychomotor impairment', *Clin. Pharmacol. Ther.*, 35: 360–6.
Endicott J. (1993). 'The menstrual cycle and mood disorders', *J. Affective Disord.*, 29: 193–200.
Endo M., Daiguji M., Asano Y. *et al.* (1978). 'Periodic psychosis occurring in association with the menstrual cycle', *Clin. Psychiatry*, 39: 456–61.
Felthous A. R., Robinson D. B. and Conroy R. W. (1980). 'Prevention of

recurrent menstrual psychosis by an oral contraceptive', *Am. J. Psychiatry*, 137: 245–6.

Fisher J. D. and Fisher W. A. (1992). 'Changing AIDS-related risk behaviour', *Psychol. Bull.*, 111: 455–74.

Frank E., Kupfer D. J., Jacob M. *et al.* (1987). 'Pregnancy-related affective episodes among women with recurrent depression', *Am. J. Psychiatry*, 144: 288–93.

Freeman E. W., Rickels K., Sondheimer S. J. *et al.* (1994). 'Nefazodone in the treatment of premenstrual syndrome: a preliminary study', *J. Clin. Psychopharmacol.*, 14: 180–6.

Gamer E., Gallant D. and Grunebaum H. (1976). 'Children of psychotic mothers: an evaluation of 1-year olds on test of object permanence', *Arch. Gen. Psychiatry*, 33: 311–17.

Goering P., Wasylenki D., St. Onge M. *et at.* (1992). 'Gender differences among clients of a case management program for the homeless', *Hosp. Community Psychiatry*, 43: 160–5.

Goldstein J. M. (1988). 'Gender differences in the course of schizophrenia', *Am J. Psychiatry*, 145: 684–9.

Gordon J. H., Borison R. L. and Diamond B. I. (1980). 'Modulation of dopamine receptor sensitivity by oestrogen', *Biol. Psychiatry*, 15: 389–96.

Gregorie A. J., Kumar S., Everitt B. (1996). 'Transdermal oestrogen for treatment of severe postnatal depression', *Lancet*, 347: 930–3.

Grunebaum H. U., Abernethy V. D., Rofman E. S. *et al.* (1971). 'The family planning attitudes, practices and motivations of mental patients', *Am. J. Psychiatry*, 128: 740–4.

Hafner H., Reicher A., Maurer K. *et al.* (1989). 'How does gender influence age at first hospitalization for schizophrenia?: a transnational case register study', *Psychol. Med.*, 19: 903–18.

Halbreich U. (1997). 'Premenstrual dysphoric disorders: a diversified cluster of vulnerability traits to depression', *Acta. Psychiatr. Scand.*, 95: 169–76.

Halbreich U. and Endicott J. (1985). 'Relationship of dysphoric premenstrual changes to depressive disorder', *Acta. Psychiatr. Scand.*, 71: 331–8.

Handel M. (1985). 'Deferred pelvic examinations: A purposeful omission in the care of mentally ill women', *Hosp. Community Psychiatry*, 36: 1070–4.

Harris B. (1994). 'Biological and hormonal aspects of postpartum depressed mood', *Br. J. Psychiatry*, 164: 288–92.

Harris B., Othman S. and Davies J. A. (1992). 'Association between postpartum thyroid dysfunction, thyroid antibodies and depression', *BMJ*, 305: 152–6.

Harrison W. M., Endicott J., Nee J. *et al.* (1989). 'Characteristics of women seeking treatment for premenstrual syndroms', *Psychosomatics*, 30: 405–11.

Hurt S. D., Schnurr P. P., Severino S. K. *et al.* (1992). 'Late luteal phase dysphoric disorder in 670 women evaluated for premenstrual complaints', *Am. J. Psychiatry*, 149: 525–30.

Kalichman S. C., Kelly J. A., Johnson J. R. *et al.* (1994). 'Factors associated with risk for HIV infection among chronic mentally ill adults', *Am. J. Psychiatry*, 151: 221–7.

Kalichman S. C., Sikkema K. J., Kelly J. A. *et al.* (1995). 'Use of a brief behavioural skills intervention to prevent HIV infection among chronic mentally ill adults', *Psychiatr. Seru.*, 446: 275–80.

Kendell R., Chalmers J. and Platz C. (1987). 'Epidemiology of puerperal psychoses', *Br. J. Psychiatry*, 150: 60–8.

Kitamura T., Shima S., Sugawara M. *et al.* (1993). 'Psychological and social correlates of the onset of affective disorders among pregnant women', *Psychol. Med.*, 23: 967–75.

Klein M. H. and Essex M. J. (1995). 'Pregnant or depressed? The effect of overlap between symptoms of depression and somatic complaints of pregnancy on rates of major depression in the second trimester', *Depression*, 2: 308–14.

Korhonen S., Saarijarvi S. and Aito M. (1995). 'Successful estradiol treatment of psychotic symptoms in the premenstrual phase', *Acta. Psychiatr. Scand.*, 92: 237–8.

Kornstein S. G. (1997). 'Gender differences in depression: implications for treatment', *J. Clin. Psychiatry*, 58 (Suppl. 15): 12–18.

Kornstein S. G., Schatzberg A. F., Yonkers K. A. *et al.* (1996). 'Gender differences in presentation of chronic major depression', *Psychopharmacol. Bull.*, 31: 711–18.

Kukopulos A., Reginaldi D., Laddomada G. *et al.* (1980). 'Course of manic-depressive cycle and changes caused by treatments', *Pharmacopsychiat.*, 13: 156–7.

Kulkarni J. (1997). 'Women and Schizophrenia—a review', *Aust. N. Z. J. Psychiatry*, 31: 46–56.

Kulkarni J., de Castella A., Smith D. *et al.* (1996). 'A clinical trial of estrogen in acutely psychotic women', *Schizophr. Res.*, 20: 247–52.

Kumar R. and Robson K. M. (1984). 'A prospective study of emotional disorders in childbearing women', *Br. J. Psychiatry*, 144: 35–47.

Leibenluft E. (1996). 'Women with bipolar illness', *Am. J. Psychiatry*, 153: 163–73.

Lier L., Kastrup M. and Rafaelson O. J. (1989). 'Psychiatric illness in relation to pregnancy and childbirth: II. Diagnostic profiles, psychosocial and perinatal aspects', *Nordisk Psykiatrisk Tidsskrift*, 43: 535–42.

McElroy S. L., Keck P. E. Jr., Pope H. G. Jr. *et al.* (1992). 'Clinical and research implications of the diagnosis of dysphoric or mixed mania or hypomania', *Am. J. Psychiatry*, 149: 1633–44.

McNeil T. F. (1987). 'A prospective study of postpartum psychoses in a high risk group: 2. Relationships to demographic and psychiatric history characteristics', *Acta. Psychiatr. Scand.*, 75: 35–43.

Meltzer H. Y., Rabinowitz J., Lee M. A. *et al.* (1997). 'Age at onset and gender of schizophrenic patients in relation to neuroleptic resistance', *Am. J. Psychiatry*, 154: 475–82.

Merkata R. B., Temple R., Sobel S. *et al.* (1993). 'Women in clinical trials of new drugs', *N. Engl. J. Med.*, 328: 292–6.

Milburn N. and D'Ercole A., (1991). 'Homeless women: moving towards a comprehensive model', *Am. Psychol.*, II. 1161–9.

Miller L. J. (1990). 'Psychotic denial of pregnancy: phenomenology and clinical management', *Hosp. Community Psychiatry*, 41: 1233–7.

Miller L. J. and Finnerty M. (1996). 'Sexuality, pregnancy and child rearing among women with schizophrenia spectrum disorders', *Psychiatr. Serv.*, 47: 502–5.

Miller Jr. W. H., Bloom J. D. and Resnick M. P. (1992). 'Prenatal care for pregnant chronic mentally ill patients', *Hosp. Community Psychiatry*, 43: 942–3.

Nicholson J. and Blanch A. (1994). 'Rehabilitation for parenting roles for people with serious mental illness', *Psychosoc. Rehab. J.*, 18: 109–19.

Nicholson J., Geller J., Fisher W. H. *et al.* (1993). 'State policies and programs that address the needs of mentally ill mothers in the public sector', *Hosp. Community Psychiatry*, 44: 484–9.

O'Hara M. W. (1986). 'Social support, life events and depression during pregnancy and the puerperium', *Arch. Gen. Psychiatry*, 43: 569–73.

Packer S. (1992). 'Family planning for women with bipolar disorder', Hosp. Community Psychiatry, 43: 479–82.

Parry B. L. (1989). 'Reproductive factors affecting the course of affective illness in women', *Psychiatr. Clin. North Am.*, 12: 207–20.

Pearce J., Hawton K. and Blake F. (1995). 'Psychological and sexual symptoms associated with menopause and the effects of HRT', *Br. J. Psychiatry*, 167: 163–73.

Prema S. V., Chandra P. S. and Chaturvedi S. K. (1991). 'Psychiatric admissions and the menstrual cycle—is there a relationship?', *NIMHANS J.*, 9: 91–6.

Price W. A. and DiMarzio L. (1986). 'Premenstrual tension in rapid-cycling bipolar affective disorder', *J. Clin. Psychiatry*, 47: 415–17.

Regier D., Farmer M., Rae D. *et al.* (1990). 'Comorbidity of mental disorders with alcohol and other drug abuse: Results from the Epidemiologic Catchment Area Study', *JAMA*, 264: 2511–18.

Riecher-Rossler A., Hafner H., Maurer K. *et al.* (1992). 'Schizophrenic symptomatology varies with serum oestradiol levels during menstrual cycle', *Schizophr. Res.*, 6: 114–15.

Rivera-Tover A. D. and Frank E. (1990). 'Late luteal phase dysphoric disorder in young women', *Am. J. Psychiatry*, 147: 1634–6.

Rosenberg S. D., Drake R. E. and Mueser K. (1996). 'New directions for treatment research of sexual abuse in persons with severe mental illness', *Community Ment. Health J.*, 32: 387–400.

Roy-Byrne P., Post R. M., Uhde T. W. *et al.* (1985). 'The longitudinal course of recurrent affective illness: life chart data from research patients at the NIMH', *Acta. Psychiatr. Scand.*, 71 (Suppl. 317) 5–32.

Rozensky R. H. and Berman C. (1984). 'Sexual knowledge, attitudes and experiences of chronic psychiatric patients', *Psychosoc. Rehab. J.*, 8: 21–7.

Rudolph B., Larson G. L., Sweeny S. *et al.* (1990). 'Hospitalised pregnant psychotic women: characteristics and treatment issues', *Hosp. Community Psychiatry*, 41: 159–63.

Sands B. F., Creelman W. L., Ciraulo D. A. *et al.* (1995). 'Benzodiazepines', in Ciraulo D. A., Shader R. I., Greenblatt D. J., Creelman W. (eds), *Drug Interactions in Psychiatry*, 2nd ed., New Delhi: B. I. Waverly Pvt Ltd, 214–48.

Sartorius N., Jablensky A., Korten A. *et al.* (1986). 'Early manifestations and first contact incidence of schizophrenia in different cultures', *Psychol. Med.*, 16: 909–28.

Seeman M. V. (1983). 'Interaction of sex, age and neuroleptic dose', Compr. Psychiatry, 24: 125–8.

——— (1996). 'The role of oestrogen in schizophrenia', *J. Psychiatry Neurosci.*, 21: 123–7.

Seeman M. V. and Lang M. (1990). 'The role of estrogen in schizophrenia: gender differences', *Schizophr. Bull.*, 16: 185–95.

Steinberg S., Annable L., Young Y. N. *et al.* (1994). 'Tryptophan in the treatment of late luteal phase dysphoric disorder: a pilot study', *J. Psychiatry Neurosci.*, 19: 114–19.

Steward D. E. (1984). 'Pregnancy and schizophrenia', *Can. Fam. Physician*, 30: 1537–41.

Stewart D. E. and Boydell K. M. (1993). 'Psychologic distress during menopause: associations across the reproductive cycle', *Int. J. Psychiatry Med.*, 23: 157–62.

Stewart D. E. and Gangbar R. (1989). 'Psychiatric assessment of competency to care for a newborn', *Can. J. Psychiatry*, 34: 34–8.

Targum S. D., Dibble E. D., Davenport Y. B. *et al.* (1981). 'The family attitude questionnaire: patients and spouses views of bipolar illness', *Arch. Gen. Psychiatry*, 38: 562–8.

Waldo M. C., Roath M., Levine W. *et al.* (1987). 'A model program to teach parenting skills to schizophrenic mothers', *Hosp. Community Psychiatry*, 38: 1110–12.

Walker E. and Emory E. (1983). 'Infants at risk for psychopathology: Offspring of schizophrenic parents', *Child Dev.*, 54: 1269–85.

Walter B. J. and Kenward H. B. (1985). 'Gender differences in living conditions found among male and female schizophrenic patients: a follow-up study', *Int. J. Soc. Psychiatry*, 31: 205–61.

Watsky E. J. and Salzman C. (1991). 'Psychotropic drug interaction', *Hosp Community Psychiatry*, 42: 247–56.

Watt B., Katz K. and Sheperd M. (1983). 'The natural history of schizophrenia: a 5-year prospective follow-up of a representative sample of schizophrenics by means of a standardized clinical and social assessment', *Psychol. Med.*, 13: 663–70.

Wehr T. A., Sack D. A., Rosenthal N. E. *et al.* (1988). 'Rapid cycling affective disorder: contributing factors and treatment responses in 51 patients', *Am. J. Psychiatry*, 145: 179–84.

Weinhardt L. S., Carey M. P. and Carey K. B. (1998a). 'HIV risk behaviour and the public health context of HIV/AIDS among women living with a severe and persistent mental illness', *J. Nerv. Ment. Dis.* 186: 276–82.

Weinhardt L. S., Carey M. P. and Carey K. B. *et al.* (1998b). 'Increasing assertiveness skills to reduce HIV risk among women with a severe and persistent mental illness', *J. Consult. Clin. Psychol.* 66: 680–4.

Weissman M. M. and Offson M. (1995). 'Depression in women: implications for health care research', *Science*, 269: 799–801.

Wilder B. J. (1992). 'Pharmacokinetics of valproate and carbamazepine', *J. Clin. Psychopharmacol.*, 12: 64S–68S.

Wisner K. L. and Perel J. M. (1988). 'Psychopharmacologic agents and electroconvulsive therapy during pregnancy and the puerperium', in Cohen R. L. (ed.). *Psychiatric Consultation in Childbirth Settings: Parent- and Child-oriented Approaches*, New York: Plenum Medical Book Company, 165–206.

Wisner K. L. and Wheeler S. B. (1994). 'Prevention of recurrent postpartum major depression', *Hosp. Community Psychiatry*, 45: 1191–6.

Yonkers K. A., Kando J. C., Cole J. D. *et al.* (1992). 'Gender differences in the pharmacodynamics and pharmacokinetics of neuroleptic drug treatments', *Am. J. Psychiatry*, 149: 587–95.

Chapter 8

Biological Treatments for Bipolar Disorder: Recent Strategies

K. N. Roy Chengappa and Joseph Levine

Introduction

The pharmacotherapy of bipolar disorder is complicated by the likelihood that the mechanisms underlying depression, mania, and the switch to either pole are different; thus, one may speak of antidepressant, antimanic, and antiswitch properties of the available drugs. At present, the extent to which the available medications display these three properties is unclear; however, prophylactic agents such as lithium and certain anticonvulsant drugs do appear to have a broad spectrum of efficacy.

Ideally, an agent used to treat bipolar illness should have the following properties:

1. It should reverse rather than merely suppress the extant pathophysiological mechanism(s).
2. It should act rapidly (in hours to days) to attenuate the relevant phase symptomatology.
3. It should have a high therapeutic index, and carry a minimal or no risk for short- and long-term adverse effects.
4. It should carry minimal or no risk for switching patients into the opposite pole of illness.
5. It should carry minimal or no risk for inducing rapid-cycling illness.
6. It should have therapeutic efficacy in both depressed and manic phases of illness.

7. It should have prophylactic efficacy in all categories of bipolar patients, including those with rapid and ultra-rapid cycling.
8. Its therapeutic and prophylactic action should be associated with high response rates.
9. Its therapeutic and prophylactic course should be easy to effect, and should not require frequent monitoring.

These requirements are not easy to fulfil. The progress made since the introduction of lithium has been disappointing; for example, although carbamazepine and valproic acid fulfil several of the requirements listed, they are not effective in all subjects, nor do they have an adequate efficacy for depressive episodes; furthermore, they occasion several adverse effects, and may require frequent monitoring.

During the last decade, however, there has been an explosion of research on potential new therapies for bipolar disorder; it is possible that certain or all of these therapies may, in the coming years, usefully augment the psychiatrist's therapeutic armamentarium. This chapter is devoted to a discussion of such new and experimental methods of treatment.

Newer Anticonvulsants

Lamotrigine

Lamotrigine (LTG) is an antiepileptic drug of the phenyltriazine class. It is a chemically novel drug, unrelated to other marketed antiepileptic agents. Its profile of action is similar to that of phenytoin and carbamazepine in that it stabilizes type II sodium channels. Neurochemical and electrophysiological studies show that LTG selectively inhibits sodium currents by interacting specifically with the slow inactivated state of the sodium channel. This enables it to affect only significantly depolarized membranes without interfering with the normal physiological activity. LTG additionally blocks the release of glutamate and aspartate (Messenheimer, 1995), which are exitatory amino acid neurotransmitters. Recently, it has been suggested that LTG may limit pathological excitation by modulating calcium and potassium channel currents (Walden *et al.*, 1997).

LTG has a broad spectrum of antiepileptic activity, with

demonstrated efficacy against partial as well as generalized seizures, and in idiopathic as well as symptomatic epilepsy. It may also be effective in the Lennox-Gastaut syndrome. LTG is used as monotherapy in epilepsy, and as an add-on drug in refractory patients.

Recent studies suggest that LTG may benefit patients with bipolar disorder (Sporn and Sachs, 1997; Labbate and Rubey, 1997). LTG was found to be effective in refractory bipolar patients, in patients with rapid-cycling bipolar illness (Fatemi *et al.*, 1997) and in patients experiencing breakthrough bipolar depression (Weisler *et al.*, 1994). Ferrier *et al.*, (1997) reported that 3 rapid-cycling patients responded to the addition of LTG after failing a trial of lithium and after responding only partially to a combination of valproic acid and carbamazepine; all 3 patients had had abnormal EEGs before the introduction of LTG.

Kusumaker and Yatham (1997) studied 22 bipolar patients in the depressed phase. All had failed to respond to a combination of divalproex sodium and another mood stabilizer, or divalproex sodium and an antidepressant drug. LTG was added to the ongoing therapy in the dose of 50 mg twice a day. Sixteen patients (73 per cent) showed response, with no switch to hypomania or mania.

A large, 21-centre, randomized, double-blind, placebo-controlled study of LTG monotherapy was conducted in the USA and in Europe on 192 depressed out-patients with bipolar I disorder. LTG was used in two doses: 50 mg/day and 200 mg/day, for 7 weeks. Preliminary results suggested an antidepressant efficacy for the 200 mg/day group; results in the 50 mg/day group were mixed (Bowden *et al.*, 1998).

Presently, it is not yet known whether LTG has antimanic and/or long-term mood-stabilizing effects (McElroy, 1997).

LTG is generally well-tolerated. Skin rash occurs in 1 per cent of treated patients, but is more common in children. The adverse effect may or may not recur on rechallenge with the drug. Rarely, more serious and life-threatening cutaneous complications may develop; an example is the Stevens-Johnson syndrome. The co-administration of valproate increases the risk for serious cutaneous rashes. Other side effects of LTG include dizziness, drowsiness, ataxia, tremors, diplopia, headache, nausea, and vomiting. There are no reported drug interactions with lithium (Freeman and Stoll, 1998).

In bipolar depression, LTG is probably best used in the same doses that are conventional in epilepsy; that is, 25–200 mg/day in two divided doses. The half-life of LTG is approximately 35 hours. This half-life is decreased to 15 hours in patients receiving enzyme-inducing drugs; in such patients, larger doses of LTG may be required. The half-life is increased to 60 hours in patients receiving sodium valproate; in such patients, a lower starting dose of 12.5 mg/day may need to be used, and upward dose titration may need to span several days to weeks.

In conclusion, preliminary reports suggest that LTG may be useful in patients with bipolar depression and rapid-cycling bipolar illness. Its role in the treatment of mania and in the long-term maintenance treatment of bipolar disorder remains to be determined.

Gabapentin

Gabapentin (GBT) is an antiepileptic drug which was synthesized as an analogue of gamma-aminobutyric acid (GABA). Recent reports suggest that GBT increases extracellular GABA, possibly by a reversal of GABA transport into the cell (Gotz *et al.*, 1993). Since GABA is an inhibitory neurotransmitter, this action may explain the action of GBT, and hence its potential applications in neuropsychiatric disorders. The effects of GBT on other neurotransmitter systems have also been reported (Beydoun *et al.*, 1995).

GBT is an approved adjunctive drug for partial seizures with or without secondary generalization; monotherapy trials with GBT are currently under way. Preliminary data suggest that GBT may be effective for the acute or prophylactic treatment of bipolar illness (Marcotte, 1997). In an open study, 28 refractory bipolar patients previously treated with lithium, valproate, and/or carbamazepine were administered GBT; 18 patients showed a positive response (Schaffer and Schaffer, 1997). Similar results were obtained in an open study of patients with bipolar depression (Young *et al.*, 1997). The use of GBT for the prophylaxis of bipolar I disorder has been examined in larger studies, but the results remain unpublished to date.

Common side effects of GBT are somnolence, ataxia, dizziness, fatigue, headache, tremors, nystagmus, and diplopia. These side effects appear early and are often transient. Three per cent of subjects show some weight gain. Some patients with epilepsy report dysphoric mood changes, including fear and irritability. Rarely, dystonias and myoclonic movements occur in patients with epilepsy.

GBT has a large therapeutic window and relatively low toxicity. It has a half-life of just 5–7 hours, and should therefore be administered in a thrice-daily schedule. Treatment is initiated at 300 mg/day, and is increased by 300 mg each day to reach 900 mg/day by the third day. Maintenance doses for epilepsy are commonly 900–1,800 mg/day, but doses up to 3,600 mg/day have also been used. Doses need to be adjusted downward if renal dysfunction is present, as renal excretion is the main route of elimination.

The optimal dose of GBT in psychiatric patients is still unknown. Patients with bipolar illness have received doses ranging from 600 mg/day to 4,800 mg/day, with a mean of 1,500 mg/day (Marcotte, 1997). Drug-drug interactions are minimal due to a lack of significant effects on hepatic mixed function oxidase enzymes and low plasma protein binding. GBT can therefore conveniently be administered in conjunction with other agents.

In conclusion, GBT may be effective during the manic and depressed phases of bipolar disorder, and in a subgroup of patients with refractory bipolar illness. Its efficacy appears to lie in co-administration with mood-stabilizing drugs and/or second generation antipsychotic agents. Its role in maintenance therapy and prophylaxis is presently uncertain.

Topiramate

Topiramate is a recently-introduced antiepileptic drug. It is a sulfamate-substituted monosaccharide derivate of D-fructose. Its antiepileptic action has been suggested to be mediated by three mechanisms:

1. The production of a state-dependent blockade of sodium channels.
2. The potentiation of GABA-mediated inhibitory neurotransmission through enhanced intraneuronal influx of chloride ions.
3. Antagonism of kainate activation of the kainate/AMPA subtype of glutamate receptors.

Topiramate has no apparent effect on the NMDA subtype

of glutamate receptor. It is a weak inhibitor of carbonic anhydrase, but this may not be of much relevance to its antiepileptic activity.

Topiramate is presently indicated as an add-on treatment in adults with partial-onset seizures. Two recent studies suggest that it may be helpful in the treatment of bipolar illness as well. Calabrese *et al.* (1998) used topiramate in 11 manic patients who were refractory to standard antimanic agents. Four weeks later, 3 patients showed more than 50 per cent improvement and 2 patients 25–49 per cent improvement.

Marcotte (1998) used topiramate in patients with bipolar I illness (n=14), bipolar II illness (n=6), mixed affective disorder (n=7), cyclothymia (n=10), bipolar disorder NOS (n=7), schizoaffective disorder (n=9), dementia (n=3), and psychoses NOS (n=2). Forty-four of these 58 patients had rapid-cycling illness, and 18 had not only failed to respond to traditional mood stabilizers, but had failed trials with LTG and/or GBT as well. The mean duration of topiramate treatment was 16 weeks. At the end of the treatment, 62 per cent of the sample was rated as markedly or moderately improved on global assessment, with response often being observed during the 1st week itself. Sixteen patients showed minimal to no response, and 6 patients worsened. Large, multicentre trials of topiramate are currently under way.

Adverse effects reported with topiramate include parathesia, anorexia and weight loss, nausea, somnolence, fatigue, impaired concentration and memory, and word-finding difficulty. In 1.5 per cent of patients, renal (phosphate) stones may develop. The effect of topiramate on appetite and weight may actually be advantageous; in bipolar disorders, weight gain is sometimes an important reason for treatment noncompliance, and in such patients topiramate may be a useful alternative drug.

Topiramate is minimally (13–17 per cent) protein bound. It undergoes little metabolism in the liver and is primarily eliminated unchanged in urine. Thus, topiramate can relatively safely be combined with other drugs; this is an advantage because polypharmacy is common in bipolar patients. Downward dose adjustment is necessary in patients with renal disorder, but not in those with mild to moderate liver dysfunction. Phenytoin and carbamazepine may decrease topiramate concentrations by 40–50 per cent, necessitating upward dose adjustments. Minimal drug interactions are noted with valproic acid. Topiramate may compromise the efficacy of concomitant oral contraceptives.

In bipolar disorder, treatment with topiramate is begun at 25 mg/day; the dose is increased by 25–50 mg/day every 3 to 4 days in in-patients and every week in out-patients. In epilepsy, doses of 200–1,000 mg/day have been used, with a dose of 400 mg/day being common; at high doses, the risk for adverse effects, such as weight loss, cognitive impairment, tremors, confusion, and depression, is increased. The ideal dose range for bipolar patients has not been established. Calabrese *et al.* (1998) used doses of 50–1,300 mg/day while Marcotte (1998) administered a mean dose of 200 mg/day. In the author's anecdotal practice, doses of 100–400 mg/day have sufficed for patients with hypomania and mania in out-patient and in-patient settings.

In epileptic patients, no correlation of topiramate levels with seizure control has been reported; therefore, therapeutic drug level monitoring is probably unnecessary.

In conclusion patients with rapid-cycling and treatment-refractory bipolar disorder are potential candidates for topiramate therapy. Large multicentre trials will commence soon, and these will demonstrate the extent to which topiramate is effective in the treatment of mania and depression, and in the prophylaxis of bipolar disorder.

Calcium Channel Blockers

Calcium channel blockers (CCBs) inhibit the flux of calcium ions into excitable cells through long-acting channels. There are four classes of CCBs:

1. Phenylalkylamines (including verapamil)
2. 1, 4-dihydropyridines (including nifedipine and nimodipine)
3. Benzothiazepines (including diltiazem)
4. Diphenylpiperazines (including flunarizine)

Besides their application in cardiovascular disorders, CCBs have been found useful in bipolar illness. Unfortunately, there is a lack of large sample, multicentre, randomized controlled clinical trials with these drugs. Verapamil is the most studied CCB; it has been suggested to be useful for manic patients who do not respond to or tolerate therapy with lithium (Bowden *et al.*, 1994; Baron and

Gitlin, 1987; Mallinger *et al.*, 1997). Nifedipine, nimodipine, diltiazem, and flunarizine have also been tried in mania, but the results are too preliminary to draw definitive conclusions (Dubovsky *et al.*, 1995). Preliminary data suggests that CCBs such as verapamil and nimodipine may function as mood stabilizers (Giannini *et al.*, 1987; Manna, 1991); while some workers believe that these agents may also be effective in rapid-cycling bipolar patients, not all agree with this viewpoint (Dubovsky and Buzan, 1995).

The results of recent studies have contradicted previous beliefs: in randomized controlled trials, verapamil was found to be inferior to lithium (Walton *et al.*, 1996), and no better than placebo (Janicak *et al.*, 1998).

The most common side effects of CCBs are dizziness, headaches, skin flushing, tachycardia, nausea, edema, and digital parasthesias (Dubovsky and Buzan, 1995). Verapamil is more likely than other CCBs to cause bradycardia and hypotension, atrioventricular block, coughing, wheezing, somnolence, rashes, and constipation. When prescribed along with lithium, verapamil may decrease serum lithium levels (Freeman and Stoll, 1998), and occasion Parkinsonian symptoms, bradycardia, or neurotoxicity. When prescribed along with carbamazepine, verapamil may increase carbamazepine levels and cause neurotoxicity. When prescribed along with neuroleptics, CCBs may increase neuroleptic levels, and hence the risk for extrapyramidal side effects.

Verapamil has generally been used in doses of 240–320 mg/day. Doses upto 320 mg/day may be well tolerated by patients with comorbid medical disorders (Dubovsky and Buzan, 1995).

In conclusion, verapamil may usefully augment lithium therapy in some patients with mania, especially when the patients have failed to respond to lithium (Mallinger *et al.*, 1997). Verapamil may also have a role in the management of bipolar women who are considering pregnancy (Goodnick, 1993) as it has already been used in pregnancy for other indications (Briggs *et al.*, 1998). At present, the available data do not recommend a broader role for the CCBs in bipolar illness.

Second Generation Antipsychotic Agents

Clozapine

Clozapine is an atypical antipsychotic agent. It is a dibenzodiazepine derivative with a broad range of neuroreceptor effects: it strongly blocks 5-HT2, muscarinic, adrenergic, and histaminic receptors, and weakly blocks dopamine D2 receptors. This profile of receptor activity, along with its spectrum of action on animal models, described its potential for antipsychotic efficacy without risk for associated extrapyramidal adverse effects.

McElroy *et al.* (1991) suggested that response rates to clozapine may be higher in patients with bipolar and schizoaffective illness (almost 85 per cent) than in those with treatment-resistant schizophrenia (46 per cent). A recent review of all published reports found that nearly 70 per cent of clozapine-treated bipolar (n=94) and schizoaffective (n=221) patients achieved clinically significant improvement (Zarate *et al.*, 1995a); however, these data must be interpreted with caution because the numbers of patients in controlled trials were small. Clozapine particularly appeared to benefit patients with rapid-cycling illness, those who were treatment–refractory, and those who had tardive dyskinesia. The rehospitalization rate for patients receiving clozapine monotherapy for refractory mood disorders was halved in one study.

Clozapine has shown benefits for patients with acute mania (Barbini *et al.*, 1997), manic psychoses (Zarate *et al.*, 1995a), and rapid-cycling bipolar illness with or without psychoses (Calabrese *et al.*, 1991; Suppes *et al.*, 1994; Frye *et al.*, 1996). Clozapine has been found useful in children and adolescents with bipolar illness (Fuchs, 1994; Kowatch *et al.*, 1995). Clozapine monotherapy has been suggested for mood stabilization in difficult-to-treat bipolar subjects (Zarate *et al.*, 1995b). Overall, the response to clozapine appears to be better in the manic and psychotic phase than in the depressed phase (Banov *et al.*, 1994).

The (albeit low) risk for agranulocytosis, a potentially life-threatening adverse effect, necessitates inconvenient weekly monitoring of blood counts during the initial 4 months of clozapine therapy. Clozapine commonly occasions other adverse effects, such as hypersalivation, sedation, and increased weight; these are tolerated even more poorly by bipolar patients than by schizophrenic patients. Seizures occur with high incidence at doses above 500 mg/day. Such problems discourage an enthusiastic use of clozapine in bipolar illness.

In schizophrenic patients, clozapine is used in the dose range of 100–900 mg/day; 250–600 mg/day is usual in adults. In the elderly and in those with Parkinson's disease and psychosis, lower doses such as 50–100 mg/day are common. The drug is best administered twice a day starting at 25 mg/day, with gradual upward dose titration over 2 to 6 weeks based on the balance between benefits and dose-limiting side effects such as sedation and orthostatic hypotension. The ideal dosing for bipolar patients is currently unknown, but the available literature suggests that most adult bipolar patients tolerate 200–500 mg/day of the drug.

Serum levels of 350–420 ng/ml have been correlated with response among patients with schizophrenia and schizoaffective disorder; however, it is unclear whether titrating the dose to these plasma levels converts non-responders to responders. Dose-response data are unavailable for bipolar patients.

In conclusion, clozapine is best reserved for bipolar patients in whom mood-stabilizing agents alone or in combination are not effective, or are not tolerated. Therefore, it is likely that clozapine will be used in treatment-resistant bipolar or schizoaffective bipolar patients with persistent psychoses, rapid-cycling illness, severe tardive dyskinesia, and/or intolerance to older agents. Clozapine may be used as monotherapy or in combination with other mood-stabilizing drugs (except carbamazepine, as there is a theoretically increased risk for bone marrow toxicity).

Risperidone

Risperidone is a newer antipsychotic agent belonging to the benzisoxazole class. An important characteristic of risperidone is that it produces more potent blockade of 5-HT2 than of D2 receptors. It also blocks adrenergic receptors, but has almost no effect on muscarinic receptors.

Case reports and open studies have documented the efficacy of risperidone in patients with mania as well as in those with bipolar schizoaffective disorder. Goodnick (1995) described two patients with mania who had not responded to previous medications and who subsequently responded to risperidone. Jacobsen (1995) reported that risperidone monotherapy/add-on therapy, in the dose of 1–6 mg/day, produced partial or complete remission in 13 of 17 patients with manic or mixed affective disorder. Sajatovic *et al.* (1996a) found that risperidone in combination with fluphenazine attenuated manic symptoms in a schizomanic patient who had been refractory to previous treatments. Several other studies have reported similar findings (Keck *et al.*, 1995; Madhusoodanan *et al.*,

1995; Tohen *et al.*, 1996; Sajatovic *et al.*, 1996b). Open studies suggest that a subgroup of bipolar patients benefit from adjunctive risperidone both during an acute episode of mania and during maintenance treatment (Ghaemi and Sachs, 1997; Ghaemi *et al.*, 1997).

Clinical predictors of response to risperidone include younger age, shorter duration of illness, and the diagnoses of bipolar or schizoaffective disorder (Keck *et al.*, 1995); in this study, among patients with bipolar schizoaffective illness, significantly more responders than non-responders were receiving concomitant mood-stabilizing drugs (lithium, divalproex sodium, or carbamazepine, alone or in combination). Tohen *et al.* (1996) reported that 12 of 15 manic patients experienced clinical improvement when risperidone was added to a mood-stabilizing drug. Vieta *et al.* (1998) found that 8 of 10 rapid-cycling bipolar patients experienced fewer affective episodes during 6 months of therapy with risperidone added to ongoing treatment with mood-stabilizing agents. A limiting factor in these open studies is that the relative contributions of risperidone and of the mood stabilizers cannot be separated.

Interestingly, there have been several reports of risperidone-induced mania, or risperidone-induced worsening of manic symptoms. Dwight *et al.* (1994) reported that risperidone, administered as a first-line treatment to 8 patients with schizoaffective disorder, reduced depressive symptoms in 2 and induced/worsened manic symptoms in 6 patients. Tomlinson (1996) described a patient with chronic schizophrenia who developed a manic syndrome when his treatment was switched from a conventional neuroleptic to risperidone. Koek and Kessler (1996) reported that a patient with psychotic depression experienced a manic switch when risperidone therapy was initiated.

Schnierow and Graeber (1996) described 3 patients who reacted adversely to risperidone: in a patient with bipolar I disorder, risperidone worsened manic symptoms; in a patient with schizoaffective disorder and another with chronic disorganized schizophrenia, risperidone precipitated a manic syndrome. Sajatovic *et al.* (1996a) administered risperidone to 5 treatment-refractory or treatment-intolerant manic patients. Two patients did not tolerate risperidone, and 2 experienced an exacerbation of manic symptoms. The last patient discontinued risperidone due to subjective complaints of insomnia and anxiety.

In many of the cases described in these reports, the manic symptoms exacerbation reported with risperidone resolved shortly after discontinuation of the drug. However, a recent study did not find induction of mania to be a problem with risperidone (McIntyre *et al.*, 1997). It is possible that the use of risperidone along with mood-stabilizing agents reduces the risk for the induction of mania.

Risperidone is a potent dopamine D2 receptor antagonist at therapeutic doses, and may induce extrapyramidal side effects in vulnerable patients. Risperidone may elevate serum prolactin and occasion amenorrhoea, galactorrhoea, and sexual dysfunction (Dickson *et al.*, 1995; Shiwach and Carmody, 1998). Antagonism at the 5-HT2 receptor site can result in sedation, increased appetite, and increased weight. In some individuals, these adverse effects may compromise long-term compliance to risperidone therapy.

Risperidone therapy may be associated with certain advantages in comparison with therapy using conventional neuroleptic drugs. Though data from well-controlled, long-term studies remain sparse, it is possible that risperidone exposes patients to a lesser risk for tardive dyskinesia than the traditional neuroleptic drugs; it is, however, unknown whether this putative benefit applies equally to subjects with schizophrenia and bipolar illness. Risperidone does not block muscarinic receptors; therefore, the risk for somatic anticholinergic adverse effects is low. For the same reason, risperidone does not impair cognitive functioning; in fact, given its greater affinity for serotonergic as compared with dopaminergic receptors, facilitation of dopaminergic neurotransmission in the frontal lobes may actually improve cognition (Kapur and Remington, 1996; Green *et al.*, 1997).

In schizophrenia, risperidone is usually prescribed in the dose of 3–6 mg/day; sometimes, higher doses are necessary despite the increased risk for adverse effects. Elderly patients generally require lower doses such as 0.5–2.0 mg/day. Twice-daily dosing is common, but the long half-life of the drug and its metabolite allow even once-daily dosing. No correlations between dose, plasma levels, and clinical response have been demonstrated.

In conclusion, risperidone may find application in the treatment of bipolar and schizoaffective bipolar patients in whom psychosis is associated with manic episodes. Risperidone combined with mood-stabilizing drugs may help patients with rapid-cycling bipolar disorder. The usefulness of risperidone in bipolar depression and in the maintenance treatment of bipolar illness remains to be determined.

Olanzapine

Olanzapine is an atypical antipsychotic agent. It is a thienobenzodiazepine derivative which blocks dopaminergic (D1, D2, D4), serotonergic (5-HT2A, 5-HT2C), muscarinic (m1, m2, m3, m4, m5), adrenergic (alpha-1), and histaminic (H1) receptors. Positron emission tomography (PET) studies indicate that in normal volunteers, olanzapine (10 mg) occupies 74–92 per cent of 5-HT2 receptors, and 59–73 per cent of D2 receptors (Nyberg *et al.*, 1997). Kapur *et al.* (1998) reported that in patients receiving olanzapine at a dose of 10–20 mg/day, D2 receptor occupancy varied from 71 per cent to 80 per cent; doses above 30 mg/day were associated with more than 80 per cent D2 receptor occupancy.

A large, multicentre study on olanzapine included 300 schizo-affective patients of whom approximately half were diagnosed with bipolar schizoaffective disorder, and half with schizoaffective depression. Response rates in these patients were comparable to those with schizophrenia, and favoured olanzapine over haloperidol. Bipolar and depressed subtypes of schizoaffective disorder showed similar responses on psychosis as well as on depression ratings (Tollefson *et al.*, 1997). Open studies published to date suggest that olanzapine benefits patients with mania and treatment-resistant bipolar disorder (Weisler *et al.*, 1997; Ravindran *et al.*, 1997; McElroy *et al.*, 1998; Zarate *et al.*, 1998).

A 3-week, double-blind, placebo-controlled, acute phase study compared olanzapine (5–20 mg/day; n=70) with placebo (n=69) in bipolar I patients with manic and mixed affective episodes. Response rates were 49 per cent with olanzapine and 24 per cent with placebo for the entire sample, and greater than 55 per cent with olanzapine and less than 30 per cent with placebo in the subgroup (n=45) with rapid-cycling bipolar illness (Tohen *et al.*, 1998). Ongoing studies are investigating the use of olanzapine in acute mania and in the long-term maintenance treatment of bipolar I disorder as an adjunct to lithium or valproic acid.

In patients with schizophrenia, olanzapine was better tolerated than haloperidol: it was found to induce fewer extrapyramidal symptoms (EPS), less treatment-emergent hyperprolactinemia, and less nausea and insomnia. Mild sedation, dizziness, and constipation were noted with olanzapine as compared with placebo (Tollefson *et al.*, 1997). During short-term trials (3–6 weeks) with olanzapine, some patients gained 2–5 kg in weight; in the long term, however, weight gain may exceed 10 kg. Anticholinergic effects, such as dry mouth, constipation, and blurring of vision, may be troublesome in vulnerable individuals.

Olanzapine is extensively metabolized in the liver, and the principal metabolic pathway is N-glucuronidation. The parent compound is responsible for the main clinical effects. The pharmacokinetics of olanzapine are dose-proportional; its half-life is 33–51 hours, and varies little with age. *In vitro* microsomal studies indicate that olanzapine is a weak inhibitor of the cytochrome P450 enzymes; this must be kept in mind when other drugs metabolized by these enzymes are concurrently prescribed. Carbamazepine and other inducers of the cytochrome P450 3A4 enzymes lower olanzapine concentrations, necessitating upward dose adjustments. Excessive smoking of tobacco acts similarly through an induction of the 1A4 cytochrome enzymes.

Olanzapine is prescribed in a once-daily schedule, in an average dose of 10–20 mg/day. No significant correlations have been found between daily doses, plasma levels, and clinical response.

In conclusion, marketing data in the USA, obtained a year after the launch of olanzapine, indicate that nearly 1 in 4 prescriptions for the drug are written for subjects with bipolar disorder. Clinical studies suggest that monotherapy with olanzapine is effective in bipolar I manic or mixed episodes with or without psychosis. Short-term data suggest that olanzapine is effective in patients with rapid-cycling bipolar mania; response rates in these patients are possibly even more favorable than those in other bipolar patients, although long-term data are needed for more definitive conclusions. Long-term studies will also indicate whether olanzapine is useful in the maintenance treatment of bipolar disorder. The use of olanzapine in bipolar depression remains to be evaluated.

Quetiapine

Quetiapine is a recently introduced atypical antipsychotic agent belonging to the dibenzothiazepine class. It produces slight to moderate blockade of D2 receptors, with minimal and transient elevation of prolactin. It prominently blocks 5-HT2, adrenergic and histaminic receptors but has little affinity for muscarinic sites.

Quetiapine has been approved of for use in patients with schizophrenia and schizoaffective disorder (Arvanitis *et al.*, 1997; Small *et al.*, 1997). An ongoing study is assessing its effects in mania, as an adjunct to ongoing treatment with mood-stabilizing drugs.

Quetiapine may produce orthostatic hypotension and sedation early during therapy but is otherwise generally well tolerated. In 1-year studies, cataracts were observed in dogs which had received quetiapine at over five times the human dose; however, cataracts did not develop in similar studies in primates and rats. In humans, the available data suggest no greater risk for cataracts with quetiapine than with older neuroleptic agents.

Quetiapine is used in doses of 300–600 mg/day in otherwise healthy psychotic adults. A titration over 3–5 days may be needed to reach the initial target dose of 300 mg/day. Elderly or medically unwell patients may require lower doses such a 50–200 mg/day, and a longer titration phase. Early during therapy, twice-daily dosing is recommended; later on, once-daily dosing can be attempted to promote compliance. Patients receiving carbamazepine may require higher initial doses due to induction of the cytochrome P450 3A4 enzyme system. Dosing guidelines for mania are currently unavailable. No correlations between dose, serum levels, and response have been noted.

In conclusion, quetiapine is likely to be useful in manic patients with or without psychotic features, and in patients with schizoaffective mania. In combination with mood stabilizers, quetiapine may also be helpful in difficult-to-treat bipolar patients. The low risks for extrapyramidal adverse effects, elevated serum prolactin, and muscarinic adverse effects are the advantages with this drug.

Dietary Supplements

Inositol

Inositol is a simple isomer of glucose, found in animals and microorganisms as inositol phospholipids, and in plants as inositol hexaphosphates. Most tissues produce inositol; the main source is the kidney, where it is synthesized from glucose in a quantity of about 4 gm/day (Holub, 1986 and 1992). Animal and plant sources contribute about 1–2 gm/day of inositol to the normal diet.

Ingested inositol is actively absorbed from the intestine much as sugars are; the process is sodium-dependent (Holub, 1986 and 1992).

Inositol was found to benefit patients with major depression (Levine *et al.*, 1995). In a preliminary, double-blind, randomized, placebo-controlled, 6-week study, Chengappa *et al.* (1998) showed that inositol may be effective in patients with breakthrough or treatment-resistant bipolar depression. The sample comprised 18 mildly to moderately depressed bipolar I and bipolar II subjects of whom 10 received inositol (12 grams/day), and 8 received placebo. Half of the inositol-treated patients but only a quarter of the placebo-treated patients showed clinical response, defined as more than 50 per cent reduction in depression ratings, and a global improvement that was at least moderate. Inositol was well tolerated and induced few or no adverse effects. No laboratory abnormalities were noted. Measures of nerve conduction were within normal limits. Of note, patients with diabetes mellitus were excluded from these clinical trials because inositol is a sugar.

Inositol is generally well tolerated. Some patients, however, experience problematic bowel disturbances that range from mild loose stools to diarrhoea; these usually stop with time. No laboratory or EKG abnormalities occur. In patients receiving inositol for several months, ophthalmic examinations do not reveal retinal pathology as was described in one rat study. Stray cases of putative inositol-induced mania have been reported.

Little specific data are available on the pharmacokinetics and pharmacodynamics of inositol. The plasma half-life is shorter than 12 hours. Spector (1988) reported that inositol crosses the blood brain barrier poorly. Levine *et al.* (1993) showed that inositol loading of 12 gm/day for 5 days raises CSF levels of the substance by 70 per cent. The kidney is the main site of catabolism of inositol: it is oxidized to D-glucuronic acid, which is catabolized to D-xylulose 5 phosphate, which in turn is degraded in the pentose phosphate cycle (Holub, 1986).

Inositol is commercially prepared from corn-steep liquor and is sold in high purity by various chemical suppliers. Suggested doses are 2 gm thrice a day during the first week, and 4 gm thrice a day during the second week. Inositol is administered orally, dissolved in water or fruit juice.

In conclusion, inositol could be useful in depressed patients with bipolar I and II disorder. It may also be useful when obsessive compulsive disorder (Fux *et al.*, 1996) or panic disorder (Benjamin *et al.*, 1995) are comorbid diagnoses.

Choline

Choline is a quaternary amine. It is an essential nutrient in humans; dietary deficiency of choline is known to cause hepatic and renal dysfunction (Ziesel, 1990). Choline is primarily ingested in the diet as phosphatidylcholine. In the CNS, choline plays a central role, both as a precursor of the neurotransmitter acetylcholine and as a precursor of phospholipids in the cell membranes of neurons and glia (Klein *et al.*, 1992).

In an open trial, Stoll *et al.* (1996) administered choline (3–8 gm/day) to 6 consecutive lithium-treated out-patients with rapid-cycling bipolar disorder. Five patients experienced a substantial reduction in manic symptoms, and 4 experienced a marked reduction in all mood symptoms. Although preliminary, this study suggests that choline may be effective in rapid-cycling bipolar patients who do not respond to lithium treatment.

Adverse effects with choline include diarrhoea and a fishy odour from the skin; the latter tends to appear when high dose are given.

In conclusion, choline may merit investigation for the treatment of patients with rapid-cycling bipolar disorder.

ADENYLATE CYCLASE INHIBITORS

Demethylchlorotetracycline, also known as demeclocycline (DMC) is a tetracycline derivative which blocks the actions of antidiuretic hormone (ADH) in the kidney much as lithium does (Forrest *et al.*, 1978). Both lithium and DMC inhibit adenylate cyclase, the enzyme responsible for the generation of cyclic adenosine monophosphate (cAMP). cAMP is the second messenger involved in neurotransmission after activation of the ADH receptor (Singer *et al.*, 1972). Since cAMP is a common second messenger in the brain, it is conceivable that DMC may have psychotropic properties mediated by the inhibition of the generation of cAMP (Belmaker, 1984).

Noradrenaline-linked elevation of cAMP is inhibited by lithium; this has been proposed as a major mechanism of action of lithium (Mork and Geisler, 1995). Noradrenaline-stimulated cAMP generation in rat brains is also inhibited by DMC (Belmaker, 1984) and by minocycline, a related tetracycline (Mork and Geisler,

1993). Kofman *et al.* (1990 and 1993) reported that DMC and minocycline inhibit amphetamine-induced hyperactivity in rats without blocking apomorphine-induced stereotypy this too is similar to the effect of lithium.

These preclinical data prompted Roitman *et al.* (1998) to design a 5-week, double-blind, placebo-controlled evaluation of DMC augmentation of haloperidol in the treatment of patients with acute excitement. Patients with mania or schizomania received DMC (n=9) in a dose of 600–1200 mg/day in 2–4 divided doses, or placebo (n=7); all patients also received haloperidol. Although the difference between the two groups did not reach statistical significance, power analysis suggested that with a sample twice as large, DMC would have emerged significantly superior to placebo.

Adenylate cyclase inhibitors combined with antipsychotic drugs may thus be effective in the treatment of excited psychosis. Interestingly, in an open study, Lerer (1985) found that manic patients did not respond to DMC alone. This study is reminiscent of reports that lithium may be ineffective as monotherapy in excited schizoaffective patients (Johnson *et al.*, 1968) but effective when used in combination with haloperidol (Biederman *et al.*, 1979). The position of DMC as monotherapy versus its position in combination therapy is at present unclear.

Adverse effects of DMC include gastrointestinal symptoms, such as anorexia, vomiting, and diarrhoea, and dermatological symptoms such as, maculopapular rashes, erythematous rashes, and hypersensitivity reactions. Polyuria may also occur (Roitman *et al.*, 1998).

Minocycline enters the CNS more readily than DMC because it is a more lipophilic drug. Minocycline may therefore be a more promising tetracycline to evaluate as an antimanic agent. A case report has suggested the efficacy of minocycline in depression (Levine *et al.*, 1996).

In conclusion, the possible efficacy of DMC and minocycline in manic states merits further investigation.

Protein Kinase C Inhibitors

Tamoxifen citrate is a nonsteroidal compound with an antiestrogenic effect. It also inhibits protein kinase C (PKC). Its current medical use lies in the prevention and treatment of breast cancer. Since lithium, valproate, and verapamil inhibit PKC isoenzymes in humans and rodents, Bebchuk *et al.* (1998) conducted an open trial of tamoxifen in 7 patients with acute mania. Patients showed a significant reduction in the severity of manic symptoms.

Women receiving tamoxifen for breast cancer experience adverse effects, such as hot flushes, nausea, and vomiting. Less frequently, vaginal bleeding and discharge, menstrual irregularities, and skin rashes occur. Osteoporosis and uterine cancer are uncommon but serious risks with long-term tamoxifen treatment.

Tamoxifen is used in a dose of 10–20 mg/day for the prevention of breast cancer; appropriate doses for bipolar disorder are unknown. Following a single dose of 20 mg, tamoxifen reaches an average peak plasma level of 40 ng/ml in 5 hours. The decline in plasma concentrations is biphasic, with a terminal elimination half-life of 5–7 days. Steady state levels are obtained 4 weeks after initiation of treatment.

In conclusion, tamoxifen may merit evalation for the treatment of acute mania.

Transcranial Magnetic Stimulation

Repetitive Transcranial Magnetic Stimulation (rTMS) is a non-invasive procedure which creates a rapidly changing focal magnetic field over the scalp and in the underlying brain tissue. This depolarizes neurons and their projections. Double-blind, controlled studies have shown the efficacy of rTMS administered to the left prefrontal cortex in patients with major depression (Pascual-Leone *et al.*, 1996; George *et al.*, 1997), and to the right prefrontal cortex in patients with mania (Grisaru *et al.*, 1999). A small report also shows beneficial result with rTMS in 2 of 3 bipolar depressed patients (Ebstein *et al.*, 1998). As an example of an rTMS treatment package, Grisaru *et al.* (1999) stimulated their patients at 20 Hz with a duration of 2 sec/train; 20 stimulus trains were administered per day for 10 treatment days.

The mechanisms whereby TMS is effective in affective disorders is unknown. Slow rTMS, given in lower frequency as compared to rapid rTMS, was suggested to induce long-term synaptic depression and to have an anticonvulsant effect in a specific model (Weiss *et al.*, 1995). And, in contrast to electroconvulsive therapy

(ECT), TMS has been suggested to induce an immediate early gene expression in restricted brain areas, especially in the thalamic paraventricular nucleus (Schlaepfer *et al.*, 1997).

Headaches are a common adverse effect of rTMS. Rarely, seizures may occur.

In conclusion, rTMS is an experimental procedure, and many technical details concerning the procedure as well as practical details concerning its administration remain to be resolved. While it is still too early to comment on the usefulness of the procedure for bipolar illness, it is possible that, in time, it may develop into an office-based alternative or complementary treatment to ECT.

REFERENCES

Arvanitis L. A., Miller B. G. and Seroquel Trial 13 Study Group (1997). 'Multiple fixed doses of seroquel in patients with acute exacerbation of schizophrenia: A comparison with haloperidol and placebo', *Biol. Psychiatry*, 42: 233–46.

Banov M. D., Zarate C. A., Tohen M. *et al.* (1994). 'Clozapine therapy in refractory affective disorders: Polarity predicts responses in long-term follow-up', *J. Clin. Psychiatry*, 55: 295–300.

Barbini B., Scherillo P., Benedetti F. *et al.* (1997). 'Response to clozapine in acute mania is more rapid than that of chlorpromazine', *Int. Clin. Psychopharmacol.*, 12: 109–12.

Baron B. M. and Gitlin M. J. (1987). 'Verapamil in treatment-resistant mania: an open trial', *J. Clin. Psychopharmacol.*, 7: 101–3.

Bebchuk J. M., Arfken C. L., Dolan-Manti S. *et al.* (1998). 'A trial of the protein kinase C inhibitor tamoxifen in the treatment of acute mania', *New Research Program Abstracts, American Psychiatric Association Annual Meeting,* Toronto, 122.

Belmaker R. H. (1984). 'Adenylate cyclase and the search for new compounds with the clinical profile of lithium', *Pharmacopsychiatry*, 17: 9–15.

Benjamin J., Levine J., Fux M. *et al.* (1995). 'Double-blind, placebo-controlled, crossover trial of inositol treatment for panic disorder', *Am. J. Psychiatry*, 152: 1084–6.

Beydoun A., Uthman B. M. and Sackellares J. C. (1995). 'Gabapentin: Pharmacokinetics, efficacy, and safety', *Clin. Neuropharmacol.*, 18: 469–81.

Biederman J., Lerner Y. and Belmaker R. H. (1979). 'Combination of lithium carbonate and haloperidol in schizoaffective disorder', *Arch. Gen. Psychiatry*, 36: 327–32.

Bowden C. L., Brugger A. M., Swann A. C. *et al.* (1994). 'Efficacy of divalproex vs lithium in the treatment of mania', *JAMA*, 271: 918–24.

Bowden C. L., Calabrese J. R., Sachs G. S. *et al.* (1998). 'Lamotrigine in bipolar depression', *New Research Program Abstracts, American Psychiatric Association Annual Meeting*, Toronto, 224.

Briggs G. G., Freeman R. K. and Yaffe S. J. (1998). *Drugs in pregnancy and lactation*, 5th ed., Baltimore: Williams and Wilkins, 1104–5.

Calabrese J. R., Meltzer H. and Markovitz P, (1991). 'Clozapine prophylaxis in rapid-cycling bipolar disorder', *J. Clin. Psychopharmacol.*, 11: 396–7.

Calabrese J. R., Shelton S., Keck P. E. *et al.* (1998). 'Topiramate in severe treatment refractory mania', *New Research Program Abstracts, American Psychiatric Association Annual Meeting*, Toronto, 121–2.

Chengappa K. N. R., Levine J., Gershon S. *et al.* (1998). 'Inositol for bipolar depression', *Abstracts, Annual New Clinical Drug Evaluation Unit Program (NCDEU) Meeting*, Boca Raton.

Dickson R. A., Dalby J. T., Williams R. *et al.* (1995). 'Risperidone-induced prolactin elevations in premenopausal women with schizophrenia', *Am. J. Psychiatry*, 152: 1102–3.

Dwight M. M., Keck P. E., Stanton S. P. *et al.* (1994). 'Antidepressant activity and mania associated with risperidone treatment of schizoaffective disorder', *Lancet*, 344: 554–5.

Dubovsky S. L. and Buzan R. (1995). 'The role of calcium channel blockers in the treatment of psychiatric disorders', *CNS Drugs*, 4: 47–57.

Ebstein C. M., Figiel G., McDonald W. M. *et al.* (1998). 'Rapid rate transcranial magnetic stimulation in young and middle-aged refractory depressed patients', *Psychiatric Annals.*, 28: 36–9.

Fatemi S. H., Rapport D. J., Calabrese J. R. *et al.* (1997). 'Lamotrigine in rapid-cycling bipolar disorder', *J. Clin. Psychiatry*, 58: 522–7.

Ferrier I. N., Potkins D. and Eccleson D. (1997). 'Lamotrigine treatment in rapid-cycling bipolar disorder: clinical and biological correlates', *Abstracts, Second International conference on Bipolar Disorder*, Pittsburgh.

Forrest J. N. Jr., Cox M., Hong C. *et al.* (1978). 'Superiority of demeclocycline over lithium in the treatment of chronic syndrome of inappropriate secretion of antidiuretic hormone', *N. Engl. J. Med.*, 298: 173–7.

Freeman M. P. and Stoll A. L. (1998). 'Mood stabilizer combinations: A review of safety and efficacy', *Am. J. Psychiatry*, 155: 12–21.

Frye M. A., Altshuler L. L. and Bitran J. A. (1996). 'Clozapine in rapid-cycling bipolar disorder', *J. Clin. Psychopharmacol.*, 16: 87–90.

Fuchs D. C. (1994). 'Clozapine treatment of bipolar disorder in a young adolescent', *J. Am. Acad. Child. Adol. Psychiatry*, 33: 1299–1302.

Fux M., Levine J., Aviv A. *et al.* (1996). 'Inositol treatment of obsessive compulsive disorder', *Am. J. Psychiatry*, 153: 1219–21.
George M. S., Wasserman E. M., Kimbrell T. A. *et al.* (1997). 'Mood improvement following daily left prefrontal repetitive transcranial magnetic stimulation in patients with depression: a placebo-controlled cross-over trial', *Am. J. Psychiatry*, 154: 1752–56.
Ghaemi S. N. and Sachs G. S. (1997). 'Long-term risperidone treatment in bipolar disorder: 6-month follow-up', *Int. Clin. Psychopharmacol.*, 12: 333–8.
Ghaemi S. N., Sachs G. S., Baldassano C. F. *et al.* (1997). 'Acute treatment of bipolar disorder with adjunctive risperidone in outpatients', *Can. J. Psychiatry*, 42: 196–9.
Giannini A. J., Taraszewski R. and Loiselle R. H. (1987). 'Verapamil and lithium as maintenance therapy of manic patients', *J. Clin. Pharmacol.*, 27: 980–2.
Goodnick P. J. (1993). 'Verapamil prophylaxis in pregnant women with bipolar disorder', *Am. J. Psychiatry*, 150: 1560.
Goodnick P. J. (1995). 'Risperidone treatment of refractory acute mania', *J. Clin. Psychiatry*, 56: 431–2.
Gotz E., Feuerstein T. J., Lais *et al.* (1993). 'Effects of gabapentin on the release of gamma-aminobutyric acid from slices of rat neostriatum', *Arzneimittelforschung*, 43: 636–8.
Green M. F., Marshall Jr. B. D., Wirshing W. C., Ames D., Marder S. R., McGurk S., Kern R. S. and Mintz J. (1997). 'Does risperidone improve verbal working memory in treatment-resistant schizophrenia?', *Am. J. Psychiatry*, 154: 799–804.
Grisaru N., Chudakov B., Yaroslavsky Y. *et al.* (1999). 'TMS in mania: A controlled study', (Submitted).
Holub B. J. (1986). 'Metabolism and function of myo-inositol and inositol phospholipid', *Ann. Rev. Nutr.*, 6: 563–97.
Holub B. J. (1992). 'The nutritional importance of inositol and the phosphoinositides', *N. Engl. J. Med.*, 326: 1285–7.
Jacobsen F. M. (1995). 'Risperidone in the treatment of affective illness and obsessive-compulsive disorder', *J. Clin. Psychiatry*, 56: 423–9.
Janicak P. G., Sharma R. P., Pandey G. *et al.* (1998). 'Verapamil for the treatment of acute mania: A double-blind, placebo-controlled trial', *Am. J. Psychiatry*, 155: 972–3.
Johnson G., Gershon S. and Hekimian L. J. (1968). 'Controlled evaluation of lithium and chlorpromazine in the treatment of manic states: An interim report', *Compr. Psychiatry*, 9: 563–73.
Kapur S. and Remington G. (1996). 'Serotonin-dopamine interaction and its relevance to schizophrenia', *Am. J. Psychiatry*, 153: 466–76.
Kapur S., Zipursky R. B., Remington G. *et al.* (1998). '5-HT2 and D2 receptor occupancy in schizophrenia: A PET investigation', *Am. J. Psychiatry*, 155: 921–8.

Keck P. E., Wilson D. R., Strakowski S. M. *et al.* (1995). 'Clinical predictors of acute risperidone response in schizophrenia, schizoaffective disorder, and psychotic mood disorders', *J. Clin. Psychiatry*, 56: 466–70.

Klein J., Koppen A., Loffelholz K. *et al.* (1992). 'Uptake and metabolism of choline by rat brain after acute choline administration', *J. Biochem.*, 58: 870–6.

Koek R. J. and Kessler C. C. (1996). 'Probable induction of mania by risperidone', *J. Clin. Psychiatry*, 57: 174–5.

Kofman O., Klein E., Newman M. *et al.* (1990). 'Inhibition by antibiotic tetracyclines of rat cortical noradrenergic adenylate cyclase and amphetamine-induced hyperactivity', *Pharmacol. Biochem. Behav.*, 37: 417–24.

Kofman O., van Embden S., Alpert C., *et al.* (1993). 'Central and peripheral minocycline suppresses motor activity in rats', *Pharmacol. Biochem. Behav.*, 44: 397–402.

Kowatch R. A., Suppes T., Gilfillan S. K. *et al.* (1995). 'Clozapine treatment of children and adolescents with bipolar disorder and schizophrenia: A clinical case series', *J. Child. Adol. Psychopharmacol.*, 5: 241–53.

Kusumakar V. and Yatham L. N. (1997). 'An open study of lamotrigine in refractory bipolar depression', *Psychiatry*, Res 72: 145–8.

Labbate L. and Rubey R. (1997). 'Lamotrigine for treatment-refractory bipolar disorder', *Am. J. Psychiatry*, 154: 1317.

Lerer B. (1985). 'Alternative therapies for bipolar disorder', *J. Clin. Psychiatry*, 46: 309–16.

Levine J., Rapaport A., Lev L. *et al.* (1993). 'Inositol treatment raises CSF inositol levels', *Brain Res.*, 627: 168–70.

Levine J., Barak Y., Gonsalves M. *et al.* (1995). 'Double-blind study of inositol versus placebo in depression', *Am. J. Psychiatry*, 152: 792–4.

Levine J., Cholestoy A. and Zimmerman J. (1996). 'Possible antidepressant effect of minocycline', *Am. J. Psychiatry*, 153: 582.

Madhusoodanan S., Brenner R., Araujo L. *et al.* (1995). 'Efficacy of risperidone treatment for psychoses associated with schizophrenia, schizoaffective disorder, bipolar disorder, or senile dementia in 11 geriatric patients: a case series', *J. Clin. Psychiatry*, 56: 514–18.

Mallinger A. G., Thase M. E., Haskett R. *et al.* (1997). 'Verapamil treatment of lithium-nonresponsive mania', *Poster Abstracts, American College of Neuropsychopharmacology Annual Meeting*, Hawaii, 131.

Marcotte D. B. (1998). 'Topiramate in bipolar and schizoaffective disorders', *New Research Program Abstracts, American Psychiatric Association Annual Meeting*, Toronto.

Marcotte D. B. (1997). 'Gabapentin: An effective therapy for patients with bipolar disorder', *Abstracts, American Psychiatric Association Annual Meeting*, San Diego, 452.

Manna V. (1991). 'Disturbi affectivi bipolar e ruolo del calcio intraneuronale. Effeti terapeutici del trattamento con cali di lito e/o calcio antagonista in pazienti con rapid a inversione di polarita', *Menerva. Med.*, 82: 757–63.

McElroy S. L. (1997). 'Update on anteipileptic drugs in bipolar disorder', *Second International Conference on Bipolar Disorder*, Pittsburgh.

McElroy S. L., Dessain E. C., Pope H. G. *et al.* (1991). 'Clozapine in the treatment of psychotic mood disorders, schizoaffective disorder, and schizophrenia', *J. Clin. Psychiatry*, 52: 411–14.

McElroy S. L., Frye M., Denicoff K. *et al.* (1998). 'Olanzapine in treatment-resistant bipolar disorder', *J. Affective Disord.*, 49: 119–22.

McIntyre R., Young L. T., Hasey G. *et al.* (1997). 'Risperidone treatment of bipolar disorder', *Can. J. Psychiatry*, 42: 88–9.

Messenheimer J. (1995). 'Lamotrigine', *Epilepsia*, 36 (Suppl. 2): S87–S94.

Mork A. and Geisler A. (1993). 'Effect of minocycline on accumulation of cyclic AMP in cerebral cortex of rat: a comparison with lithium', *Eur. Neuropsychopharmacol.*, 32: 793–8.

Mork A. and Geisler A. (1995). 'Effects of chronic lithium treatment on agonist-enhanced extracellular concentrations of cyclic AMP in the dorsal hippocampus of freely moving rats', *J. Neurochem.*, 65: 134–9.

Nyberg S., Farde L. and Halldin C. (1997). 'A PET study of 5-HT2 and D2 receptor occupancy induced by olanzapine in healthy subjects', *Neuropsychopharmacol.*, 16: 1–7.

Pascual-Leone A., Rubio B., Pallardo F. *et al.* (1996). 'Beneficial effect of rapid-rate transcranial magnetic stimulation on the left dorsolateral prefrontal cortex in drug-resistant depression', *Lancet*, 348: 233–7.

Ravindran A. V., Jones B. W., Al-Zaid K. *et al.* (1997). 'Effective treatment of mania with olanzapine: two case reports', *J. Psychiatry Neurosci.*, 22: 345–6.

Roitman G., Levine J. and Belmaker R. H. (1998). 'An adenylate cyclase inhibitor in the treatment of excited psychosis', *Hum. Psychopharmacol.*, 13: 121–5.

Sajatovic M., DiGiovanni S. K., Bastani B. *et al.* (1996a). 'Risperidone therapy in treatment refractory acute bipolar and schizoaffective mania', *Psychopharmacol. Bull.*, 32: 55–61.

Sajatovic M., Ramirez L. F., Vernon L. *et al.* (1996b). 'Outcome of risperidone therapy in elderly patients with chronic psychosis', *Int. J. Psychiatry Med.*, 26: 309–17.

Schaffer C. B. and Schaffer L. C. (1996). 'The use of risperidone in the treatment of bipolar disorder', *J. Clin. Psychiatry*, 57: 136.

Schaffer C. B. and Schaffer L. C. (1997). 'Gabapentin in the treatment of bipolar disorder', *Am. J. Psychiatry*, 154: 291–2.

Schleapfer T. E., Rupp F. and Ji R-R (1997). 'Effects of rTMS and electroconvulsive stimulation on expression of immediate early genes', *Abstracts, American College of Neuropsychopharmacology Annual Meeting*, Hawaii.

Schnierow B. J. and Greaber D. A. (1996). 'Manic symptoms associated with initiation of risperidone', *Am J. Psychiatry*, 153: 1235–6.

Shiwach R. S. and Carmody T. J. (1998). 'Prolactogenic effects of risperidone in male patients—a preliminary study', *Acta. Psychiatr. Scand.*, 98: 81–3.

Singer I., Rotenberg D. and Puschett J. B. (1972). 'Lithium-induced nephrogenic diabetes insipidus: *In vivo* and *in vitro* studies', *J. Clin. Investigation*, 51: 1081–91.

Small J. G., Hirsch S. R., Arvanitis L. A. *et al.* (1997). 'Quetiapine in patients with schizophrenia: A high and low dose double-blind comparison with placebo', *Arch. Gen. Psychiatry*, 54: 549–57.

Spector R. (1988). 'Myo-inositol transport through the blood-brain barrier', *Neurochem. Res.*, 13: 785–7.

Sporn J. and Sachs G. (1997). 'The anticonvulsant in treatment-resistant manic-depressive illness', *J. Clin Psychopharmacol.*, 17: 185–9.

Stoll A. L., Sachs G. S., Cohen B. M. *et al.* (1996). 'Choline in the treatment of rapid-cycling bipolar patients', *Biol. Psychiatry*, 40: 382–8.

Suppes T., Phillips K. A. and Judd C. R. (1994). 'Clozapine treatment of nonpsychotic rapid-cycling bipolar disorder: A report of three cases', *Biol. Psychiatry*, 36: 338–40.

Tohen M., Zarate C., Centorrino F. *et al.* (1996). 'Risperidone in the treatment of mania', *J. Clin. Psychiatry*, 57: 249–53.

Tohen M., Sanger T. M., Tollefson G. D. *et al.* (1998). 'Olanzapine versus placebo in the treatment of acute mania', *Annual New Clinical Drug Evaluation Unit Program (NCDEU) Meeting*, Boca Raton, Poster 23.

Tollefson G. D., Beasley C. M., Tran P. V. *et al.* (1997). 'Olanzapine versus haloperidol in the treatment of schizophrenia, schizoaffective and schizophreniform disorders: results of an international collaborative trial', *Am. J. Psychiatry*, 154: 457–65.

Tomlinson W. C. (1996). 'Risperidone and mania', *Am. J. Psychiatry*, 153: 132–3.

Vieta E., Gasto C., Colom F. *et al.* (1998). 'Treatment of refractory rapid-cycling bipolar disorder with risperidone', *J. Clin. Psychopharmacol.*, 18: 172–4.

Walden J., Wegerer J., Berger M. *et al.* (1997). 'The antiepileptic drug lamotrigine may limit pathological excitation by modulating calcium and potassium currents: Update on antiepileptic drugs in bipolar disorder', *Second International Conference on Bipolar Disorder*, Pittsburgh.

Walton S. A., Berk M. and Brook S. (1996). 'Superiority of lithium over

verapamil in mania: A randomized controlled single-blind trial', *J. Clin. Psychiatry*, 57: 543–6.
Weisler R. H., Rinser M. E., Ascher J. A. *et al.* (1994). 'Use of lamotrigine in the treatment of bipolar disorder', *New Research Program Abstracts, American Psychiatric Association Annual Meeting*, NR611.
Weisler R. H., Ahearn E. P., Davidson J. R. T. *et al.* (1997). 'Adjunctive use of olanzapine in mood disorders: Five case reports', *Ann. Clin. Psychiatry*, 9: 259–62.
Weiss S. R. B., Li X. L., Rosen J. B. *et al.* (1995). 'Quenching: inhibition of the development and expression of amygdala kindled seizures with low frequency stimulation', *Neuro. Report*, 6: 2171–6.
Young L. T., Robb J. C., Patelis-Siotis I. et al. (1997). 'Acute treatment of bipolar depression with gabapentin', *Biol. Psychiatry*, 42: 851–3.
Zarate C. A., Tohen M. and Baldessarini R. J. (1995a). 'Clozapine in severe mood disorders', *J. Clin. Psychiatry*, 56: 411–17.
Zarate C. A., Tohen M., Banov M. D. *et al.* (1995b). 'Is clozapine a mood stabilizer?', *J. Clin. Psychiatry*, 56: 108–12.
Zarate C. A., Narendran R., Tohen M. *et al.* (1998). 'Clinical predictors of acute response with olanzapine in psychotic mood disorders', *J. Clin. Psychiatry*, 59: 24–8.
Zeisel S. H. (1990). 'Choline deficiency', *J. Nutr. Biochem.*, 1: 332–49.

Chapter 9

Themes: A Pot-Pourri

CHITTARANJAN ANDRADE AND
ALAN J. GELENBERG

The last few years have witnessed the development of several interesting themes in psychiatry and related disciplines, and the publication of many articles of importance. This chapter addresses certain of these articles and themes without pretence of being comprehensive in scope. A further purpose of this chapter is to sensitize readers to developments that may otherwise pass unnoticed. The emphasis is on subjects that are likely to remain topical for some time to come. Accordingly, this chapter presents, as titled, a pot-pourri of themes.

ALCOHOL CONSUMPTION AND MORTALITY

There is a large body of literature which demonstrates that men and women who consume alcohol regularly have higher death rates from injury, violence, suicide, poisoning, cirrhosis, cancer, and possibly haemorrhagic stroke. There is also a large body of literature which shows that such men and women have lower death rates from coronary heart disease and thrombotic stroke.

What is the net impact of these favourable and unfavourable alcohol-mediated effects on individuals who consume alcohol regularly? Unfortunately, no reliable answers are available. Since the incidence of different alcohol-related events varies between men and women, across age groups, and across other sociodemographic

Acknowledgments: Certain of the themes in this chapter have been modified from *Psychiatry Update, Psychiatry Review,* and *Biological Therapies in Psychiatry*; these are private and independent newsletters that are written and circulated by the authors.

and clinical categories, it is evident that any study of the balance of risk will need to take subpopulations into account. Such an epidemiologic study was described by Thun *et al.* (1997). The sample comprised nearly half a million Americans aged 30 years or more who provided complete information about smoking and drinking habits. There were totally of 238, 206 men and 251, 420 women aged 30–104 years (mean = 56 years). About 98 per cent of these men and women could be followed up for 9 years, during which period 12 per cent died. Death certificates were obtained for all but 2 per cent of those who died.

Using questionnaires, alcohol consumption was assessed at baseline and at endpoint, and was categorized as none, less than daily but at least thrice a week, 1 drink/day, 2–3 drinks/day, and 4 or more drinks/day. For operational purposes, one drink was considered as 12 g of absolute alcohol; this amounts to about one small peg (30 ml) of 75 degree proof spirit.

On the surface, it appears that this classification is somewhat weak on several counts; useful quantitative indices, for example, might have been average daily consumption of absolute alcohol, lifetime consumption of absolute alcohol, and quantity of absolute alcohol consumed per drinking occasion. However, such indices can be reliably calculated only from data obtained through direct interview; furthermore, such quantitative indices may not be more helpful when the relationship between alcohol consumption and mortality variables is U-shaped (as actually transpired for several variables). Therefore, considering the epidemiologic nature of the investigation, Thun *et al.* probably did the best that was possible under the circumstances.

After excluding former drinkers and patients with baseline cancer or cirrhosis from the analysis, it was discovered that the results in general supported existing literature:

1. In men, consumption of alcohol was found to significantly increase the risk for mortality due to the following: cirrhosis, alcoholism, or both; injuries and external causes; alcohol-related cancers (mouth, oesophagus, pharynx, larynx, liver); colorectal cancer; all other cancers.
2. In women, consumption of alcohol was found to significantly increase the risk for mortality due to the following: cirrhosis, alcoholism, or both; alcohol-related cancers; breast cancer. Risk

for death due to colorectal cancer, all other cancers, injuries, and external causes was not significantly elevated.

3. In both sexes, consumption of alcohol was found to significantly decrease the risk for mortality due to the following: coronary heart disease when the disease did not pre-exist; coronary heart disease when such disease did pre-exist; stroke; other circulatory disease; all cardiovascular diseases; all other causes. In patients with pre-existing coronary heart disease and with the diagnosis of stroke, benefits with alcohol were evident at all levels of consumption for women, but only with moderate consumption for men.

Thun *et al.* presented relative risk data for each mortality variable in each drinking category for men and women separately. A few interesting observations were:

1. The risk for death due to all cardiovascular diseases was lowered by 30 per cent (in men) to 40 per cent (in women) in persons who consumed at least one drink a day, as compared with non-drinkers.
2. The risk for death due to breast cancer was 30 per cent higher in women who consumed at least one drink a day, as compared with women who did not drink.
3. The risk for death from all causes was 20 per cent lower in persons who consumed one drink a day, as compared with non-drinkers; for above one drink per day, the advantage for alcohol was progressively attenuated.

Subjects were grouped into those at low and high cardiovascular risk. The former group reported no heart disease, hypertension, stroke, or diabetes mellitus at baseline; the latter group reported at least one of these conditions. Multivariate-adjusted death rates from all causes were calculated for both sexes. The results were:

1. In low-risk subjects aged 30–60 years, one drink a day or less lowered the risk for death by about 10 per cent, in comparison with not drinking at all; in contrast, four drinks a day or more increased the risk for death by 20 per cent.
2. In high-risk subjects aged 30–60 years, three drinks a day or less lowered the risk for death by 10–20 per cent, in comparison with not drinking at all.

3. In low-risk subjects aged 60–79 years, three drinks a day or less lowered the risk for death by 10–20 per cent, in comparison with not drinking at all.
4. In high-risk subjects aged 60–79 years, drinking at all levels lowered the risk for death by 20 per cent, in comparison with not drinking at all.

Thus, in middle-aged subjects and in those at low risk for cardiovascular disease, moderate consumption of alcohol moderately reduces the risk for mortality while high consumption moderately increases the risk. As age and risk for cardiovascular disease increase, increased levels of alcohol consumption also appear to moderately protect against death.

Smokers, defined as those smoking at least a pack a day, were compared with non-smokers. In both men and women aged 35–69 years, continued smoking approximately doubled the risk for death. Since persons who consume alcohol often smoke as well, clinicians who counsel patients about drinking habits should also offer guidance about smoking habits.

Unanswered questions are the duration for which a subject must drink to experience the benefit of reduced risk for death, and the duration for which this benefit continues after cessation of drinking.

The lessons that it conveys notwithstanding, this study has several limitations. An obvious limitation is that the findings are applicable predominantly to middle-class Caucasian subjects aged 30 years and more; it is uncertain as to what extent these findings can be generalized to patients of different races in different socioeconomic strata. Another limitation is that the study examined only mortality data, not morbidity data. It is conceivable that even moderate alcohol consumption may result in psychosocial or medical morbidity, and hence impaired quality of life. Furthermore, such morbidity may have an impact on mortality statistics in follow-up periods which exceed that described by Thun *et al.*

The Harmful Effects of Smoking During Pregnancy

The harmful effects of smoking during pregnancy are well known; for example, such smoking increases the risk for pediatric problems such as low birth weight, prematurity, and infant mortality. Two recent studies on the behavioural teratogenicity of smoking merit attention. Milberger *et al.* (1996) found that maternal smoking during pregnancy increased the risk for attention deficit hyperactivity disorder (ADHD) and, irrespective of the presence or absence of ADHD, was also associated with a decrease in mean IQ by 10.5 points.

Wakschlag *et al.* (1997) studied the effects of maternal cigarette smoking during pregnancy in 177 boys aged 7–12 years, of whom 105 were diagnosed with DSM-III-R conduct disorder. Mothers who had smoked more than half a pack of cigarettes daily during pregnancy were 4.4 times more likely to have a child with conduct disorder than mothers who did not smoke during pregnancy. This association remained statistically significant even after controlling for variables that are known to influence the risk for the development of conduct disorder. Variables that were controlled for included maternal age, socioeconomic status, parental antisocial personality, substance abuse during pregnancy, and maladaptative parenting.

What might be the mechanism of nicotine-induced harm to the foetus? Nicotine reduces uteroplacental blood flow and increases carboxyhaemoglobin in foetal blood. Nicotine also crosses the placental barrier and directly affects the developing foetus. Preclinical studies, reviewed by Wakschlag *et al.* (1997), indicate that maternal smoking during pregnancy produces changes in the offspring's neural functioning. These changes include a reduction in serotonin reuptake, alterations in dopaminergic neurotransmission, alterations in peripheral and central noradrenergic neurons, inhibition of cholinergic brain cell growth, and changes in brain synthesis of DNA and RNA. Functional deficits following nicotine exposure persist well after effects on receptor binding have attenuated, and occur even at levels that are not generally considered toxic. An unresearched area is the behavioural teratogenicity of passive smoking.

It is of course uncertain whether cigarette smoking *directly* influences risks; an alternate explanation for the findings reported by Milberger *et al.* (1996) and Wakschlag *et al.* (1997) is that a maternal trait or an unmeasured environmental characteristic may independently predispose to both maternal smoking and the risk for ADHD, lower IQ, and conduct disorder in the offspring.

Discounting such a possibility, these studies suggest that a woman who smokes during pregnancy may deliver a healthy baby; however, the child will be at an increased risk for developmental problems related to intelligence and behaviour.

USE OF ANTIDEPRESSANT DRUGS DURING PREGNANCY: RECENT EVIDENCE

Maternal depression during pregnancy poses risks to the foetus; these risks arise from poor nutrition, poor hygiene (leading to the possibility of infection), and attempts at suicide. While most clinicians therefore agree that depression during pregnancy needs to be actively treated, there is much dissatisfaction with the treatment options (Robert, 1996). Cognitive therapy is effective, but is unsuitable for severely depressed patients. Electroconvulsive therapy is safe, but is preferred only for major depression; the procedure may require elaborate maternal and foetal monitoring.

Drug therapy is the most convenient option, but is associated with an increased risk for teratogenicity, stillbirths, or neurodevelopmental abnormalities. In this context, it is particularly notable that the period of highest risk lies during weeks 4–10 of intrauterine life (this is when organogenesis begins), when a woman receiving antidepressant drugs may not even realize that she is pregnant.

SSRIs and the Outcome of Pregnancy

The effects of fluoxetine on the outcome of pregnancy were reported by Pastuszak *et al.* (1993) and Chambers *et al.* (1996). In summary, while the administration of fluoxetine during pregnancy was not associated with major malformations or behavioural teratogenicity, the use of this drug all through the period of gestation was linked to an increased incidence of perinatal complications and minor malformations.

Results of maternal intra-gestational use of the newer Selective Serotonin Reuptake Inhibitors (SSRI) were reported by Kulin *et al.* (1998). In a prospective, controlled, multicentre study, the authors examined the outcome of pregnancy in 267 women who had been treated for depression with sertraline (n = 147), paroxetine (n=97), or fluvoxamine (n=26) during the first trimester; three women had used more than one SSRI. The modal doses used were 50 mg/day for sertraline, 30 mg/day for paroxetine, and 50 mg/day for fluvoxamine.

These 267 women were matched with an equal number of control women who had been exposed to nonteratogenic agents. The incidence of spontaneous abortions, elective abortions, major malformations, and stillbirths did not differ between the experimental and control groups. Gestational age at delivery and mean birth weight also did not differ between the two groups. Pregnancy outcome also did not differ between the 49 women who took an SSRI all through pregnancy, and the remaining women who took the SSRI during the first trimester and for a varying period thereafter. Although SSRI users were significantly more likely to be smokers, there were no differences within the SSRI group based on use of tobacco.

These data provide preliminary evidence that sertraline, paroxetine, and fluvoxamine do not adversely influence the outcome of pregnancy when used in their recommended doses. More data are of course required before firm conclusions become possible.

Antidepressant Drugs and Neurodevelopment

Drug use during pregnancy may occasion a subtle adverse influence, the impact of which does not become apparent until many years of life have passed. This is because although weeks 4–10 of gestation are the most important for development, the brain continues to develop, and hence remains vulnerable to adverse influences all through pregnancy (and even after birth). Thus, in addition to studying the teratogenic effects of pharmacological agents, and the effects of these agents on the course and outcome of pregnancy, it is necessary to study the neurodevelopmental effects of drugs. Behavioural teratogenicity is a term that is sometimes used in this context. This term has a somewhat narrower frame of reference, and describes the effects which a drug (used during pregnancy) exerts on behaviour during postnatal life.

Nulman *et al.* (1997) studied the neurodevelopmental effects of antidepressant drug use during pregnancy in a sample of 219 children. There were 80 children whose mothers had received a tricyclic antidepressant (TCA) during pregnancy, 55 children whose mothers had received fluoxetine during pregnancy, and 84 children whose mothers had not been exposed during pregnancy to any agent known to adversely affect the foetus. The TCAs included several different drugs, most commonly amitriptyline (n=29) and imipramine (n=20). Other TCAs included clomipramine, desipramine, nortriptyline, doxepin, amoxapine, and trimipramine. The doses of TCAs and fluoxetine were not specified, but were presumably in the recommended range. In the majority of women, the indication for treatment was depression.

Assessment of pregnancy outcome and of other variables was conducted at various time points. The global IQ and language development of these children were assessed between 16 and 86 months after birth.

Mothers in the two drug groups reported significantly greater use of alcohol and tobacco during pregnancy than did the mothers in the control group. Nevertheless, the general conclusion was that the three groups did not differ on any outcome variable. There was no significant difference between the three groups in the gestational age at birth, in the incidence of major malformations, or in perinatal complications. At birth as well as at the time of testing, height, weight, and head circumference were similar in the three groups.

When neurodevelopmental variables were considered, it was found that the mean global IQ scores were in the narrow range of 115–118 in the three groups; and the differences between groups were not statistically significant. Language development scores were likewise similar in the three groups. There were also no significant differences between the three groups in variables such as temperament, mood, arousability, activity level, distractability, or behaviour problems. Finally, children whose mothers had taken the drugs during the first trimester (n=81) did not differ from those who had taken the drugs all through pregnancy (n=54).

Considering the large number of drugs that were pooled together in the TCA group, and considering the many variables that might have confounded the results of such a study, the sample sizes were too small for firm conclusions; nevertheless, the study appears to suggest that the use of antidepressant drugs during the first trimester or at other times during pregnancy is not associated with adverse developments during pregnancy or in early childhood.

This information is likely to prove reassuring to women who have taken or who are taking antidepressant drugs during pregnancy.

NEUROLEPTIC DOSING FOR SCHIZOPHRENIA: INSIGHTS FROM A MATHEMATICAL MODEL

All clinicians know that different patients require different neuroleptic doses, and that there is no way of knowing beforehand what the ideal dose is for any particular case. Variables such as age, sex, and body weight may affect drug kinetics or distribution, but do not lend themselves to the prediction of the ideal dose. In consequence, therapeutics with neuroleptic drugs is largely a matter of trial and error with clinicians adjusting doses within a window of efficacy. This window is conventionally considered to lie between 400 and 1000 chlorpromazine equivalents per day (CPZ/day); doses below this range are unlikely to be effective while doses above this range are unlikely to offer further benefit (Kane, 1994).

Clinicians often respect the lower limit of this window, but disregard the upper limit. Why is this? One consideration is that in an individual case, a generalization may not be applicable; hence, in order to be as certain as possible that the patient will respond to therapy, clinicians may use higher doses than are warranted under the circumstances. Another consideration is that clinicians may use high doses of drugs to 'chemically straitjacket' the patient for his own safety, and for the safety and satisfaction of others (such as the nursing staff or family members).

Such practices notwithstanding, a meta-analysis of 22 published randomized controlled trials found that at neuroleptic doses in excess of 375 CPZ/day during maintenance therapy in adults with psychosis, adverse reactions significantly increased without a corresponding increment in clinical improvement; doses below 165 CPZ/day were, however, less effective (Bollini *et al.*, 1994).

The Consensus Panel of the Royal College of Psychiatrists defined high-dose antipsychotic therapy (in the context of nearly 30 oral and injectable preparations), suggested several alternatives to high-dose therapy, and provided guidelines to be adopted in case the high-dose therapy was considered necessary; there did not appear to be adequate justification for megadose therapy (Thompson, 1994). Discussing the subject, Hirsch and Barnes

(1994) and Kane (1994) opined that there is no evidence that high-dose neuroleptic therapy is superior to continued therapy with conventional doses; higher doses are in fact counter-productive because they are more expensive, occasion dose-dependent adverse effects, and often lead to behavioural and biological withdrawal syndromes when reduced to conventional doses. There is also the risk that if a patient does show improvement, he/she may be continued indefinitely on the high dose when, in fact, a persistence of therapy with a conventional dose may have occasioned the same degree of improvement.

Hirsch and Barnes (1994) concluded that the use of very high doses is a last resort; such treatment should be regarded as an individual trial in each patient, to be carried out advisedly, under specialist guidance, and with caution. This is because of the risk for serious behavioural and medical adverse effects, certain of which (for example, cardiac conduction abnormalities) may even be life-threatening.

Recently, there has been a useful contribution to the discussion on the subject. Mossman (1997) used previously published data to derive a dose-response curve through mathematical modelling. He observed that response rates fit a sigmoid curve that flattens out at 500 CPZ/day. Another curve, describing adverse effects, was hyperbolic and flattened out at much higher doses. Thus, higher drug doses yield diminishing returns, because as the dose increases, adverse effects increase without an equal increase in therapeutic potential.

Table 9.1 summarizes the predictions made from Mossman's equations. The predictions are tabled under two headings: the percentage of patients likely to respond to a given neuroleptic dose, and the percentage of patients likely to experience significant adverse effects with maintenance therapy at that dose.

Table 9.1: Predictions Based on Mossman's Equation

CPZ/Day	Response %	Adverse effect %
200	59.8	5.5
300	65.2	12.6
400	67.3	15.6
600	68.9	20.3
800	69.4	23.9
1000	69.6	26.8

From the table, it is apparent that 200 CPZ/day is associated with response in 59.6 per cent of patients; at this dose, 5.5 per cent of patients experience significant adverse effects during maintenance therapy. At 300 CPZ/day, 65.2 per cent of patients respond, and 12.6 per cent experience significant adverse effects. With further increases in the neuroleptic dose, the percentage of response increases marginally, while the percentage of adverse effects increases substantially.

These predictions represent generalizations across clinical practice, and need not influence decision-making in the individual case. In other words, this study suggests that clinicians aim for a dose of 300–400 CPZ/day. The decision to raise the dose should be carefully made, keeping in mind Mossman's equations, and the need of the situation; thus, for example, if psychosis is severe, the clinician may consider it worthwhile to expose the patient to a substantially increased risk for adverse effects in order to obtain a slightly increased chance of response.

Ample data exist to suggest that there are ethnic/racial differences in the way patients metabolize (Lin *et al.*, 1996) as well as respond to psychopharmacologic agents; Asian patients generally appear to require lower doses of psychotropic medication than Caucasians (Jeste *et al.*, 1996). There may be several explanation for these differences: genetic factors, diet, clinicians' prescribing practices, etc. (Turner and Cooley-Quille, 1996). Since Mossman's data were obtained from Western literature, may one conclude that Asian patients require still lower CPZ/day doses than Mossman recommends?

Mossman's conclusions, while salient, must be viewed with a degree of caution. Firstly, Mossman made various assumptions during calculations (such as for the values of the response rates for drug and placebo); these assumptions are not necessarily valid. Secondly, the studies on which Mossman's calculations were based may not necessarily be representative of contemporary clinical practice in terms of diagnostic criteria, definitions of outcome, definitions of significant adverse effects, etc. Thirdly all mathematical models best fit the data from which they were derived; therefore, such models need to be prospectively validated. Fourthly, the relationship between dose of drug and response to treatment may differ for positive and negative symptoms. Finally, these equations are applicable only to the treatment of psychosis with conventional neuroleptics; many atypical antipsychotic agents are now available, but the mathematical rules which these agents follow (for positive and negative symptoms) are so far unknown. A positive aspect of Mossman's thesis is that it provides a method whereby the reader may construct a table for himself based on definitions and studies of his own choice.

Dose ranging comparisons against placebo have been conducted with the newer antipsychotic agents; such studies indicate the likely minimum and maximum therapeutic doses for the average patient. For example, Peuskens (1995) found that the response rate to risperidone was 54.4 per cent at 2 mg/day, 63.4 per cent at 4 mg/day, 65.8 per cent at 8 mg/day, 58.2 per cent at 12 mg/day and 60.5 per cent at 16 mg/day; the difference between groups was not statistically significant even though the sample size, averaging about 225 patients per group, was large. These data suggest that at a risperidone dose of 2–16 mg/day, *irrespective of the actual dose*, a patient has an approximately 60 per cent chance of showing therapeutic response. If higher doses are truly associated with a higher rate of response, a much larger sample size would be required to detect the difference. This suggests that the response rate differs only marginally between doses, and that the likelihood of the average patient requiring a higher (as compared with a lower) dose is very small.

In another study, Zimbroff *et al.* (1997) compared three doses of sertindole (12, 20, and 24 mg/day) and three doses of haloperidol (4, 8, and 16 mg/day) with placebo. The results with haloperidol were that the three doses did not differ significantly between themselves; the two higher doses were superior to placebo on all measures of efficacy, and the lowest dose was superior to placebo on almost all measures. These results suggest that, for the average patient, the maximum effective dose of haloperidol probably lies between 4 and 8 mg/day.

Clozapine and Time of Response

How long should a clinician wait before deciding that a treatment-refractory, positive-symptom schizophrenic patient is refractory to clozapine as well? A few years ago, the answer was 'Six to twelve months'. This was partly because certain researchers held the view that in a few patients clinical gains accrue gradually, and partly because it was considered that as clozapine was the last resort, the patient might just as well remain on clozapine (in the hope of experiencing a delayed response) as change to a drug that had already been proven ineffective (Meltzer, 1992 and 1995).

There have however been several publications expressing contrary opinions. Owen *et al.* (1989) studied 37 patients with chronic psychosis. Response to clozapine, including in those patients who were treatment-resistant, was obtained within the first three months; subsequently, no significant changes in ratings were noted. In an open study of 14 chronic schizophrenics treated for up to 2 years, Mattes (1989) reported that significant improvement was obtained within 3 months; this improvement appeared to be an ongoing process, for the patients continued to improve over the further course of clozapine therapy.

Lieberman *et al.* (1994) studied 66 treatment-refractory and 18 neuroleptic-intolerant schizophrenics for up to a year. The response rate was 50 per cent and 76 per cent respectively. The authors observed that neuroleptic-intolerant patients respond early to therapy. For treatment-refractory patients, they suggested that an optimal clozapine trial should last for 3–6 months; however, they found that even in late responders (that is, patients who met the criteria for response after the third month), more than 70 per cent of the total reduction in illness ratings had already occurred by the third month of treatment.

Wilson (1996) reviewed the case records of 100 consecutive adults treated with clozapine in a state hospital. Of the 73 patients who met the criteria for global social improvement, 55 demonstrated initial improvement within 6 months; the remainder showed improvement by 11 months. The response at the third month correlated with the response at the eighteenth month of therapy. Wilson concluded that while initial response to clozapine appears to occur within the initial months of therapy, gross social improvement appears to lag behind clinical improvement in psychopathology.

Carpenter *et al.* (1995) reviewed the literature on the time course and pattern of response of schizophrenia to clozapine, and observed that response is rapid once a therapeutic dose is reached; the data did not support the opinion that some patients respond only after 3–12 months of therapy. How then might one explain the delayed response reported by some clinicians? Carpenter *et al.*, citing several studies that supported their stance, offered the following views:

1. The 'late' improvement may have comprised a slowly evolving change which developed early but met the clinical criteria for improvement late as with the late responders in the Lieberman *et al.* (1994) study.
2. The 'late' improvement may have comprised an idiosyncratic fluctuation in the severity of the illness; such fluctuations are known to occur in schizophrenic patients when the period of evaluation is as long as a year.
3. The improvement in the 'late' responders may not have been robust and clinically meaningful.
4. The 'late' improvement may have been due to factors other than clozapine therapy.

In the most recent and most influential study, Conley *et al.* (1997) examined the antipsychotic response to clozapine in 50 treatment-refractory schizophrenic in-patients. Over a period of at least a year (irrespective of clinical response), all patients received a standardized, increasing dose schedule of clozapine. According to this schedule, doses of 400–450 mg/day were attained by weeks 2–3. Subsequently, doses were raised (subject to tolerance) to 600 mg/day, then 700 mg/day, and finally 800–900 mg/day. Each dose was held constant for at least 6 weeks, pending assessment of results with that dose. It's assets notwithstanding, one disadvantage of this dosing schedule is that it does not allow for the identification of responders to clozapine as doses below 400–450 mg/day.

Patients were assessed monthly. Thirty-four (68 per cent) of subjects responded to treatment, maintaining at least 20 per cent reduction in psychosis ratings for at least 2 months. Most of these patients (n=30) showed a response within a dose of 600 mg/day; the mean dose at which response was achieved was 468 mg/day. It took an average of 2 months for patients to reach the dose of clozapine at which response occurred; in a few patients, however, the experience of adverse effects slowed the upward titration process, and it took around a year to reach the dose at which response was obtained. Once this dose was reached, response developed in an average of 17 (range=2–56) days. In non-responders, no 'late' response to clozapine was observed, despite a follow-up period of an average of 75 weeks.

The intriguing results of this study provide no guidance about the overall duration of an adequate clozapine trial. However, the results suggest a very important conclusion: if a patient does not respond at least moderately within 2 months to a particular dose of clozapine, either the clozapine trial should be considered a failure or the dose should be raised and held constant for another two months pending reassessment. This process can be repeated until the maximum recommended or the maximum tolerated dose is reached, however long the upward titration process may take.

If the patient shows partial response that does not meet response criteria, the cautious clinician may wish to be guided by Lieberman *et al.* (1994) and Wilson's (1996) results, which recommend that the trial be extended by a few more months to identify an ongoing but slowly evolving improvement. Curiously, the American Psychiatric Association's (1997) Practice Guidelines for the treatment of schizophrenia contain no advice on the ideal duration of such a clozapine trial.

Clozapine For Childhood Schizophrenia

Several case reports and open studies had earlier documented the efficacy of clozapine in childhood/adolescent schizophrenia. There have been three recent articles on the subject; these are briefly reviewed.

Kumra *et al.* (1996) studied 21 severely ill patients with DSM-III-R schizophrenia that began by 12 years of age. All patients were intolerant of and/or non-responsive to at least two neuroleptic drugs. Most patients had received high doses of several standard neuroleptics, risperidone, and augmenting agents such as mood stabilizers and antidepressants.

The patients' medication regime was tapered over 2 weeks. After a further 4-week drug-free interval, patients were randomized to receive clozapine and placebo (n = 10) or haloperidol and benztropine (n = 11). Starting doses of clozapine were 6.25–25 mg/day, while those of haloperidol were 0.25–1.0 mg/day. Doses were gradually increased every 3–4 days, depending on need. Average doses at the end of the 6-week trial were 176 mg/day with clozapine (239 mg/day, disregarding the three treatment drop outs) and 16 mg/day with haloperidol.

On measures evaluating positive symptoms, negative symptoms, and overall severity of illness, clozapine was found to be substantially superior to haloperidol. In at least two patients, the response to clozapine was pronounced. For negative symptoms, the superiority of clozapine over haloperidol was not due to greater extrapyramidal symptoms in haloperidol patients; extrapyramidal symptoms were similar in the two groups, no doubt because the haloperidol patients also received benztropine. It is possible, however, that the greater improvement of negative symptoms may have arisen from the greater improvement of positive symptoms in the clozapine group.

Three clozapine patients and one haloperidol patient dropped out of the study due to adverse effects. Five clozapine patients developed neutropenia; in three, blood counts stabilized while in the other two, discontinuation of clozapine was necessary. Two clozapine patients developed seizures which did not respond to the addition of anticonvulsant drugs; clozapine was ultimately withdrawn from these patients' drug regime after the 6-week trial. Several other adverse events with clozapine were also recorded.

Clozapine was prescribed to the haloperidol patients and was continued in the clozapine patients after the conclusion of the 6-week trial. Follow-up of these patients for up to 2 years essentially showed a similar pattern of efficacy and adverse effects.

Turetz *et al.* (1997) studied 11 patients aged 9–13 years, diagnosed with childhood-onset schizophrenia (DSM-III-R). All the patients had failed trials with at least two different antipsychotic drugs belonging to at least two different chemical classes, prescribed for at least 6–8 weeks in the range of accepted therapeutic doses. After a 2-week drug washout, patients were commenced on clozapine. The initial dose was 12.5–25 mg/day. Doses were gradually increased by 12.5 mg/day every 5 days. At week 16, the mean dose was 227 mg/day. All the patients showed substantial improvement in both positive and negative symptoms; most of the improvement developed during the first 6–8 weeks of therapy. The magnitude of response was greater in patients with fairly normal premorbid development.

Important adverse events were: drowsiness (90 per cent), hypersalivation (90 per cent), non-specific, subclinical excitatory EEG changes (82 per cent), transient psychomotor agitation during the first 3 weeks (27 per cent), transient eosinophilia during the initial weeks (18 per cent). Agranulocytosis did not develop in any patient during the 16-week trial. Tardive dyskinesia, present in two patients at the start of the trial, disappeared during clozapine therapy. Follow-up of these cases for up to 3 years revealed that these clinical gains with clozapine were maintained in all but one patient.

In the only Indian article on the subject, Srinivasan and Latha (1997) described a 10-year-old female schizophrenic (ICD-10) who had failed to tolerate or respond to previously prescribed neuroleptics. She was treated with clozapine in a dose that reached 200 mg/day over the course of a month. Clinical response was excellent, and the therapeutic gains with clozapine were maintained over a year. Adverse effects with clozapine included hypersalivation, drowsiness, and slurring of speech.

Schizophrenia in childhood or adolescence is associated with disturbed normal development, poor response to drug therapy, and an increased risk for drug induced adverse effects (including tardive dyskinesia). It appears that clozapine is a useful drug for children or adolescents with treatment-refractory schizophrenia; clozapine, however, occasions its own spectrum of adverse effects, which is possibly more severe in children than in adults, a matter of much concern.

Cognitive Therapy for Chronic Schizophrenia

Antipsychotic drugs and electroconvulsive therapy are (ECT) established treatments for schizophrenia, and particularly benefit positive symptoms. Family therapy and social support reduce the risk for relapse. Occupational therapy improves various aspects of behaviour related to everyday life. Cognitive retraining may improve cognitive functioning. In special cases, behaviour therapy may benefit individual symptoms (such as delusions or hallucinations) that are otherwise drug-resistant. Various other forms of intervention have also been attempted in schizophrenic patients with varying degrees of success.

In recent times, cognitive therapy has been shown to be a powerful tool in disorders such as depression and anxiety, with demonstrated efficacy during both acute and maintenance phases of treatment (see Blackburn and Moore (1997) for recent results). Cognitive therapy has also been attempted in schizophrenic patients; although the results during the past decade had been encouraging, general conclusions were difficult to draw because the research available largely comprised small case series or uncontrolled studies.

Recently, however, the picture has changed. Several controlled investigations have shown that cognitive therapy effectively augments the efficacy of antipsychotic drugs during both acute (Drury *et al.*, 1996a and b) and chronic (Tarrier *et al.*, 1993; Kuipers *et al.*, 1997) phases of psychotic illness; patients with drug-resistant symptoms are also benefited (Garety *et al.*, 1994; Kuipers *et al.*, 1997), and the benefit does not appear to depend on the expectations from therapy (Tarrier *et al.*, 1993). Interestingly, cognitive therapy appears to attenuate specific symptoms (Tarrier *et al.*, 1993) as well as hasten recovery (Drury *et al.*, 1996b). A limitation of the cited studies, however, is that they were small and non-blind; some studies had other, more serious limitations (see Johnson, 1996).

What are the cognitive behaviour therapy interventions for psychotic patients? Most of these are actually similar to those applied in depression and other contexts. The therapist, for example, identifies dysfunctional cognitions; these include delusions. The dysfunctional cognitions are challenged in a non-confrontational non-threatening manner, and the client is encouraged to review his beliefs in these cognitions, and to seek alternate explanations. Assistance is also obtained from family members to provide reality-oriented information in a manner that is acceptable to the patient.

Other common elements of cognitive therapy programmes overlap with techniques that have been described in family therapy programmes for schizophrenia. For example, the patient is taught coping skills that enhance his ability to deal with the impairments that result from his symptoms. He is taught methods of handling difficult situations in everyday life. He is instructed in problem-solving processes that help him deal with various practical difficulties that he faces, including those resulting from his illness. He is educated about medication compliance, and how he can reduce the risk for relapse, etc. An important caveat in this as in any psychotherapeutic intervention for schizophrenia is that the patient must never be overstimulated, pressurized, or otherwise stressed; this can be counter-therapeutic.

The latest, largest and most rigorous (from a methodological perspective) of studies on cognitive behaviour therapy was published by Tarrier *et al.* (1998). The sample comprised 87 patients diagnosed with schizophrenia, schizoaffective disorder, or delusional disorder on DSM-III-R. All patients had persistent delusions, hallucinations, or both for at least 6 months, despite stabilization on antipsychotic medication. No patient was in acute exacerbation. These patients were randomized to receive cognitive behaviour therapy (n=33), supportive counselling (n=26), or routine clinical care (n=28).

The 20-session cognitive therapy package comprised three important elements: training in strategies intended to assist in coping with illness symptoms, training in problem-solving, and training in strategies intended to reduce the risk for relapse. The 20-session supportive counselling package provided emotional support through the development of a therapeutic relationship that fostered rapport and unconditional regard for the patient; general counselling skills were used to maximize the impact of non-specific factors in psychotherapy. The supportive counselling group was therefore a control group which sought to ascertain whether benefits (if any) with cognitive therapy were specific to the therapeutic technique or secondary to non-specific factors. Routine clinical care comprised standard psychiatric management. The entire study was conducted on an out-patient basis or in the patients' homes.

The mean age of the sample was 38.6 years; 79 per cent of the patients were males. Schizophrenia was the main diagnosis (90 per cent of cases). The median duration of illness was 11 years. The three groups were receiving a mean of 425–517 chlorpromazine equivalents per day; there was no significant difference between groups. Medication was held constant during the study.

Seventy-two patients completed the study. The cognitive therapy group showed the maximum improvement in both number and severity of psychotic symptoms, while the routine care group showed deterioration in both these indices; the supportive counselling group showed intermediate results. For both the indices of improvement, the difference between the groups was statistically significant. Eleven patients receiving cognitive therapy showed more than 50 per cent improvement in psychotic symptoms as compared with only seven patients in the other two groups combined; the difference was again statistically significant.

The use of cognitive therapy, shorter duration of illness, and lesser initial severity of symptoms predicted greater likelihood of more than 50 per cent improvement. In comparison with routine clinical care, the use of cognitive therapy was associated with an eight times greater chance of responding by more than 50 per cent.

A particular strength of this study is that it was double-blind; raters were unable to guess which patient had been receiving which form of treatment. Furthermore, videotaped assessments confirmed the conformity of the sessions to the nature of the intervention planned.

Strictly speaking, the positive symptoms in the patients in this study were not treatment-refractory. Tarrier *et al.* did not furnish evidence to demonstrate that these patients had failed several medication trials of adequate dosage and duration, nor was there evidence that these patients had failed trials with the atypical antipsychotics and electroconvulsive therapy. Readers must, therefore, keep these circumstances in mind when generalizing from the conclusion of this study. Nevertheless, the Tarrier *et al.* (1998) study conveys several important lessons for the management of chronically ill psychotic patients who experience persistent psychotic symptoms despite pharmacotherapy:

1. Routine clinical care will only maintain the status quo.
2. Supportive psychotherapy, comprising commonsense counselling and the establishment of a sound therapeutic relationship with the patient, will produce modest clinical gains. It is presumed that non-specific factors of psychotherapy will mediate clinical gains in such circumstances.
3. Cognitive therapy, comprising training in strategies that seek to enhance coping and problem-solving skills, and reduce the risk for relapse, are associated with convincing clinical gains.

Good clinical care does not stop with a prescription. A combination of somatic therapy, cognitive therapy, psychoeducational therapy, occupational therapy, family therapy, and social support (tailored to individual requirements) will surely prove to be the most effective treatment programme for patients diagnosed with schizophrenia.

Religion and Remission of Depression

Koenig *et al.* (1998) examined the influence of religion on the remission of depressive symptoms in medically ill elderly patients admitted to a university hospital. The sample comprised consecutive patients aged 60 years and over who, on the basis of a structured psychiatric interview, were diagnosed to have depression.

After discharge, patients were reassessed by telephone at a frequency of once in 12 weeks for 48 weeks. In this manner, data were obtained for a total of 87 patients. Depression remitted in 54 per cent of these patients, and the median time to remission was 30 weeks.

Religious variables were examined as predictors of time to remission after controlling for demographic, psychosocial, physical health and treatment variables. Intrinsic religiosity significantly and independently predicted time to remission, but church attendance and private religious activities did not; that is, patients who were fundamentally more religious recovered faster from their depressive episode than those who were fundamentally less religious; and, external exhibitions of religious behaviour had no influence on recovery time.

It remains to be determined whether these findings are demonstrable in other (non-medical) contexts in which depression occurs. It also needs to be ascertained whether these findings hold across cultures. And finally, it is a moot point whether fundamental religiosity can be manipulated as a therapeutic strategy.

Hormone Replacement Therapy for Alzheimer's Disease

HRT in Medicine and Psychiatry

Hormone replacement therapy (HRT) during or after menopause is a much discussed treatment, with proponents both for and against its use. On the positive side, HRT eliminates the symptoms of menopause, reduces osteoporosis (Schneider *et al.*, 1997), and decreases the risks for major coronary heart disease (Grodstein *et al.*, 1996). On the negative side, HRT increases the risks for breast and endometrial cancers (Colditz *et al.*, 1995; Grodstein *et al.*, 1997), gall bladder disease, migraine, and venous thrombosis. Overall, HRT is associated with a 10–50 per cent reduction in the risk for mortality, depending on the risk factors in the population being treated (Grodstein *et al.*, 1997). Therapeutic implications of HRT have been discussed by Brinton and Schairer (1997), and a mathematical model for identification of women likely to benefit from HRT has been proposed by Col *et al.*, (1997).

What is the relevance of HRT to psychiatry? The conventional application lies in the attenuation of the psychological symptoms of menopause; these are otherwise treated with benzodiazepines or antidepressant drugs. An experimental application for HRT, specifically with oestrogen, is now being mooted: the prophylaxis and treatment of Alzheimer's disease.

HRT in Alzheimer's Disease: Mechanisms

Oestrogen receptors have been identified in the hypothalamus, anterior pituitary, preoptic area, CA1 region of the hippocampus, and several other brain regions. Several theoretical oestrogen-dependent pro-cognitive mechanisms have been proposed on the basis of animal research; these have been discussed by Burns and Murphy (1996), Wickelgren (1997), Morrison and Hof (1997), Seeman (1997), Birge (1997), McEwen *et al.* (1997), and Yaffe *et al.* (1998).

1. Oestrogens enhance the activity of neurotrophins in the brain by upregulating neurotrophin receptors and by facilitating second messenger signalling between the neurotrophin receptor and the genes in the nucleus of the cell. Neurotrophins are proteins that promote the growth of neurons, nurture axons and dendrites, and facilitate the formation of synapses. Nerve Growth Factor (NGF) is an example of a neurotrophin which interacts with oestrogens.
2. Oestrogens are antioxidants and mop up toxic free radicals that are potentially neurotoxic. Through this mechanism, oestrogens protect neurons from the effects of excessive glutaminergic stimulation. Also through this mechanism, oestrogens protect neurons against beta-amyloid, which is a protein which accumulates in Alzheimer's patients' brains and causes neuronal degeneration.
3. Oestrogens facilitate the secretion of acetylcholine in the hippocampus and in the basal forebrain through an increase in

the levels of choline acetyltransferase in these brain loci. Choline acetyltransferase is an enzyme involved in the synthesis of acetylcholine.

4. Oestrogens protect brain cells from the neurotoxic effects of glucocorticoids in loci such as the hippocampus.
5. Oestrogens improve cerebral blood flow by diminishing the reduced vessel-wall compliance that is associated with menopause and aging. Oestrogens may also reduce the central arterial smooth muscle injury response, and reduce platelet aggregation.
6. Oestrogens modulate the expression of the apolipoprotein E gene; this gene is involved in Alzheimer's disease. Oestrogens also promote the non-amyloidogenic metabolism of amyloid precursor protein.

Through such mechanisms, oestrogens increase the survival of cholinergic neurons that are involved in cognitive processes. Oestrogens also maintain or promote neuronal circuitry in the hippocampus, an area important to cognition.

It is conceivable that the loss of oestrogen in postmenopausal women is partly or wholly responsible for the accelerated cognitive decline and the greater risk of Alzheimer's disease in women as compared with men. In this context, it should be noted that testosterone continues to be secreted (albeit in lesser quanta) even in older men; this testosterone is converted to some extent to oestradiol in the brain. Thus, men, unlike women, do not lose the benefits purveyed by oestrogen to brain functioning.

There is growing evidence for the beneficial effect of oestrogen in Alzheimer's disease. Too many studies have been published for these to be exhaustively reviewed; therefore, selected examples from different categories of research will be presented, and for a detailed discussion the reader is referred to Yaffe *et al.* (1998), and Farlow and Evans (1998).

Observational Studies of Oestrogen and Cognition in Non-Demented Postmenopausal Women

Paganini-Hill and Henderson (1996) designed a case-control study with a sample of 8,877 non-demented postmenopausal women. Of the 3,760 women who died over a 15-year follow-up period, 248 women with likely Alzheimer's disease were identified. Five controls were individually matched to each case according to the years of birth and death. It was found that the risk for Alzheimer's disease and related dementia was significantly reduced (by 35 per cent) in oestrogen users as compared with non-users. The risk was reduced for oral, parenteral as well as topical (creams) users of oestrogen. The risk decreased significantly with both increased dose and increased duration of therapy. These findings suggest that HRT may be useful for preventing or delaying the onset of Alzheimer's disease in postmenopausal women.

Yaffe *et al.* (1998) listed four other studies in this category, of which three described small but significant gains associated with oestrogen use. In a study not examined by Yaffe *et al.*, Resnick *et al.* (1997) described a possible protective effect of oestrogen on visual memory: non-demented postmenopausal women (n = 116) who reported that they were receiving oestrogen replacement therapy during a cognitive assessment performed significantly better on several visual memory tasks than did similar women (n = 172) who had never received oestrogen replacement.

Trials of Oestrogen Therapy on Cognition in Non-Demented Postmenopausal Women

Sherwin (1988) described a 3-month, double-blind, randomized, crossover trial with 5 groups: oestrogen, androgen, oestrogen combined with androgen, placebo, and control. The sample comprised 50 women who were postmenopausal as a result of recent surgery. The mean age of the sample was 45 years. There was significant improvement with oestrogen as compared with placebo on all four cognitive tests employed; a confounding variable, however, was that many women had menopausal symptoms which might have compromised their cognitive performances during the placebo phase.

Yaffe *et al.* (1998) described seven other studies in this category. Of these, two showed gains with oestrogen on most of the outcome variables, while three more showed gains on a few variables only. Results were negative for oestrogen in the remaining two studies.

Case-Control and Observational Studies of the Association of Oestrogen Use and Dementia

Henderson *et al.* (1994) designed a case-control study to examine the use of HRT and the possible consequences thereof in women with Alzheimer's disease as compared with normal controls. There were 143 elderly women in the community who met the criteria for probable Alzheimer's disease, and 92 non-demented controls; 70 women who later died met the histopathological criteria for Alzheimer's disease. Among eligible cases, there were 10 oestrogen users and 128 non-users. The findings were that Alzheimer's patients were significantly less likely to be using oestrogen replacement; those who were using oestrogen, however, performed significantly better on the Mini-Mental Status Examination than those who were not. The authors concluded that postmenopausal HRT may be associated with a decreased risk for Alzheimer's disease, and that HRT may improve cognition in women with this illness.

Yaffe *et al.* (1998) listed seven other studies in this category; all the studies failed to demonstrate a significant role for oestrogen. In a study not reviewed by Yaffe *et al.*, Lerner *et al.* (1997) reported a protective effect for oestrogen. In another study, Baldereschi *et al.* (1998) used data from the Italian Longitudinal Study on Aging to show that there was an inverse relationship between oestrogen use and Alzheimer's disease; this suggests that oestrogen protects against the development of this disorder. The protective effect remained significant even after controlling for possible confounding variables, such as age, education, age at menarche, age at menopause, smoking, alcohol use, body weight at age 50, and number of children. Waring *et al.* (1999) reported an inverse association between the use of oestrogen and Alzheimer's disease in postmenopausal women (n=222); this association remained significant even after adjusting for education and age at menopause, and was dependent on both duration of oestrogen therapy and cumulative dose. Finally, in an abstract, Mayeux *et al.* (1997) reported that the postmenopausal use of oestrogen appeared to protect against dementia in women with Parkinson's disease.

Prospective Cohort Studies of the Association of Oestrogen Use and Dementia

Tang *et al.* (1996) studied 1,124 mentally healthy elderly women who were initially free of Alzheimer's disease, Parkinson's disease, and stroke, and who were taking part in a longitudinal study on health and aging. Overall, 156 (12.5 per cent) women reported taking oestrogen after the onset of menopause. During a 1–5 year follow-up, 9 (5.8 per cent) of these women developed Alzheimer's disease in contrast with 158 (16.3 per cent) of the 968 women who had not used oestrogen. The age of onset of Alzheimer's disease was significantly later in women who had taken oestrogen than in those who had not. Oestrogen use reduced the relative risk for Alzheimer's disease by 60 per cent. These findings remained significant even after adjusting for differences in education, ethnic origin, and apolipoprotein-E genotype. Women who had used oestrogen for longer than a year had a greater reduction in risk for Alzeimer's disease.

Yaffe *et al.* (1998) listed one other study in this category; the results again favoured the role of oestrogen in the prevention of development of Alzheimer's disease (Kawas *et al.*, 1997).

Trials of Oestrogen in Alzheimer's Disease

There have been only four studies in this category, all with very small samples; the total number of subjects in the four trials was just 58. Only one study employed a double-blind, randomized, placebo-controlled design. In these four studies, modest gains favouring oestrogen were recorded (Yaffe *et al.*, 1998).

In an unusual study, Schneider *et al.* (1996) reported that women with Alzheimer's disease who were receiving tacrine improved significantly more if they were also receiving oestrogen than if they were receiving placebo or tacrine alone.

Birge (1997) reported preliminary data from an ongoing 9-month double-blind, randomized, placebo-controlled study: Alzheimer's patients ($n=10$) receiving oestrogen showed improvement while those receiving placebo ($n=10$) deteriorated.

General Conclusions

It thus appears that the postmenopausal use of oestrogen may improve cognitive performance in healthy women, and may delay the onset of or decrease the risk for Alzheimer's disease; a meta-analysis of observational studies found that oestrogen decreased the risk for dementia by 29 per cent (Yaffe *et al.*, 1998). It is possible that the benefit with oestrogen may be dependent on both the dose and the duration of therapy.

Overall, the results are not sufficiently convincing to recommend the routine postmenopausal use of oestrogen for the prophylaxis or treatment of dementia. This does not mean to say that oestrogen does not work; rather, it indicates that many studies with unsatisfactory design and heterogeneous results have been published, from which no firm conclusions can be drawn. Until large sample, double-blind, randomized, placebo-controlled studies are conducted, oestrogen replacement therapy for the prevention and/or treatment of dementia will remain an experimental treatment. Two large studies are currently under way (Skolnick, 1997).

Scope for the Future

If the beneficial effects of oestrogen on cognition can be confirmed, oestrogen replacement therapy in postmenopausal women will receive a further boost; the treatment might find application in the prophylaxis as well as in the treatment of age-related cognitive decline and of Alzheimer's disease. It is conceivable that appropriate drugs can then be designed that have the beneficial effects of oestrogen without causing feminization or other unwanted side effects (including carcinogenesis); such drugs could be useful in men with cognitive problems as well. Preliminary leads towards the development of such drugs have already been obtained (Wickelgren, 1997).

The extent to which oestrogen-mediated cognitive benefits (in non-demented postmenopausal women) are contingent on oestrogen-mediated improvements in mood requires to be determined (Stahl, 1997). Since oestrogens are often used along with progesterone, particularly in women with a uterus, studies might evaluate the application of the oestrogen—progesterone combination as well.

Lastly, an ethical issue may need to be resolved: if oestrogen does slow down the progression of Alzheimer's disease, would it be justified to provide a treatment that prolongs suffering in patients and their caregivers? A consensus needs to be reached on when exactly during the course of the disease it becomes ethical to withdraw the treatment.

Further Reading

The subject of oestrogen replacement for the prophylaxis or treatment of dementia has been much discussed in recent years. Interested readers may consult the following reviews and commentaries: Burns and Murphy (1996), Wickelgren (1997), Morrison and Hof (1997), Seeman (1997), Birge (1997), McEwen *et at*. (1997), and

Yaffe *et al.* (1998). During 1997, two entire supplements (Suppl. 6 and Suppl. 7) of *Neurology* were devoted to Alzheimer's disease and the use of hormones as treatment; these too make excellent reading.

Ginkgo Biloba for Dementia

Herbal extracts are touted for psychopharmacological efficacy in many countries across the world. Le Bars *et al.* (1997) recently addressed the efficacy of Ginkgo biloba for dementia in a randomized, double-blind, placebo-controlled, 1-year, 6-centre prospective trial conducted in the USA.

The sample comprised patients diagnosed with mild to moderately severe, uncomplicated dementia according to DSM-III-R and ICD-10. Patients were excluded if they had any other (significant) primary medical or psychiatric diagnosis, or if the dementia was secondary to a brain tumour or haemorrhage. Existing medications were kept unchanged during the period of the study.

Ginkgo was administered in the dose of 40 mg thrice a day; placebo was administered likewise. Assessments were conducted at baseline, and again at weeks 12, 26, and 52; these evaluated cognitive functioning, daily living and social behaviour, and general psychopathology. A number of physical and other investigations were also performed at baseline and endpoint.

A total of 166 patients were assigned to the Ginkgo group, and 161 to the placebo group. The two groups were similar at baseline on a variety of sociodemographic and clinical measures. The mean age of the groups was 69 years, and the sex distribution was predominantly female. About 76 per cent of the sample was diagnosed with Alzheimer's disease. The mean duration of illness was about 4 years.

Significantly more Ginkgo patients (n=78; 50 per cent) than placebo patients (n=59; 38 per cent) completed the trial. The commonest reasons for drop out were caregivers' requests, non-compliance with treatment, and inefficacy of treatment. Drop out due to inefficacy was commoner with placebo (n=21) than with Ginkgo (n=12) while drop out due to adverse effects was commoner with Ginkgo (n=10) than with placebo (n=4).

The average patient receiving Ginkgo showed no cognitive deterioration, and improved in social behaviour and activities of daily living. In contrast, the average patient receiving placebo manifested deterioration in both measures. The difference between the two groups was statistically significant. The two groups, however, did not differ on ratings of global psychopathology. Similar results were obtained when patients with Alzheimer's disease were analyzed separately.

Statistically significant differences notwithstanding, the average differences between the groups were small. However, when patients were recategorized on the basis of magnitude of improvement, significantly more Ginkgo than placebo patients showed mild to moderate improvement. The authors did not provide information on the percentage of patients in each group which showed a specified percentage of improvement; therefore, the general conclusion that can be drawn is that some but not all patients will benefit from Ginkgo.

Adverse events were comparable between the two groups in nature, number, and severity.

While the results of this study are encouraging, they provoke questions that need to be addressed in future research:

1. Will lower or higher doses of Ginkgo (than those used in this study) be less or more effective in terms of the number of patients responding and the magnitude of clinical benefit?
2. What is the minimum duration for which treatment is necessary to determine whether or not the patient will respond?
3. What are the clinical subtypes of cognitive impairment that can be expected to respond to Ginkgo?
4. Are the benefits limited to the period of therapy or are they sustained for a longer period (indicating a change in the course of the disease)?

How does Ginkgo work? Nobody knows, but at least one viable hypothesis has been suggested. Constituents of ginkgo such as the flavonoids, the terpenoids (ginkgolides, bilobalide) and the organic acids act synergistically to produce an antioxidant effect. These compounds, to varying degrees, scavenge free radicals which have been considered to mediate the excessive lipid peroxidation and cell damage observed in Alzheimer's disease. Ginkgo constituents have also been suggested to provide membrane protection, modulate neurotransmission, and regulate inflammation; these mechanisms may also be germane to improved cognitive functioning.

A caveat that needs to be noted is that Le Bars *et al.* studied the extract of Ginkgo biloba referred to as EGb 761. This extract is widely used in Europe to alleviate cognitive dysfunction, and has been approved of in Germany for the treatment of dementia. The composition of this extract is not necessarily the same as the composition of the Ginkgo that is commercially available in other parts of the world. Clinicians are reminded that the chemical contents of medicinal herbs vary from place to place, from season to season, and from one part of the plant to another; therefore, standardization of the extract for commercial use is difficult, especially when one is uncertain of the identity of the clinically-relevant ingredients. The bottomline is that the herbal extract of each pharmaceutical company must be tested for efficacy and safety; afterwards, it is to be hoped that the company will be able to standardize the product for uniformity of composition.

LIDOCAINE FOR ACUTE MIGRAINE

Migraine is a common condition, with a 1-year prevalence of 17 per cent in women and 6 per cent in men (Stewart *et al.*, 1994). Serotonergic mechanisms have been implicated in migraine. Drugs used in the prophylaxis of migraine include 5-HT2 antagonists such as cyproheptadine, and selective serotonin reuptake inhibitors such as fluoxetine. Drugs used for pain relief in migraine include sumatriptan, a potent and selective 5-HT1D agonist.

Several non-serotonergic agents have also been used with success for both treatment and prophylaxis in patients who experience this type of headache. The therapeutic agents include analgesics such as aspirin, and vasoconstrictors such as ergot derivatives. The prophylactic agents include beta blockers such as propranolol, anticonvulsants such as sodium valproate, calcium channel blockers such as verapamil and flunarizine, and tricyclic antidepressants such as imipramine.

Sumatriptan is one of the recent therapies offered for acute migraine. Cerebral vasoconstriction is its likely mechanism of action. The disadvantage of oral sumatriptan is that response is delayed as it depends on the quantum and rate of absorption of the drug. Parenteral sumatriptan probably offers the fastest avenue of pain relief in acute migraine; however, this treatment is expensive and does not always work; when it does work, relapse of headache is not uncommon (The Subcutaneous Sumatriptan International Study Group, 1991). A further disadvantage of parenteral sumatriptan is that few patients will be able to avail of its benefits if they live far from medical facilities, or if they experience migraine on a public holiday, or during the night, when the accessibility to medical staff is restricted.

Maizels *et al.* (1996) provided evidence for the efficacy of an alternate emergency treatment. Adults with acute migraine (n=81) were randomized 2:1 to receive either intranasal lidocaine (n=53) or normal saline (n=28). Lidocaine was administered in the form of a 4 per cent topical solution, 0.5 ml of which was instilled over 30 secs into the nostril while the patient lay with his head hyperextended to 45 degrees, and rotated 30 degrees to the side of the headache. The instillation was effected into the nostril ipsilateral to the headache; in the case of bilateral headaches, the instillation was effected into both nostrils. The procedure was repeated after 2 mins if the benefit was inadequate. Saline-treated patients underwent the same procedure. Neither patients nor raters were aware of the treatment assignment.

Twenty-nine patients (55 per cent) treated with intranasal lidocaine reported 50 per cent or greater relief from headache, nausea, and photophobia; this improvement occurred within 5 mins. Only 6 patients (21 per cent) treated with saline reported similar benefit. Complete or near complete resolution of headache occured in 21 per cent of lidocaine-treated patients, and in 7 per cent of saline-treated patients. No headache characteristic (either duration of symptoms or presence/absence of lateralization) predicted response to lidocaine.

Only 28 per cent of lidocaine-treated patients as compared with 71 per cent of saline-treated patients required rescue medication for the headache. Among the patients who showed initial response to treatment, 10 relapsed in the lidocaine group and 5 relapsed in the saline group. Relapse usually occurred within the first hour of treatment. Adverse effects were noted almost exclusively in the lidocaine group; these included burning or numbness in the nose or in and around the eye, an unpleasant taste, and numbness of the throat, often associated with a sense of gagging. Experience of these adverse effects contributed to a loss of blinding in the assessments.

Maizels *et al.* hypothesized that intranasal lidocaine aborts acute migraine through its action on the sphenopalatine ganglion. They discussed mechanisms whereby this ganglion is relevant to migraine.

It thus appears that intasnasal lidocaine has the potential to become a convenient home remedy for acute migraine. At least half of the patients so treated can expect rapid relief from headache, nausea, and photophobia. However, nearly half of patients who respond can expect relapse of headache within an hour. The adverse effects of treatment are minor and transient.

Zolmitriptan (Zolmig, Zeneca Pharmaceuticals; 311C90), a 5-HT1B/1d agonist, is currently being investigated in the treatment of migraine. Preliminary evidence suggests that zolmitriptan is both effective and safe (Ferrari, 1997; Zagami, 1997; Dawson, 1997).

Vagal Stimulation for Epilepsy

At the 22nd International Epilepsy Congress held at Dublin, Ireland, during 1997, the Vagus Nerve Stimulator emerged as a treatment option for patients with severe, treatment-refractory epilepsy. Vagal stimulation has long been known to control seizures, possibly by modulating the abnormal neuronal firing associated with seizures through its projections to the nucleus solitarius in the brainstem, and thence to the hippocampus and cerebral cortex.

In 1988, Cybernetics Inc, a firm in Texas, developed the NeuroCybernetic Prosthesis (NCP) System for epileptic patients. This system includes an implantable generator and stimulating lead that can deliver electrical impulses to the vagus. The generator is implanted in the upper left chest and the lead is attached to the left vagus in the neck. The entire surgery lasts about 2 hours, and is conducted under general anaesthesia. After implantation, the NCP generator is programmed to deliver regular stimuli to the vagus. In addition, a hand-held magnet is available for use by the patient or by an attendant to stimulate the nerve at the onset of a seizure.

The NCP generator has a battery life of about 5 years when the device is used at the recommended stimulation parameters. These parameters are the same as those considered in brief-pulse ECT, and describe pulse amplitude, pulse width, pulse frequency, the duration of stimulation (on-time), and the duration of break (off-time). A typical high-dose setting involves 30 secs on and 5 mins off. When the battery life approaches its end, the generator can be replaced in an out-patient procedure that lasts 30–60 mins.

In a 3-month, 20-centre, randomized controlled trial conducted in the USA, 199 patients with refractory epilepsy were treated with high- or low-dose vagal stimulation. High-dose stimulation involved treatment with optimal doses of current, while low-dose stimulation involved the administration of current in a dose that was perceptible to the patient but was not therapeutic. All patients had had at least 6 complex partial seizures a month for at least 3 consecutive months, and were taking up to 3 antiepileptic drugs.

In the high-dose group, 26 per cent of patients had a 25–50 per cent reduction in seizures, 13 per cent had a 50–75 per cent reduction, 11 per cent had over 0.75 per cent reduction, and one patient became seizure-free. The mean seizure reduction in this group was 28 per cent. The mean seizure reduction in the control group was 15 per cent. The difference between the two groups was not large, but was nevertheless statistically significant.

Adverse effects of vagal stimulation included transient hoarseness during stimulation, tingling in the neck, muscle quivering, and a sensation of dyspnoea. Overall, the device was well-tolerated and well-accepted by the patients.

More than 2000 patient-years of experience with vagal stimulation have now been recorded. The vagal stimulator received regulatory approval for marketing and use in the European Union during 1995, in Canada during March 1997, and in the USA during July 1997. The stimulator is used along with and not instead of conventional medical and other therapies for epilepsy. A discussion on the subject has been provided by Phillips (1997).

Recent data suggest that uagal stimulation may benefit patients with refractory depression as well. The issue is currently being investigated in clinical trials.

REFERENCES

American Psychiatric Association (1997). 'Practice guideline for the treatment of patients with schizophrenia', *Am. J. Psychiatry*, 154 (suppl. 4): 1–63.

Baldereschi M., Di Carlo A., Lepore V. *et al.*, for the Italian Longitudinal Study on Aging Working Group (1998). 'Estrogen-replacement therapy and Alzheimer's disease in the Italian Longitudinal Study on Aging', *Neurology*, 50: 996–1002.

Birge S. J. (1997). 'The role of estrogen in the treatment of Alzheimer's disease', *Neurology*, 48 (Suppl. 7): S36–S41.

Blackburn I. M. and Moore R. G. (1997). 'Controlled acute and follow-up trial of cognitive therapy and pharmacotherapy in out-patients with recurrent depression', *Br. J. Psychiatry*, 171: 328–34.

Bollini P., Pampallona S., Orza M. J. *et al.* (1994). 'Antipsychotic drugs: is more worse? A meta-analysis of the published randomized control trials', *Psychol. Med.*, 24: 307–16.

Brinton L. A. and Schairer C. (1997). 'Postmenopausal hormone-replacement therapy—time for a reappraisal?', *New Engl. J. Med.*, 336: 1821–2.

Burns A., and Murphy D. (1996). 'Protection against Alzheimer's disease', *Lancet*, 348: 420–1.

Carpenter W. T., Conley R. R., Buchanan R. W. *et al.* (1995). 'Patient response and resource management: another view of clozapine treatment of schizophrenia', *Am. J. Psychiatry*, 152: 827–32.

Chambers C. D., Johnson K. A., Dick L. M. *et al.* (1996). 'Birth outcomes in pregnant women taking fluoxetine', *N. Engl. J. Med.*, 335: 1010–15.

Col N. F., Eckman M. H. and Karas R. H. (1997). 'Patient-specific decisions about hormone replacement therapy in postmenopausal women', *JAMA*, 277: 1140–7.

Colditz G. A., Hankinson S. E. and Hunter D. J. (1995). 'The use of oestrogens and progestins and the risk of breast cancer in postmenopausal women', *N. Engl. J. Med.*, 332: 1589–93.

Conley R. R., Carpenter W. T. and Tamminga C. A. (1997). 'Time to clozapine response in a standardized trial', *Am. J. Psychiatry*, 154: 1243–7.

Dawson A. J. (1997). '311C90: Patient profiles and typical case histories of migraine management', *Neurology*, 48 (suppl. 3): S29–S33.

Drury V., Birchwood M., Cochrane R. *et al.* (1996a). 'Cognitive therapy and recovery from acute psychosis. I: Impact on symptoms', *Br. J. Psychiatry*, 169: 593–601.

——— (1996b). 'Cognitive therapy and recovery from acute psychosis. II: Impact on recovery time', *Br. J. Psychiatry*, 169: 602–7.

Farlow M. R. and Evans R. M. (1998). 'Pharmacologic treatment of cognition in Alzheimer's dementia', *Neurology*, 51 (suppl. 1): S36–S44.

Ferrari M. D. (1997). '311C90: Increasing the options for therapy with effective acute antimigraine 5-HT1B/1D receptor agonists', *Neurology*, 48 (suppl. 3): S21–S24.

Garety P., Kuipers L., Fowler D. *et al.* (1994). 'Cognitive behavioural therapy for drug resistant psychosis', *Br. J. Med. Psychol.*, 67: 259–71.

Grodstein F., Stampfer M. J., Manson J. E. *et al.* (1996). 'Postmenopausal oestrogen and progestin use and the risk of cardiovascular disease',

N. Engl. J. Med., 335: 453–61. (Erratum, *N. Engl. J. Med.*, 1996, 335: 1406)

Grodstein F., Stampfer M. J., Colditz G. A. *et al.* (1997). 'Postmenopausal hormone therapy and mortality', *N. Engl. J. Med.*, 336: 1769–75.

Henderson V. W., Paganini-Hill A., Emanuel C. K. *et al.* (1994). 'Oestrogen replacement therapy in older women', *Arch. Neurol.*, 51: 896–900.

Hirsch S. R. and Barnes T. R. E. (1994). 'Clinical use of high-dose neuroleptics', *Br. J. Psychiatry*, 164: 94–6.

Jeste D. V., Lindamer L. A., Evans J. *et al.* (1996). 'Relationship of ethnicity and gender to schizophrenia and pharmacology of neuroleptics', *Psychopharmacol. Bull.*, 32: 243–51.

Johnson D. A. W. (1996). 'Peer review of cognitive therapy and recovery from acute psychosis', *Br. J. Psychiatry*, 169: 608–9.

Kane J. M. (1994). 'The use of higher-dose antipsychotic medication: Comment on the Royal College of Psychiatrists' consensus statement', Editorial, *Br. J. Psychiatry*, 164: 431–2.

Kawas C., Resnick S., Morrison A. *et al.* (1997). 'A prospective study of oestrogen replacement therapy and the risk of development of Alzheimer's disease: The Baltimore Longitudinal Study of Aging', *Neurology*, 48: 1517–21.

Koenig H. G., George L. K. and Peterson B. L. (1998). 'Religiosity and remission of depression in medically ill older patients', *Am. J. Psychiatry*, 155: 536–42.

Kuipers E., Garety P., Fowler D. *et al.* (1997). 'The London-East Anglia randomized controlled trial of cognitive behaviour therapy for psychosis: effects of the treatment phase', *Br. J. Psychiatry*, 171: 319–25.

Kulin N. A., Pastuszak A., Sage S. R. *et al.* (1998). 'Pregnancy outcome following maternal use of the new selective serotonin reuptake inhibitors: A prospective controlled multicenter study', *JAMA*, 279: 609–10.

Kumra S., Frazier J. A., Jacobsen L. K. *et al.* (1996). 'Childhood-onset schizophrenia: a double-blind clozapine-haloperidol comparison', *Arch. Gen. Psychiatry*, 53: 1090–7.

Le Bars P. L., Katz M. M., Berman N. *et al.* (1997). 'A placebo-controlled, double-blind, randomized trial of an extract of Ginkgo Biloba for dementia', *JAMA*, 278: 1327–32.

Lerner A., Koss E., Debanne S. *et al.* (1997). 'Smoking and oestrogen-replacement therapy as protective factors for Alzheimer's disease', *Lancet*, 349: 403–4.

Lieberman J. A., Safferman A. Z., Pollack S. *et al.* (1994). 'Clinical effects of clozapine in chronic schizophrenia: response to treatment and predictors of outcome', *Am. J. Psychiatry*, 151: 1744–52.

Lin K. M., Poland R. E., Wan Y. J. Y *et al.* (1996). 'The evolving science of pharmacogenetics: clinical and ethnic perspectives', *Psychopharmacol. Bull.*, 32: 205–17.

Maizels M., Scott B., Cohen W. *et al.* (1996). 'Intranasal lidocaine for treatment of migraine: a randomized, double-blind, controlled trial', *JAMA*, 276: 319–21.

Mattes J. A. (1989). 'Clozapine for refractory schizophrenia: an open study of 14 patients treated up to 2 years', *J. Clin. Psychiatry*, 50: 389–91.

Mayeux R., Tang M. X., Marder K. *et al.* (1997). 'Postmenopausal oestrogen use and Parkinson's disease with and without dementia', *Neurology*, 48 (suppl. 2): A79.

McEwen B. S., Alves S. E., Bulloch K. *et al.* (1997). 'Ovarian steroids and the brain', *Neurology*, 48 (suppl. 7) S8–S15.

Meltzer H. Y. (1992). 'Dimensions of outcome with clozapine', *Br. J. Psychiatry*, 160 (suppl.): 46–53.

——— (1995). 'Clozapine: Is another view valid?', Editorial, *Am. J. Psychiatry*, 152: 821–5.

Milberger S., Biederman J., Faraone S. V. *et al.* (1996). 'Is maternal smoking during pregnancy a risk factor for attention deficit hyperactivity disorder in children?', *Am. J. Psychiatry*, 153: 1138–42.

Morrison J. H. and Hof P. R. (1997). 'Life and death of neurons in the aging brain', *Science*, 278: 412–19.

Mossman D. (1997). 'A decision analysis approach to neuroleptic dosing: Insights from a mathematical model', *J. Clin. Psychiatry*, 58: 66–73.

Nulman I., Rovet J., Stewart D. E. *et al.* (1997). 'Neurodevelopment of children exposed in utero to antidepressant drugs', *N. Engl. J. Med.*, 336: 258–62.

Owen R. R., Beake B. J., Marby D. *et al.* (1989). 'Response to clozapine in chronic psychotic patients', *Psychopharmacol. Bull.*, 25: 253–6.

Paganini-Hill A. and Henderson V. W. (1996). 'Oestrogen replacement therapy and risk of Alzheimer's disease', *Arch. Intern. Med.*, 156: 2213–17.

Pastuszak A., Schick-Boschetto B., Zuber C. *et al.* (1993). 'Pregnancy outcome following first-trimester exposure to fluoxetine (Prozac)', *JAMA*, 269: 2246–8.

Peuskens H., on behalf of the Risperidone Study Group (1995). 'Risperidone in the treatment of patients with chronic schizophrenia: a multinational, multi-centre, double-blind, parallel-group study versus haloperidol', *Br. J. Psychiatry*, 166: 712–26.

Phillips P. (1997). 'Current view of advances in epilepsy', *JAMA*, 278: 883–6.

Resnick S. M., Metter E. J. and Zonderman A. B. (1997). 'Oestrogen replacement therapy and longitudinal decline in visual memory: A possible protective effect?', *Neurology*, 49: 1491–7.

Robert E. (1996). 'Treating depression in pregnancy', Editorial, *N. Engl. J. Med.*, 335: 1056–8.

Schneider L. S., Farlow M. R., Henderson V. W. *et al.* (1996). 'Effects of oestrogen replacement therapy on response to tacrine in patients with Alzheimer's disease', *Neurology*, 46: 1580–4.

Schneider D. L., Barrett-Connor E. L. and Morton D. J. (1997). 'Timing of postmenopausal oestrogen for optimal bone mineral density: the Rancho Bernado Study', *JAMA*, 277: 543–7.

Seeman M. V. (1997). 'Psychopathology in women and men: focus on female hormones', *Am. J. Psychiatry*, 154: 1641–7.

Sherwin B. B. (1988). 'Oestrogen and/or androgen replacement therapy and cognitive functioning in surgically postmenopausal women', *Psychoneuroendocrinology*, 13: 345–57.

Skolnick A. A. (1997). 'Evaluating oestrogen for Alzheimer's disease poses ethical and logistical challenges', *JAMA*, 277: 1831–3.

Srinivasan T. N. and Latha S. (1997). 'Use of clozapine in childhood schizophrenia', *Indian J. Psychiatry*, 39: 262–4.

Stahl S. M. (1997). 'Sex therapy in psychiatric treatment has a new partner: reproductive hormones', *J. Clin. Psychiatry*, 58: 468–9.

Stewart W. F., Shechter A. and Rasmussen B. K. (1994). 'Migraine prevalence: a review of population-based studies', *Neurology*, 44 (suppl. 4): S17–S23.

Tang M-X, Jacobs D., Stern Y. *et al.* (1996). 'Effect of oestrogen during menopause on risk and age at onset of Alzheimer's disease', *Lancet*, 348: 429–32.

Tarrier N., Beckett R., Harwood S. *et al.* (1993). 'A trial of two cognitive-behavioural methods of treating drug-resistant residual psychotic symptoms in schizophrenic patients. 1: Outcome', *Br. J. Psychiatry*, 162; 524–32.

Tarrier N., Yusupoff L., Kinney C. *et al.* (1998). 'Randomized controlled trial of intensive cognitive behaviour therapy for patients with chronic schizophrenia', *BMJ*, 317: 303–7.

The Subcutaneous Sumatriptan International Study Group (1991). 'Treatment of migraine attacks with sumatriptan', *N. Engl. J. Med.*, 325: 316–21.

Thompson C. (1994). 'The use of high-dose antipsychotic medication', *Br. J. Psychiatry*, 164: 448–58.

Thun M. J., Peto R., Lopez A. D. *et al.* (1997). 'Alcohol consumption and mortality among middle-aged and elderly U.S. adults', *N. Engl. J. Med.*, 337: 1705–14.

Turetz M., Mozes T., Toren P. *et al.* (1997). 'An open trial of clozapine in neuroleptic-resistant childhood-onset schizophrenia', *Br. J. Psychiatry*, 170: 507–10.

Turner S. M. and Cooley-Quille M. R. (1996). 'Socioecological and sociocultural variables in psychopharmacological research: methodological considerations', *Psychopharmacol. Bull.*, 32: 183–92.

Wakschlag L. S., Lahey B. B., Loeber R. *et al.* (1997). 'Maternal smoking during pregnancy and the risk of conduct disorder in boys', *Arch. Gen. Psychiatry*, 54: 670–6.

Waring S. C., Rocca W. A., Petersen R. C. *et al.* (1999). 'Postmenopausal oestrogen replacement therapy and risk of AD: a population-based study', *Neurology*, 23; 52: 965–70.

Wickelgren I. (1997). 'Estrogen stakes claim to cognition', *Science*, 276: 675–8.

Wilson W. H. (1996). 'Time required for initial improvement during clozapine treatment of refractory schizophrenia', *Am. J. Psychiatry*, 153: 951–2.

Yaffe K., Sawaya G., Lieberburg I *et al.* (1998). 'Estrogen therapy in postmenopausal women: Effect on cognitive function and dementia', *JAMA*, 279: 688–95.

Zagami A. S., for the International 311C90 Long-Term Study Group (1997). '311C90: Long-term efficacy and tolerability profile for the acute treatment of migraine', *Neurology*, 48 (suppl. 3): S25–S28.

Zimbroff D. L., Kane J. M., Tamminga C. A. *et al.* (1997). 'Controlled, dose-response study of sertindole and haloperidol in the treatment of schizophrenia', *Am. J. Psychiatry*, 154: 782–91.

Index